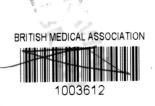

Neurorehabilitation Therapy and Therapeutics

Neurorehabilitation Therapy and Therapeutics

Edited by

Krishnan Padmakumari Sivaraman Nair
Sheffield Teaching Hospitals NHS Foundation Trust

Marlís González-Fernández
Department of Physical Medicine and Rehabilitation Johns Hopkins University School of Medicine

Jalesh N. Panicker
National Hospital for Neurology and Neurosurgery

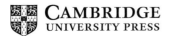

CAMBRIDGE
UNIVERSITY PRESS

University Printing House, Cambridge CB2 8BS, United Kingdom

One Liberty Plaza, 20th Floor, New York, NY 10006, USA

477 Williamstown Road, Port Melbourne, VIC 3207, Australia

314–321, 3rd Floor, Plot 3, Splendor Forum, Jasola District Centre, New Delhi – 110025, India

79 Anson Road, #06–04/06, Singapore 079906

Cambridge University Press is part of the University of Cambridge.

It furthers the University's mission by disseminating knowledge in the pursuit of
education, learning, and research at the highest international levels of excellence.

www.cambridge.org
Information on this title: www.cambridge.org/9781107184695
DOI: 10.1017/9781316882290

© Krishnan Padmakumari Sivaraman Nair, Marlís González-Fernández, and Jalesh N. Panicker 2019

First published 2019

Printed in the United Kingdom by TJ International Ltd. Padstow Cornwall

A catalogue record for this publication is available from the British Library.

Library of Congress Cataloging-in-Publication Data
Names: Nair, Krishnan Padmakumari Sivaraman, editor. | Gonzalez-Fernandez, Marlis, editor. |
Panicker, Jalesh N., editor.
Title: Neurorehabilitation therapy and therapeutics / edited by Krishnan Padmakumari Sivaraman
Nair, Marlis Gonzalez-Fernandez, Jalesh Panicker.
Description: New York, NY : Cambridge University Press, 2018. | Includes bibliographical references and index.
Identifiers: LCCN 2018015380 | ISBN 9781107184695 (alk. paper)
Subjects: | MESH: Neurological Rehabilitation | Nervous System Diseases – therapy
Classification: LCC RC349.8 | NLM WL 140 | DDC 616.8/046–dc23
LC record available at https://lccn.loc.gov/2018015380

ISBN 978-1-107-18469-5 Hardback

To Dr Anisya Vasanth (20 May 1959–9 February 2003), who struggled stoically with a smile on her lips and kindness in her heart to lighten the burden of those in distress.

Krishnan Padmakumari Sivaraman Nair

To the patients who allow me to partner with them as they work to get their life back;

to my colleagues, the rehabilitation staff, clinicians, and therapists who work every day to help patients on the path to recovery; to family and friends who always support my endeavours;

and to my husband, Justin, for whom I strive to be efficient and get home every day.

Marlís González Fernández

Dedicated to our patients, whose never-ending resolve to get better is a constant source of inspiration.

Jalesh N. Panicker

Contents

Contributors

Anna V. Agranovich PhD
Georgetown University Medical Center,
Washington, DC, USA

Alba Azola MD
Department of Physical Medicine and Rehabilitation,
Johns Hopkins University School of Medicine,
Baltimore, MD, USA

Apurba Barman MBBS, MD, DNB (PMR)
Department of Physical Medicine and Rehabilitation,
All India Institute of Medical Sciences (AIIMS),
Bhubaneshwar, Odisha, India

Amit Batla MD, DM
Luton and Dunstable University Hospital,
UCL Institute of Neurology,
London, UK

Andreas Bender MD
Therapiezentrum Burgau, Burgau, Germany,
University of Munich,
Munich, Germany

Rohit Bhide MBBS, DNB (PMR)
Princess Royal Spinal Injuries Centre, Northern
General Hospital,
Sheffield, UK

Gila Bronner MD
Sexual Medicine Center, Movement Disorders
Institute, Sheba Medical Center,
Tel-Hashomer, Israel

Adolfo M. Bronstein MD, PhD, FRCP
Imperial College,
London, UK

Pierre Denys MD
Raymond Poincaré Hospital, Department of
Neurology, University of Versailles Saint Quentin,
Versailles, France

Anton Emmanuel MD, FRCP
GI Physiology Unit, University College London
Hospital, and National Hospital for Neurology and
Neurosurgery,
London, UK

Marlís González-Fernández MD, PhD
Department of Physical Medicine and Rehabilitation,
Johns Hopkins University School of Medicine,
Baltimore, MD, USA

Tanya Gurevich MD
Division of Neurology, Tel-Aviv Medical Center,
The Sackler Faculty of Medicine, Tel Aviv
University,
Tel-Aviv, Israel

Ellen Merete Hagen MD, PhD
National Hospital for Neurology and Neurosurgery,
London, UK

Ramaswamy Hariharan MBBS, DNB
Princess Royal Spinal Injuries Centre, Northern
General Hospital,
Sheffield, UK

Simon J. Hickman MA, PhD, FRCP
Royal Hallamshire Hospital,
Sheffield, UK

Korey Kennelty PharmD, PhD
Division of Health Services Research, Department of
Pharmacy Practice and Science, University of Iowa,
College of Pharmacy,
Iowa City, IA, USA

Fiona Lindop MCSP
Derby Teaching Hospitals NHS Foundation Trust
Specialist Assessment and Rehabilitation Centre,
London Road Community Hospital,
Derby, UK

Jonathan F. Marsden FCSP, BSc (Hons), MSc, PhD
Plymouth University,
Plymouth, UK

Lewys Morgan MRCPsych
Sheffield Health and Social Care NHS Foundation
Trust, The Longley Centre,
Sheffield, UK

Rachel Mulheren PhD
Department of Neuroscience and Department of
Physical Medicine and Rehabilitation, John Hopkins
University School of Medicine,
Baltimore, MD, USA

**Krishnan Padmakumari Sivaraman Nair MBBS,
MD, DM, FRCP**
Sheffield Teaching Hospitals NHS Foundation Trust,
Sheffield, UK

Mahreen Pakzad MBBS, BSc, MRCS
University College London Hospital and National
Hospital for Neurology and Neurosurgery,
London, UK

Marousa Pavlou PhD, BA, MCSP
King's College,
London, UK

Diane Playford MD, FRCP
University of Warwick,
Warwick, UK

Preeti Raghavan MD
Department of Rehabilitation Medicine, NYU
Langone Medical Center,
New York, NY, USA

Martin J. Rhodes BMedSci, MSc
Royal Hallamshire Hospital,
Sheffield, UK

Nicole Rogus-Pulia PhD, CCC-SLP
Departments of Medicine and Surgery, University of
Wisconsin's School of Medicine and Public Health
(UWSMPH)
Swallowing Research Laboratory, Swallow
STRengthening OropharyNGeal (Swallow STRONG)
Program, Geriatric Research Education and Clinical
Center (GRECC), William S. Middleton Memorial
Veterans Hospital,
Madison, WI, USA

Rajani Sebastian PhD
Department of Neurology, Johns Hopkins University
School of Medicine,
Baltimore, MD, USA

Abhijeeth Shetty MRCPsych
Sheffield Health and Social Care NHS Foundation
Trust, The Longley Centre,
Sheffield, UK

David M. Simpson MD, FAAN
Clinical Neurophysiology Laboratories,
Neuromuscular Division, Neuro-AIDS Program,
Icahn School of Medicine at Mount Sinai,
New York, NY, USA

Valerie L. Stevenson MBBS, MRCP, MD
National Hospital for Neurology and Neurosurgery,
London, UK

Donna C. Tippett MPH, MA, CCC-SLP
Department of Otolaryngology, Head and Neck
Surgery, Department of Neurology, Department of
PM&R, Johns Hopkins University School of
Medicine,
Baltimore, MD, USA

Pegah Touradji PhD
Department of Physical Medicine and
Rehabilitation, Johns Hopkins University School of
Medicine,
Baltimore, MD, USA

Anand Viswanathan MBBS, MD
Princess Royal Spinal Injuries and
Neurorehabilitation Centre, Northern General
Hospital,
Sheffield, UK

Manuel Wilfred PT, DPT
Rehabilitation Department, NYU Langone Hospital,
New York, NY, USA

Joanne Yee MS, CF-SLP
Swallow STRONG program, Geriatric Research
Education and Clinical Center (GRECC), William
S. Middleton Memorial Veterans Hospital,
Madison, WI, USA

Elina Zakin, MD
Department of Neurology, Mount Sinai Hospital,
New York, NY, USA

Chapter 1

An Introduction to Neurological Rehabilitation

Diane Playford and Krishnan Padmakumari Sivaraman Nair

1.1 Introduction

Advances in diagnosis and therapeutics have resulted in better survival of subjects with neurological disorders [1]. However, they are often left with permanent impairments which in turn result in limitations in daily activities and difficulty performing social roles [1, 2]. These changes in function may be classified using the World Health Organization (WHO) International Classification of Function (ICF). Using this framework, impairment is any loss or abnormality of psychological, physiological or anatomical structure or function [3]. Common neurological impairments include aphasia, weakness, involuntary movements, ataxia, loss of sensations, and loss of vision. Activity limitation is any restriction or lack of ability to perform an activity in a manner or within the range considered normal. Restriction in participation is any disadvantage for a given individual resulting from an impairment or disability that limits or prevents the fulfilment of a role that is normal for that individual [4]. The relationship between impairment, activity limitation, and participation is not linear. It is moderated by environmental and personal factors which are also captured in the ICF framework. Relatively minor impairments can lead to significant difficulties maintaining social roles; for example, loss of dexterity in the left hand may not have a significant impact on many roles but may be devastating to a professional musician.

The aim of neurological rehabilitation is restoration of the individual to the highest feasible functional level. The process of neurological rehabilitation involves assessment, goal planning, and interventions (Figure 1.1).

1.2 Assessments

Assessments in neurological rehabilitation include identification, measurement, and recording of impairment, activity limitation, participation, and the identification of patients' goals. The advantage of the ICF framework is that it allows a shared language for people from different disciplines to describe an individual's abilities and disabilities and to design interventions which are tailored to an individual's social roles based on their impairments, and sensitive to their environment and personal factors, including their values and beliefs. Multidisciplinary assessment results in a more accurate assessment of the underlying impairments and allows rehabilitation planning, which can be complex as the individual may have multiple interacting problems [5].

For example, an individual with multiple sclerosis may present with poor work performance because of a combination of fatigue, anxiety, and cognitive impairment. Anxiety aggravates fatigue, fatigue aggravates cognitive errors, cognitive errors aggravate impairment. The fatigue may be due to workload, domestic commitments, medication, poor physical fitness, and the multiple sclerosis itself. Analysing this complex situation requires skilled assessment from a multidisciplinary team. Designing a rehabilitation intervention also depends on a clear understanding of the individual's wants. In this case, they may be 55, and want to retire because their partner has already retired. If this is their primary driver, then any intervention to improve work performance, which is not the individual's preferred outcome, may fail.

1.3 Goal Planning

A goal is the state or change in state that is hoped or intended for an intervention or course of action to achieve [6]. Goal setting is a process of discussion and negotiation in which the patient, family, and the treating team determine the key priorities for that individual and agree on the performance level to be attained by the patient for defined activities within a specified time frame. It involves assessment of current functional status, identification of potential for

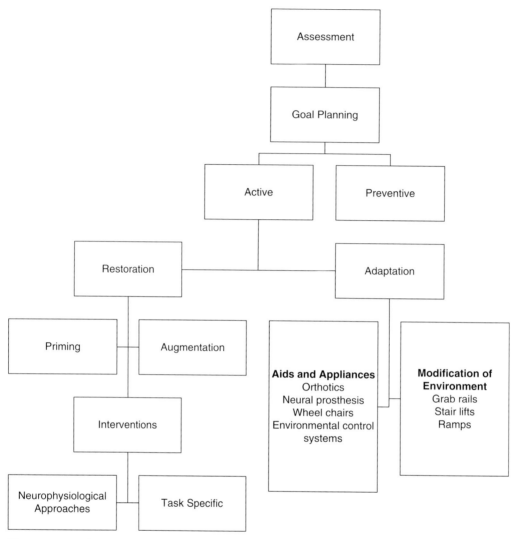

Figure 1.1 Neurological rehabilitation: The process

improvement, and setting short-, medium-, and long-term goals [6]. There are two elements to this definition. First is the process of discussion and negotiation.

Negotiation takes place between equals. Many studies demonstrate that in conversations between clinicians and patients, clinicians dominate the conversation. Recognition is increasing of the importance of shared decision-making in medicine. This is particularly important when individual preference informs the decision, which is true of many rehabilitation interventions. The steps in shared decision-making have been articulated by a number of authors but may be summarized as [7]:

A. Building trust and empathy
B. Negotiated agenda setting and prioritizing
C. Information sharing
D. Communicating and managing risk
E. Supporting deliberation
F. Summarizing and making the decision.

These steps are facilitated by the use of clear goal-setting processes and goal-setting materials. Steps may include a clear explanation of the rehabilitation process, the role of the multidisciplinary team, and the approach to goal setting, followed by an invitation to consider how their injury/disease has impacted different aspects of their lives.

Life goals are desired states that people seek to obtain, maintain, or avoid [8]. These goals take shape in childhood and adolescence as an idealized self-image and are influenced by age, gender, personality, experiences, and society and environment. Pursuit and attainment of life goals affect sense of well-being. Life goals are accessible to conscious awareness and can be identified. Several questionnaires are available for assessment of life goals [8]. Impairments and activity limitations interfere with goal striving and result in emotional distress. Motivation to participate in a rehabilitation programme depends on concurrence between patient's life goals and treatment goals.

Having identified the key goal domains, the patient needs to prioritize the areas that are most important, and then work with the rehabilitation team to identify potential solutions. It is at this point that clinicians can describe any knowledge about the diagnosis, nature and extent of impairment, activity limitation and restrictions in participation, available interventions, and information about the patient's environment and how that individual has responded to interventions undertaken so far. The team can identify the most likely outcomes and the reasoning behind that prediction.

During this negotiation stage, the rehabilitation team need to support patient self-efficacy [9, 10] by highlighting progress that has already been made, providing vicarious experience which models success by describing similar patients who have improved using a particular approach (often during inpatient rehabilitation patients will provide this support to other patients), verbal persuasion, and emotional support. Patients then need to write goals down in their own words. There is no point in the only record of the goals being in the clinical notes where patients cannot see them or share them with their families. Finally, goals need to be reviewed, so progress is monitored. During this review stage, it is helpful to identify what worked for an individual and what did not.

The second part of the goal-setting definition stated that patient and staff agree on the performance level to be attained by the patient for defined activities within a specified time frame. This is making goals 'SMART' (specific, measurable, achievable, relevant, and timely). These concepts originally derived from the organizational psychology literature of the 1970s, which aimed to increase workplace productivity [11, 12]. This work featured three key findings. First, challenging goals lead to better performance [11, 12]. Second, participative goals tend to be more demanding than assigned goals [13–16], and, third,

goal setting is more effective when goals are specific [12]. The goals should be clearly defined in terms of both purpose and duration. It is of interest that it was never stated that goals have to be achievable, and recent consensus conferences have highlighted they should, at least, be 'possible'. This confusion over the need for SMART goals lies in the fact that two types of goals are being set. Good practice dictates that the patients have both short-term goals which are reviewed every two to three weeks, and long-term goals. However, the long-term goals often contain elements which are not the patient's goal but an organizational goal around discharge from hospital. It is important that the rehabilitation team communicate clearly the planned discharge, including the date of discharge and the destination, but this is not a patient-centred goal. Organizational goals need to be achievable within the resources available. Patient goals merely need to be 'possible'. There is concern that patients can be demoralized by the failure to achieve goals. Patients are able to cope with setbacks, and an important part of the goal-setting process is the development of 'coping' or 'contingency' plans which will operate if barriers to goal achievement occur [10].

Goal setting has many other advantages. Subjects with neurological disorders often have multiple deficits and require input from different professionals. A major risk of this team approach is that individual professionals work independently without coordination, often with conflicting goals [17]. A process of goal planning is essential to ensure cooperation and coordination between different team members.

Despite the fact that goal setting in rehabilitation practice has been established for many years, the evidence base is very limited. A recent Cochrane review suggested that there is some very low-quality evidence that goal setting may improve some outcomes for adults receiving rehabilitation for acquired disability, with the best of this evidence appearing to favour positive effects for psychosocial outcomes (i.e., health-related quality of life, emotional status, and self-efficacy) rather than physical ones [18].

Family and carers should also be involved throughout the rehabilitation process, including goal setting, if that is acceptable to the patient. People with neurological disability often depend on their family members for emotional and physical support. Family members have to support a patient with disabilities in spheres of locomotion, self-care, communication, cognition, and depression and personality changes.

Factors associated with high degrees of depression in caregivers are disability in spouses, lack of social support, the presence of physical problems in caregivers, and the presence of depression, cognitive impairment, and abnormal behaviour in the patient. It is essential to take family and carers' views into account while planning for long-term care of people with severe permanent disabilities.

1.4 Outcome Measurement

In some cases, assessments using outcome measures help in communication between team members, evaluating effectiveness of interventions, and discharge planning. Assessment tools must be valid, reliable, sensitive to changes, simple, short, and applicable by all members of the rehabilitation team. Traditional psychometric approaches measure validity, reliability, and responsiveness [19, 20].

Validity measures the extent to which the scale measures what it is designed to measure. There are different ways to consider validity. Face validity is the most basic approach and asks whether the items in the measure appear to measure what they are meant to. For example, in a questionnaire about mobility, a question about whether an individual is able to leave the house when he wants to may measure mobility, but may also capture agoraphobia or fatigue. Only if it specifies 'does your mobility prevent you leaving the house when you want to?' would the item have face validity. Other forms of validity include content validity, which identifies whether the scale covers the range of relevant content. A scale aimed at capturing the mobility of a wheelchair user might differ from a scale aimed at capturing the mobility of an elite athlete with a prosthetic limb. Construct validity refers to the extent to which the scale measures the construct in relationship to other measures. This includes convergent validity, which occurs when two scales which aim to measure the same thing correlate. For example, the Barthel Index [21, 22], a measure of dependency, should correlate with the Functional Independence Measure [23], which also measures dependence, but not with the Hospital Anxiety and Depression Scale [4]. Discriminant validity measures the extent to which the measure is not associated with things that differ from the construct. Known groups validity measures the extent to which a measure can discriminate between two groups who are known to differ on the construct in question. For example, one would anticipate that the scores for

people with schizophrenia differ on the Barthel Index from the scores for those with stroke.

Reliability is how consistent a measure is of the construct over a period of time, and between different users. Test-retest reliability occurs when the measure obtains the same test score on two different occasions when the patient has not changed clinically. Inter-rater reliability occurs when two or more individuals obtain comparable ratings on the same patient [19]. Responsiveness captures whether the patient has changed with time [19].

Item response theory (IRT) was first proposed in the field of psychometrics for the purpose of ability assessment. Most measures capture ordinal but not interval data [20, 21]. This theory allows the calibration of items in tests and the scoring of subjects on the domain being measured. The likelihood of an item being endorsed is dependent on the difficulty of the item and the 'ability' of the person. Many measures in rehabilitation have been developed or subject to Rasch analysis [20], which is one approach to item response theory, and this allows the ranking of patients depending on the extent of their ability, or otherwise, in the domain under question, attitudes, or other latent traits.

A wide range of scales is in use in rehabilitation. Various scales measure different impairments like motor power, tone, sensations, language, cognition, range of motion, visual fields, and ataxia. Commonly used impairment scales include the Medical Research Council (MRC) grading of motor power, the National Institutes of Health stroke scale, the Glasgow coma scale, and the Modified Ashworth scale for spasticity. Assessments of limitation activity include activities of daily living (ADL), social functioning, intellectual functioning, perception, speech, mobility, gait, and arm functions [2]. Scales used in the assessment of activities include the Barthel Index [21], the Functional Independence Measure [22], and the Spinal Cord Independence Measure. Scales to measure participation include the Ghent Participation Scale [24], the WHO Handicap Scale [2], and the Impact on Participation and Autonomy Questionnaire [25].

1.5 Interventions

Rehabilitation interventions are typically delivered by a team including physicians, nurses, physiotherapists, occupational therapists, speech and language

Table 1.1 Neurological rehabilitation: The team

Team member	Role
Rehabilitation physician	Medical assessment and interventions, prognostication
Rehabilitation nurse	Skin care, bowel and bladder management, liaison with family and carers, coordinates the team
Physiotherapist	Strengthening of muscles, improve endurance, optimize functional movements
Occupational therapist	Training in activities of daily living assessment and remediation of impact of cognition on functional activities
Speech therapist	Assessment and treatment of communication issues, swallowing issues, and salivary control
Neuropsychologist	Assessment and management of cognitive issues, coping with loss of function, management of mood and behaviour
Social worker	Identification of community resources, help with benefits, housing, and home modifications, reintegration into community
Orthotist	Assessment, fabrication, and maintenance of orthoses and prostheses
Dietician	Nutritional assessment and advice, home enteral feeding, parenteral nutrition
Activity coordinator	Coordinate social and recreational activities like sports, arts and crafts, community reintegration, provide psychological support
Biomedical engineer	Maintenance and provision of devices like environmental controls, wheelchairs, and functional electrical stimulation systems

therapists, psychologists, rehabilitation engineers, orthotists, dieticians, and social workers (Table 1.1).

Rehabilitation teams tend to follow one of three models: multidisciplinary, interdisciplinary, and transdisciplinary [5]. Multidisciplinary rehabilitation involves members from different disciplines working individually with the patient towards separate goals. Interdisciplinary rehabilitation refers to the activities of a group of rehabilitation professionals who work towards common goals. The objectives are set jointly by the members of the team and may require joint therapy sessions. In transdisciplinary rehabilitation, a single team member acts as a primary therapist with other members providing information and advice [5]. This approach is cost-effective and useful in delivering rehabilitation services at patients' homes and for patients with cognitive behavioural issues who may find it difficult to deal with different therapists.

Rehabilitation interventions can be grouped as 'active' and 'preventive' processes. Active rehabilitation includes a process to facilitate recovery from impairments and adaptive strategies to cope with limitations in activities. People with neurological disabilities are prone to develop complications secondary to impairments and activity limitations like pressure ulcers, pain, and contractures. The interventions to maintain function and prevent these complications are grouped here as preventative rehabilitation.

1.5.1 Active Rehabilitation

Potential for recovery is maximal early on after injury. During the early phases emphasis should be on restoration of functions. Recovery from neurological disorders is often incomplete. Later in the course the rate of recovery slows and reaches a plateau. As the time from the injury lapses, the emphasis should shift from restoration to adaptation.

1.5.1.1 Restorative Interventions

Restorative interventions aim to rectify neurological impairments by facilitating recovery through modification of the neural networks. These can be divided into priming techniques, augmenting techniques, and specific interventions (Table 1.2) [26].

1.5.1.2 Priming Interventions

Priming interventions try to make the nervous system more receptive to rehabilitation interventions. For example, imagery is used to 'rehearse' the motor, sensory, and visual consequences of movement [27]. When a patient mentally rehearses a specific task, the motor areas associated with the planning,

5

Table 1.2 Interventions to promote recovery

Priming interventions	Augmenting interventions	Specific interventions
Motor and visual imagery	Robotics	**Neurophysiological approaches**
Tactile stimulation	Biofeedback	
Passive movements	Treadmill with body weight support	Bobath's neurodevelopmental approach
Action observation and mirror therapy	Constraint-induced movement therapy	
Transcranial magnetic stimulation		Brunnstrom's technique
Transcranial direct current stimulation		Proprioceptive neuromuscular facilitatory approach
		Task-specific training

preparation, and execution of the movement get activated. Repeated imagination strengthens the cortical movement templates and facilitates the effects of interventions. Tactile stimulation and passive movements provide sensory input that may act by improving attention and prime the neural circuits for the desired movement. Action observation and mirror therapy use visual input for priming. The patient observes specific movements of their non-affected limb reflected in a mirror placed at the body's midline. This activates the frontal and parietal circuits involved in the movements and may facilitate recovery [28]. Repetitive transcranial magnetic stimulation (rTMS) and transcranial direct current stimulation (tDCS) are non-invasive techniques for priming the brain. Using these techniques, it is feasible to improve or reduce the excitability of the specific cortical neural circuits. Five sessions of rTMS could improve upper limb dysfunction following stroke [29].

1.5.1.3 Augmentative Interventions

Augmentative interventions are used to augment the effects of rehabilitation interventions. Robot-assisted therapy is using robots to deliver therapy [30]. This is a less expensive way of accurately delivering multiple repetitions of standard therapy exercises. Some of these devices can also vary torque and provide feedback. Functional electrical stimulation activates the muscles to produce the desired movement. This can be used to augment the weak muscles and can be combined with the robot-assisted therapy to enhance limb movements [31]. Biofeedback provides the patient with visual and auditory feedback about the timing, accuracy, and strength of the movements [32].

This can help the patient to identify errors and learn the correct movement patterns. Constraint-induced movement therapy (CIMT) aims to reduce the inhibition of the affected cortex from the non-affected side by restricting the activity of the non-paretic arm. This involves wearing a mitten to constrain the normal arm with high-intensity task-specific training of the paretic arm. Several studies, including randomized controlled trials, validate this approach in rehabilitation of upper limb function in people with stroke [32]. Treadmill training with body weight support involves walking on a treadmill with a harness to support part or all of the body weight. The proportion of the body weight supported is incrementally reduced. This can increase the amount of walking practice and has been tried to improve gait in people with stroke [32].

1.5.1.4 Specific Interventions

Specific interventions seek to facilitate recovery from impairments. They are broadly divided into neurophysiological approaches and task-specific practice.

Neurophysiological Approaches

These techniques are based on neurophysiological principles of motor control and recovery. The basic principles of neurophysiological approaches are: (a) application of sensory stimuli to facilitate or inhibit an activity; (b) patient evaluation and treatment plans based on milestones of developments; (c) utilization of reflexes to facilitate or inhibit any motor activity; (d) utilization of concepts of motor relearning such as repetition; (e) focus on the patient as a whole; and (f) close interaction between the therapist and the patient. These approaches stress enhancement of the natural recovery process. Neurophysiological approaches include the proprioceptive neuromuscular facilitation technique (PNF), Bobath's neurodevelopmental approach, Brunnstrom's technique, and Rood's approach.

Task-Specific Practice

Repeated performance of a specific task facilitates learning and improves performance. Task-specific practice can induce experience-dependent plasticity in the cortex. Task-specific training includes breaking down of the meaningful task into simple individual components. The training starts with the patient performing multiple repetitions of a small component of a specific task. It gives the brain opportunities to identify errors and correct them. As the patient masters this step, further components are added, leading to the performance of the complex task. A meta-analysis showed that task-specific training may have a positive effect on the hand function after stroke [32]. None of these therapies have any proven superiority over others. Each of these techniques try to facilitate recovery of motor control through different strategies. They can be integrated and used based on the requirements of the patient, experience of the rehabilitation team and stage of motor recovery.

1.5.1.5 Adaptive Interventions

Adaptive strategies facilitate recovery of function through training, use of aids and appliances, or modification of environment. One of the major objectives of rehabilitation is to regain functional independence. Patients can be taught dressing techniques with adapted clothing like Velcro closures, pullovers, and front-buttoning clothing. Similarly, self-feeding can be helped with the use of friction plates, rocker knives, and other modified utensils. For grooming also different techniques and assistive devices are available. An occupational therapist can train the patient in ADL and the use of various assistive devices.

Orthotic devices like ankle or foot orthoses help to facilitate movement or to maintain alignment of joints and relieve pain. Neural prostheses are devices that substitute or augment functions lost due to neurological injury. Commonly used neural prosthesis include cochlear implants and the functional electrical stimulation systems for upper and lower limb movements. Environmental control systems, also known as electronic aids to daily living, enable people with neurological disabilities to access everyday electronic devices in their environment such as navigating through television channels, operating remote-controlled doors, and using mobile phones and computers. Environmental control systems are devices that help a person with a limitation in an activity to control his or her surroundings. Some individuals may also require environmental adaptations like stair lifts and ramps to facilitate functional independence.

1.5.2 Preventive Rehabilitation

Around 56–95% of patients undergoing inpatient rehabilitation develop medical complications [33]. These complications adversely affect outcome and prolong hospital stays. These complications include pressure sores, deep venous system thrombosis, shoulder pain, and contractures. Most of these complications are preventable. Techniques like proper positioning of the limbs and passive exercises may help to prevent complications. Protocols for prevention, early detection, and treatment of common medical complications should be an integral part of any rehabilitation programme.

Traditional exercise programmes are interventions to prevent complications from immobilization and can be divided into a passive range of motion exercises and active joint-by-joint exercises. In the passive range of motion exercises, the therapist or the caregiver moves various joints passively through their entire range of motion. This helps in preventing disuse atrophy, contractures, and development of abnormal postures. In active exercises, the patient actively moves the joints. These may be either isotonic or isometric exercises. Initially, the patient attempts simple movements, and subsequently complex movements and actions are tried.

1.6 Outcome

Rehabilitation helps in promoting natural recovery, preventing complications due to disabilities and adapting to disabilities. A well-planned coordinated strategy towards rehabilitation is bound to yield good results. Factors favouring a good outcome are good family support and financial status, higher social and educational levels, early initiation of a rehabilitation programme, and the expertise of the centre. Patients with low motivation, confusion and disoriented thinking, withdrawn and apathetic behaviour, previous medical illness, gross perceptual deficits, low levels of education, old age, and prolonged unconsciousness do not improve with rehabilitation programmes. However, currently, it is not possible to predict the outcome of an individual patient and therefore all patients should be given a trial of rehabilitation.

References

1. Cumberland Consensus Working Group. Cheeran B, Cohen L, Dobkin B, Ford G Greenwood R, Howard D, Husain M, Macleod M, Nudo R, Rothwell J, Rudd A, Teo J, Ward N, Wolf S. The future of restorative neurosciences in stroke: Driving the translational research pipeline from basic science to rehabilitation of people after stroke. *Neurorehabil Neural Repair* 2009; **23**: 97–107. doi:10.1177/1545968308326636.

2. Wade DT, de Jong BA. Recent advances in rehabilitation. *BMJ* 2000; **20**(320): 1385–8.

3. World Health Organization. *International classification of functioning, disability and health.* Geneva, Switzerland: World Health Organization, 2001.

4. Van de Velde D, Coorevits P, Sabbe L, et al. Measuring participation as defined by the World Health Organization in the International Classification of Functioning, Disability and Health: Psychometric properties of the Ghent Participation Scale. *Clin. Rehabil.* 2017; **31**: 379–93.

5. Nair KPS, Wade DT. Satisfaction of team members with interdisciplinary rehabilitation team meetings. *Arch. Phys. Med. and Rehabil.* 2003; **84**: 1710–13.

6. Wade DT. Goal setting in rehabilitation: An overview of what, why and how. *Clin. Rehabil.* 2009; **23**: 291–5.

7. Coulter A, Collin A. *Making shared decision making a reality: No decision about me without me.* London, UK: Kings Fund, 2011.

8. Nair KPS. Life goals: The concept and its relevance to rehabilitation. *Clin. Rehabil.* 2003; **17**: 191–201.

9. Bandura A. Self-efficacy mechanism in human agency. *American Psychologist* 1982; **37**: 122–47. doi:10.1037/0003-066X.37.2.122.

10. Scobbie L, McLean D, Dixon D, Duncan E, Wyke S. Implementing a framework for goal setting in community based stroke rehabilitation: A process evaluation. *BMC Health Serv. Res.* 2013; **13**: 190. doi:10.1186/1472–6963-13-190.

11. Locke EA. Effects of knowledge of results, feedback in relation to standards, and goals on reaction-time performance. *Am. J. Psychol.* 1968; **81**: 566–74.

12. Locke EA, Latham GP. Building a practically useful theory of goal setting and task motivation. A 35-year odyssey. *Am. Psychol.* 2002; **57**: 705–17.

13. Latham GP, Mitchell TR, Dossett DL. Importance of participative goal setting and anticipated rewards on goal difficulty and job performance. *Journal of Applied Psychology* 1978; **63**: 163–71.

14. Dachler HP, Wilpert B. Conceptual dimensions and boundaries of participation in organizations: A critical evaluation. *Adm. Sci. Q.* 1978; **23**: 1–39.

15. Tjosvold D. Effects of shared responsibility and goal interdependence on controversy and decision making between departments. *Journal of Social Psychology* 1988; **128**: 7–18.

16. Tjosvold D. Performance appraisal of managers: Goal interdependence, ratings, and outcomes. *Journal of Social Psychology* 1992; **132**: 629–39.

17. Schut HA, Stam HJ. Goals in rehabilitation teamwork. *Disabil. Rehabil.* 1994; **16**: 223–6.

18. Levack WM, Weatherall M, Hay-Smith EJ, Dean SG, McPherson K, Siegert RJ. Goal setting and strategies to enhance goal pursuit for adults with acquired disability participating in rehabilitation. *Cochrane Database Syst. Rev.* 2015; **20**(7): CD009727. doi:10.1002/14651858.CD009727.pub2.

19. Wade DT. *Measurements in neurological rehabilitation.* Oxford, UK: Oxford University Press, 1998.

20. Hobart J, Cano S. Improving the evaluation of therapeutic interventions in multiple sclerosis: The role of new psychometric methods. *Health Technol. Assess.* 2009; **13**: 1–177. doi:10.3310/hta13120.

21. Wade DT, Collin C. The Barthel ADL Index: A standard measure of physical disability? *Int. Disabil. Stud.* 1988; **10**: 64–7.

22. Collin C, Wade DT, Davies S, Horne V. The Barthel ADL Index: A reliability study. *Int. Disabil. Stud.* 1988; **10**: 61–3.

23. Hobart JC, Lamping DL, Freeman JA, Langdon DW, McLellan DL, Greenwood RJ,Thompson AJ. Evidence-based measurement: Which disability scale for neurologic rehabilitation? *Neurology* 2001; **28**(57): 639–44.

24. Bjelland I, Dahl AA, Haug TT, Neckelmann D. The validity of the Hospital Anxiety and Depression Scale. An updated literature review. *J. Psychosom. Res.* 2002 Feb; **52**: 69–77.

25. Cardol M, de Haan RJ, de Jong BA., et al. Psychometric properties of the Impact on Participation and Autonomy Questionnaire. *Arch. Phys. Med. Rehabil.* 2001; **82**(82): 210–16.

26. Pomeroy V, Aglioti SM, Mark VW, et al. Neurological principles and rehabilitation of action disorders: Rehabilitation interventions. *Neurorehabilitation and Neural Repair* 2011; **25** (Suppl.): 33S–43S.

27. Carrasco DG, Cantalapiedra JA. Effectiveness of motor imagery or mental practice in functional recovery after stroke: A systematic review. *Neurología* 2016; **31**: 43–52.

28. Thieme H, Mehrholz J, Pohl M, et al. Mirror therapy for improving motor function after stroke. *Stroke*. 2013. doi:10.1161/STROKEAHA.112.673087.

29. Zhang L, Xing G, Fan Y, et al. Short and long term effects of repetitive transcranial magnetic stimulation on upper limb motor function after stroke: A systematic review and meta-analysis. *Clin. Rehabil.* 2017; **31**: 1137–53.

30. Liao W, Wu C, Hsieh Y, et al. Effects of robot-assisted upper limb rehabilitation on daily function and real-world arm activity in patients with chronic stroke: A randomized controlled trial. *Clin. Rehabil.* 2012; **26**: 111–20.

31. Langhorne P, Coupar F, Pollock A. Motor recovery after stroke: A systematic review. *Lancet Neurol.* 2009; **8**: 741–54.

32. Wattchow KA, McDonnell MN, Hillier SL. Rehabilitation interventions for upper limb function in the first four weeks following stroke: A systematic review and meta-analysis of the evidence. *Arch. Phys. Med. Rehabil.* 2017. doi:10.1016/j.apmr.2017.06.014.

33. Nair KPS, Taly AB, Maheshwarappa BM, Kumar J, Murali T, Rao S Nontraumatic spinal cord lesions: A prospective study of medical complications during in-patient rehabilitation. *Spinal Cord.* 2005; **43**: 558–64.

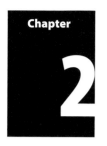

Chapter 2

Management of Disorders of Cognition in Neurorehabilitation

Pegah Touradji and Anna V. Agranovich

2.1 Introduction

Impaired cognitive functioning is a hallmark consequence of acquired/traumatic brain injuries, leading to potential disruptions in all aspects of life functioning. Many factors impact cognitive functioning following brain injuries and illnesses, including pre-morbid intellectual functioning, nature and severity of injury or illness, and biopsychosocial factors impacting cognitive functioning and the recovery process. Thus, planning effective neurorehabilitation interventions first relies on a comprehensive evaluation of cognitive functioning status, biopsychosocial barriers to cognitive functioning, and therapeutic engagement, as well as patient-specific goals for community reintegration. In an interdisciplinary model of neurorehabilitation, various providers work within their expertise but with collaborative goals of improving cognitive functioning and promoting functional independence.

Neurorehabilitation is conceptualized here as a collaborative, interdisciplinary, rehabilitation model of care to serve those with acquired brain injuries, which not only addresses specific areas of cognitive dysfunction but also helps improve associated barriers to cognitive functioning and establish goals to maximize functional independence. A key component of neurorehabilitation is cognitive rehabilitation. The Cognitive Rehabilitation Task Force of the Brain Injury Interdisciplinary Special Interest Group (BI-ISIG) of the American Congress of Rehabilitation Medicine (ACRM) has developed evidence-based clinical guidelines for cognitive rehabilitation [1, 2, 3]. Cognitive rehabilitation interventions are intended to facilitate progress towards maximizing safety, independence, daily functioning, and overall quality of life through targeted approaches for ameliorating neurocognitive deficits [4]. Cognitive rehabilitation can be carried out by various trained rehabilitation specialists, including occupational therapists (OT), speech-language pathologists (SLP), and rehabilitation neuropsychologists.

Comprehensive neuropsychological rehabilitation interventions, in conjunction with cognitive rehabilitation interventions, facilitate therapy engagement, provide targeted interventions to reduce the impacts of emotional, behavioural, interpersonal, and injury-related difficulties (e.g., sleep, fatigue, pain) on cognitive status and functional independence, and assist in navigating reintegration into appropriate community settings.

This chapter reviews evidence-based cognitive rehabilitation interventions for specific areas of neurocognitive impairments. Furthermore, neuropsychological rehabilitation considerations and interventions are described as they relate to impacts on cognitive functioning and disability status.

2.2 Treatment: Evidence-Based Cognitive Rehabilitation

Evidence-based cognitive rehabilitation practice recommendations have been established by the BI-ISIG Cognitive Rehabilitation Task Force of the ACRM [1, 2, 3]. Systematic reviews of the cognitive rehabilitation literature have informed empirically supported cognitive rehabilitation treatment strategies primarily for stroke and traumatic brain injury (TBI) populations [1, 2, 3]. Recommendations are categorized as 'Practice Standard' if shown to have 'substantive evidence of effectiveness', 'Practice Guideline' if shown to have 'probable effectiveness', and 'Practice Option' for strategies that are thought to have 'possible effectiveness' but require further investigation [2]. The *Cognitive Rehabilitation Manual: Translating Evidence-Based Recommendations into Practice* was developed based on the empirical evidence from these systematic reviews to provide clinicians with specific evidence-based interventions for addressing specific neurocognitive deficits [4].

Cognitive rehabilitation intervention initially relies on formal evaluation, such as a comprehensive neuropsychological evaluation to identify cognitive and neurobehavioral impairments impacting daily functioning, as well as relative strengths to utilize in the rehabilitation intervention process [4]. Neuropsychological assessment can also help identify cognitive barriers to rehabilitation and help prioritize treatment recommendations. The neuropsychological evaluation also takes into account patient-specific factors that may impact rehabilitation outcomes (e.g., psychological distress, sleep disturbance, pain, fatigue, social support).

Following a comprehensive evaluation to identify goals and priorities, treatment planning takes place and emphasizes cognitive interventions that are relevant to patients' life goals and addresses specific underlying cognitive impairments. Cognitive rehabilitation intervention is ideally carried out in three hierarchical stages [5]. The acquisition stage involves bringing awareness to the patients about their cognitive impairments and the need for intervention, establishing collaborative short- and long-term meaningful goals, and teaching the treatment model for cognitive rehabilitation interventions. In the application stage, patients initially work closely with therapists to apply strategies to simple tasks, typically within the therapeutic setting. Early in this stage, strategies are usually external or compensatory (e.g., use of planners, calendars, technology aids) and are structured by the therapist, who provides consistent cues and supervision. With therapist cues and feedback, the goal is for increased patient internalization of strategies (i.e., increased automaticity of practised strategies with improved independence through consistent use of compensatory strategies). This is achieved by providing ample practice of strategies with gradual removal of external cues to promote internal or self-generated cues for strategy use. For individuals with more pronounced cognitive impairments, the therapy goal is procedural learning through structure, practice, and repetition. Finally, in the adaptation stage, patients learn to apply strategies to more complex, functional, and non-structured tasks outside of the therapeutic environment. Generalization is promoted and refers to the process of applying learned skills across a variety of settings. Again, not all patients are able to generalize, given the severity of their cognitive deficits, and thus the use of external cues for these individuals is necessary long term.

The following sections review evidence-based cognitive rehabilitation interventions across the cognitive domains of attention, memory, executive functioning, visuospatial skills, and language. For comprehensive systematic reviews of the cognitive rehabilitation literature, refer to Cicerone et al. [1, 2, 3], and for comprehensive clinical guidance for evidence-based cognitive rehabilitation protocols, refer to the *Cognitive Rehabilitation Manual: Translating Evidence-Based Recommendations into Practice* [4].

2.2.1 Executive Functioning

Executive functions determine goal-directed and purposeful behaviours and include abilities to formulate goals, problem-solve, think abstractly, think flexibly, plan and organize, initiate behaviours, anticipate consequences of behaviours and actions, and self-monitor and adjust behaviours according to the situation and environment [4].

Executive dysfunction is a common outcome of brain injury and can manifest in disruptions of cognitive functioning as well as emotional and behavioural regulation. Cognitive impairments in executive functioning can result in problems with awareness, difficulties planning out and organizing daily activities, being able to problem-solve effectively in new situations, anticipating and analysing situations, and self-monitoring responses to tasks at hand. Impairments in awareness after brain injury are multifactorial and can involve right hemispheric or parietal damage, frontal injury, diffuse brain injury, and impairments in executive functions, as well as contributing causes of psychological or emotional readiness and social-environmental factors impacting the opportunity for meaningful learning about brain injury [6].

Emotional dysregulation after brain injury can range from non-reactivity (apathy) and lability in emotional reactivity, to over-reactivity with heightened emotional responsiveness. Behavioural manifestations of executive dysfunction can be characterized by 'positive symptoms' or behaviours overly influenced by the environment (e.g., impulsivity, disinhibition, stimulus-bound behaviours), or 'negative symptoms' such as abulia, poor initiation, task impersistence, or lack of spontaneity [4].

Cognitive rehabilitation interventions for executive functioning. Practice Standard recommendations for evidence-based cognitive rehabilitation of executive functioning deficits include training of metacognitive strategies after TBI to help with emotional dysregulation and as a component of cognitive interventions for attention, neglect, and memory [3]. During post-acute rehabilitation after TBI, problem-solving strategies to help with dealing with everyday situations and functional activities are recommended as Practice Guidelines. Group-based interventions can also be considered as a Practice Option to help with remediation of executive and problem-solving impairments after TBI.

Studies show that strategies focused on enhancing metacognitive skills are beneficial for improved self-awareness after moderate to severe TBI, and can facilitate treatment of attention, memory, language deficits, and social skills impaired in those with TBI or stroke [3]. Metacognition is defined as 'thinking about thinking' with metacognitive knowledge representing awareness about cognitive abilities, and metacognitive control representing self-monitoring and adaptive change to environmental demands [7]. Metacognitive training goals involve helping the patient enhance and internalize awareness to then exert greater behavioural and emotional control through a process of learning self-monitoring and self-control through education, feedback and cuing, modelling, external directions, and instructional aids [4].

Problem-solving strategies in cognitive rehabilitation aim to teach individuals to apply consistent, general strategies to each new problem across situations through a framework of identifying the problem, goal-setting, planning a solution, executing the solution, then monitoring feedback to make appropriate changes [4]. Practice and repetition are implemented to help with internalizing problem-solving strategies so that individuals can generalize the use of strategies across situations with less external cues, though external cuing remains optimal for those who cannot demonstrate internalization [4].

2.2.2 Memory

Several cognitive functions are required for memory processes. Attention, encoding, storage, and retrieval are all involved in memory functioning [5]. Attention is required to attend to and process the information to be encoded and stored into long-term memory, usually through repetition and association for later retrieval or acquisition of stored information [4].

Long-term memory is conceptualized as declarative or non-declarative. Declarative or episodic memory refers to conscious and intentional recall of episodic (i.e., autobiographical) and semantic memory (concept-based knowledge) [8]. Non-declarative or implicit memory refers to recall of information learned through repeated performance without conscious effort and is often seen in motor learning (e.g., brushing teeth, riding a bike) [8].

Memory functions can easily be disrupted by brain injury given the reliance on the complex network of brain pathways involved in memory functioning. Memory retrieval is thought to involve the frontal lobes and subcortical regions, impacting free recall but with benefit from the provision of cues. Subcortical damage (e.g., hippocampus, amygdala, or striatum) may impact declarative memory. Procedural memory can be disrupted with damage to the cerebellum or basal ganglia, though it is less commonly seen in TBI [4].

Cognitive rehabilitation interventions for memory. Based on Cicerone et al.'s [3] evidence-based cognitive rehabilitation review, the Practice Standard recommendation for remediation of memory deficits involves both internalized and external memory compensatory strategies for mild memory impairments following TBI. External memory compensatory strategies are recommended for individuals with severe memory deficits following TBI or stroke as a Practice Guideline. Practice Options include errorless learning for specific skill/knowledge learning (but not for novel tasks or functional memory problems in TBI-related severe memory impairments), as well as group interventions for remediation of memory deficits after TBI.

The severity of injury impacts practice recommendations given that severe memory impairments and/or limitations in self-awareness impact the utility of internalized memory strategies. Rather, for severe impairments, external compensatory strategies or the use of external devices to aid in memory is recommended. Given that executive functioning impacts learning and the utility of external memory strategies, executive functioning difficulties must also be addressed in the treatment of memory disorders. External memory aids may include a Memory Notebook (e.g., written notebook or planner, electronic planner, smartphone). Orientation Books are beneficial to those with very severe memory impairments, including during post-traumatic amnesia, and help with reducing confusion by orientating to basic, relevant personal information. Agitation can also be reduced by having providers routinely redirect patients to simple orientation cues. Procedural memory techniques, including errorless learning, spaced retrieval, and chaining techniques, are employed by clinicians to optimize the functional use of external memory aids [4].

Memory strategy training is intended for those with milder memory impairments. Explicit memory and self-instruction are methods of training with external strategies used to facilitate explicit memory for those with more moderate impairments. Association strategies pair verbal information with personally relevant visual stimuli or imagery to help with acquisition and recall. Organizational strategies are also evidence-based memory training strategies [4].

2.2.3 Attention

Attention is conceptualized in a hierarchical model for the treatment of impairments in attention following brain injury and stroke [9]. Focused attention is the most basic aspect of attention that requires the ability to recognize specific sensory information. Sustained attention involves the ability to maintain attention during a continuous, repetitive activity over time. Working memory is the highest level of sustained attention and refers to the ability to sustain information in the mind while manipulating that information. Selective attention requires the ability to focus attention on target stimuli while inhibiting distractions. Alternating attention involves the ability to shift attention or between tasks requiring different cognitive demands. Finally, divided attention requires the ability to attend to two or more tasks or stimuli simultaneously.

Impairments of attention are prevalent following acquired brain injuries. Subcortical injuries can result in impairments in focused and sustained attention, right parietal injuries may lead to sensory-specific attention impairments (neglect), and frontal lobe injuries can result in disturbances of higher-level attentional processes (e.g., selective, alternating, and divided attention) that often relate to executive functioning impairments [4].

Cognitive rehabilitation interventions for attention. According to Cicerone et al. [3], Practice

Standard guidelines for remediation of brain injury-related attention impairments include direct attention training and metacognitive training in the post-acute phase of rehabilitation. Attention Processing Training (APT) [9, 10], Time Pressure Management (TPM) [11], and strategy training in working memory skills [12] have been identified as effective remediation-strategy training in brain injury rehabilitation [3]. Adjunctive computer-based interventions can be considered as a Practice Option in addition to clinician-guided evidence-based interventions [3].

APT is a structured attention training programme based on the theoretical hierarchical model of attention. This technique has revealed empirical evidence of efficacy for brain injury–related attention deficits [10]. Initially, assessment is used to identify the specific type of attention impairment(s). APT training corresponds to one of the five types of attention impairment (focused, sustained, selective, alternation, and divided attention) and intervention is first targeted on the most fundamental or basic area of attention found to be impaired. The treatment is further individualized with a goal-driven approach to tasks (home, work, or community) targeted for generalization.

TPM was designed to address difficulties with brain injury–related cognitive slowing through a structured problem-solving strategy to assist with control and regulation of information input [11]. TPM strategies help patients with a decision-making and problem-solving approach [13]. 'Strategic' decisions help with planning ahead prior to a task in order to minimize potential problems, 'tactical' decisions help with troubleshooting types of decisions when executing tasks, and 'operational' decisions help manage problems that arise during tasks that require urgent or rapid decision-making [13].

Rehabilitation of working memory utilizes metacognitive training to address difficulties with mental manipulation of complex information, particularly pronounced in situations with rapid time demands and/or in situations with multiple task demands [12]. Treatment is individualized with initial treatment focused on increased awareness of attention difficulties in the context of contributing factors (e.g., slowed processing, mood, fatigue). Subsequent treatments involve strategies (e.g., verbal mediation, rehearsal, anticipation of task demands, self-pacing, self-monitoring, prioritizing) to allow for more effective management of attentional resources and rate of cognitive demands.

2.2.4 Hemispatial Neglect

Hemispatial neglect occurs with injury to the right cerebral cortex and manifests as inattention to the contralateral side of space. Presence of visual hemispatial neglect can co-occur with tactile, proprioceptive, and auditory inattention or neglect. Furthermore, in the acute phase of injury, there may be lack of awareness of the presence of neglect [4].

Cognitive rehabilitation interventions for hemispatial neglect. The Practice Standard for left visual neglect after right hemisphere stroke involves visuospatial rehabilitation with visual scanning training. The Practice Standard guideline for apraxia following left hemisphere stroke is for specific gestural or strategy training during acute rehabilitation. Practice options include limb activation or electronic technologies for visual scanning training for neglect associated with right hemisphere stroke, systematic training of visuospatial deficits and visual organization skills for visual perceptual deficits without visual neglect in those with right hemisphere stroke in acute rehabilitation, and computer-based interventions for persons with TBI or stroke with visual field damage [3].

Visual scanning training often uses visual cancellation tasks to intervene with left visual neglect or inattention. Anchoring strategies provide verbal or visual cues to start the cancellation task at the extreme left side of the page. Once anchoring is established, pacing strategies are employed to slow down performance as a tendency remains to rapidly drift attention back to the right side of space. Modifications used to help reduce errors include increased distance between targets or increased font size. Strategies for increasing complexity include simultaneous search for two targets, as well as conditional target cancellation (e.g., crossing out one target while circling the second target). Computer-based visual scanning training can be used in conjunction with traditional paper-pencil cancellation tasks, but they are not recommended as stand-alone interventions. Visual scanning interventions for visual hemineglect also include visual scanning for reading, copying prose, and describing pictures. Spatial-motor strategies for limb activation involve prompting the use of the left upper extremity immediately before or during visual training tasks, while visuospatial-motor strategies involve simultaneously anchoring visual scanning training with visuomotor cuing for limb activation [4].

2.2.5 Language and Communication

Disorders of language tend to be lateralized to the left hemisphere, with anterior left hemisphere injury leading to expressive aphasia characterized by non-fluent output, but adequate comprehension and posterior left hemisphere lesion, resulting in receptive aphasia characterized by poor comprehension and fluent but impoverished output [14]. Aphasias can also be classified as conduction aphasia (fluent output, adequate comprehension, difficulty with repetition and auditory-verbal memory span), global aphasia (significant impairment in both expressive and receptive language), and anomic aphasia (primary deficits in word finding) [14].

In TBI, cognitive, behavioural, and emotional disruptions related to frontally mediated brain systems can result in social communication impairments, negatively impacting interpersonal relationships, community integration, adjustment to disability, and quality of life. Social communication deficits may emanate from executive dysfunction, resulting in disinhibited and impulsive behaviours impacting social boundaries. Impairments in judgment may impact the ability to benefit from social and emotional cues to help guide behaviour. Affective adjustment difficulties following brain injury can also exacerbate social communication difficulties through further maladaptive behaviours and/or social withdrawal [4].

Cognitive rehabilitation interventions for social communication. In persons with left hemisphere stroke, both during acute and post-acute rehabilitation, traditional cognitive-linguistic SLP therapy is recommended as a Practice Standard to address language deficits. In persons with TBI, the Practice Standard recommendation is for specific interventions for functional communication deficits, including pragmatic conversational skills to help with social communication skills. Practice Guidelines for those with left hemisphere stroke include considerations for treatment intensity of language-based rehabilitation and recommendations for cognitive interventions to address specific language impairments (e.g., reading comprehension or language formulation). Also for those with left hemisphere stroke, the Practice Option cognitive rehabilitation intervention is consideration of group-based interventions for language remediation. Computer-based interventions in conjunction with evidence-based, clinician-guided, cognitive-linguistic rehabilitation interventions are also Practice Option recommendations for TBI and stroke patients with language deficits. However, sole reliance on computer-based tasks is not recommended [3].

Group Interactive Structured Treatment (GIST) for Social Competence was developed as a social communication cognitive rehabilitation intervention to help with skill development in listening and comprehension, communicating needs and thoughts, using and interpreting nonverbal language, regulating emotional reactions, conforming to social boundaries, collaborating with others to problem-solve, and asserting oneself as appropriate [15]. Group intervention has also been developed to train pragmatic communication and social perception in conjunction with individual psychotherapy to facilitate emotional adjustment and social adaptation [16]. These group-based interventions follow a structured format, recognizing a high need for structure to accommodate cognitive difficulties in those with TBI. Further, the group format provides opportunities for structured interactions, feedback, and practice of social skills [4].

2.3 Treatment: Psychological Rehabilitation Intervention

Evidence-based Practice Standard recommendations based on cognitive rehabilitation systematic reviews also support engagement in comprehensive holistic neuropsychological rehabilitation in post-acute rehabilitation [3]. Studies show that engagement in a neuropsychological rehabilitation programme can improve patient outcomes in community reintegration, functional independence, productivity, cognitive and emotional symptom management, and quality of life satisfaction compared to just receiving conventional rehabilitation interventions [3].

Rehabilitation neuropsychologists are typically integrated into both inpatient and outpatient or post-acute rehabilitation settings treating individuals with acquired brain injuries or illnesses. In the inpatient setting, rehabilitation neuropsychological assessments and interventions can assist with issues related to cognitive capacity for decision-making and discharge disposition recommendations, as well as cognitive, emotional, and behavioural recommendations and interventions to help maximize rehabilitation participation. Further, psychoeducation for families can help with better understanding of cognitive behavioural manifestations of brain injury that will impact caregiver and supervision needs, as well as behavioural strategies to help with cognitive functioning. In early stages of recovery, strategies may involve modifying the environment to reduce cognitive overstimulation leading to confusion and agitation and promoting regular sleep-wake cycles. Problems with awareness deficits may be most pronounced in acute phases of recovery and thus primary recommendations are for metacognitive interventions [4].

In post-acute or outpatient neurorehabilitation settings, treatment begins with an evaluation involving a clinical interview with the patient and preferably family members and care providers to assess pre- and post-injury biopsychosocial risk factors to cognitive functioning status, adjustment to disability, and engagement in rehabilitation. A comprehensive neuropsychological evaluation provides specific evidence of deficits across various neurocognitive domains to inform ideal cognitive rehabilitation interventions, as well as help with insight into emotional and behavioural difficulties warranting further psychological interventions. Evaluations further assess life goals and ability to return to community activities (e.g., driving [17], employment [18]). Neuropsychological rehabilitation interventions may involve the patient, family, caregivers, and treatment team. Within a cognitive rehabilitation approach, the overarching goal of neuropsychological rehabilitation intervention is to maximize rehabilitation engagement and reduce the impact of emotional and behavioural factors that may compete with depleted cognitive resources. The following sections review common issues (emotional functioning, sleep, fatigue, pain) related to brain injury/illness that may impede cognitive functioning status and benefit from neuropsychological rehabilitation interventions.

2.3.1 Emotional Functioning

Emotional difficulties following brain injury can result from neuropathological changes, difficulties with affective adjustment to disability, and/or exacerbation of pre-injury psychiatric disorders. Psychiatric disturbances in neurorehabilitation populations appear regardless of injury severity, and can involve personality changes, maladaptive social behaviours, psychosis, depressed mood, poor disability adjustment, reduced coping skills, and anxiety [19]. Most common psychiatric diagnoses after TBI include major depression, substance abuse, and post-traumatic stress disorder (PTSD). The prevalence of mental health diagnoses after brain injury is reported to range from 28% to 43% [19, 20]. Following brain injury, emotional distress may be related to feelings of loss, confusion, lack of independence, uncertainty about the future, and suffering related to fatigue, pain, and sleep difficulties. The combination of emotional and physical suffering tends to further negatively impact cognitive function, hindering the ability to focus and sustain attention and engage in new learning. Furthermore, psychological distress and physical suffering may occupy already limited cognitive resources and exacerbate both fatigue symptoms and the magnitude of cognitive difficulties. Emotional distress may also hinder engagement in structured rehabilitation, further impeding functional outcomes.

Rehabilitation engagement has been conceptualized as the interplay between internal (e.g., effects of injury, psychological adjustment to injury, and personality traits) and external (e.g., rehabilitation environment, social support system, and cultural variables) in determining rehabilitation outcomes [21]. Key determinants of engagement in rehabilitation are perceived need for treatment (as it is related to self-awareness and anticipation of improvements and perceived benefits of the activity), perceived self-efficacy, and outcome expectancies [21]. Thus, psychological interventions to facilitate cognitive rehabilitation efforts must address emotional and physical suffering (e.g., pain, fatigue, sleep disturbance) that may exacerbate cognitive difficulties, as well as help with engagement strategies to maximize rehabilitation benefits.

Interventions for psychological engagement and mood management. Among the preferred approaches for psychological interventions focused on improving engagement and facilitating psychological adjustment after neurological injury or illness are cognitive behavioural therapy (CBT) for anxiety and depression, along with motivational interviewing (MI) and mindfulness-based therapies.

CBT strategies for adjustment to disability and mood management include developing adaptive coping strategies through changing maladaptive cognitions (e.g., thoughts, attitudes, and beliefs), behaviours, and feelings. CBT has been shown to improve quality of life for adults with persistent post-concussive symptoms in the context of outpatient brain injury rehabilitation services [22]. A systematic review of studies that investigated the application of CBT in neurorehabilitation samples for treatment of depression and anxiety reported partial reduction in anxiety and depression symptoms with targeted treatment [23].

Motivational interviewing is an intervention to facilitate engagement in treatment, improve health behaviours, and promote positive change [24]. It is a person-centred approach that involves a collaborative conversation between providers and patients to facilitate the move from ambivalence to change and enhance commitment. MI involves four processes, including engaging (building a working relationship), focusing (developing and maintaining a specific focus on change), evoking (eliciting the client's own motivation for change), and planning (developing commitment to and a plan for change). MI has been applied to promote engagement in neurorehabilitation. The initial phase of MI is focused on building a collaborative therapeutic context for establishing a positive alliance between the patient and rehabilitation team, which creates the optimal conditions to conduct the assessment of cognitive function, activities of daily living, emotional well-being, and personal values and aspirations [25]. The focusing stage provides the foundation for constructive feedback and structured experiences to promote self-awareness and perceived self-efficacy, mastery, and control [26]. The evoking stage corresponds to forming of and committing to personally meaningful goals while being supported through feelings of loss and grief associated with neurological injury. Regardless of the patient's cognitive limitations associated with brain injury, interventions that seek to maximize therapeutic alliance and collaboration are more likely to promote enhanced cognitive and emotional gains. The maintenance stage utilizes MI techniques targeted at eliciting personal strengths and a sense of control, self-efficacy, and renewed coping resources [25]. MI has also been used as a prelude to CBT in randomized controlled trials for anxiety after brain injury to facilitate treatment response. Patients with TBI who were offered MI demonstrated better engagement in CBT and improved outcomes [27].

2.3.2 Sleep

Sleep impairments and disorders of arousal are common and pervasive sequelae of acquired brain injury that often hinder cognitive function and recovery. Symptoms of sleep disturbance, insomnia, and excessive daytime sleepiness have been documented across all levels of brain injury severity and across stages of recovery. After TBI, sleep disturbance was reported to impact from 40% to 70% of survivors [28]. The aetiology of sleep disturbances after a brain injury is likely multifactorial and may be attributed to a combination of neurological factors, such as damage to the basal forebrain, the reticular activating system, endocrine changes associated with injury, alterations in the circadian rhythm due to injury of the suprachiasmatic nuclei of the anterior hypothalamus [29], and co-morbid depression, pain, substance abuse, poor sleep hygiene, and reduced physical activity post injury [30]. In addition, some individuals present with premorbid sleep problems in addition to those triggered by the brain injury. Insomnia, excessive daytime sleepiness, narcolepsy, and circadian rhythm disturbances can occur independently from TBI and/or be exacerbated by injury.

Disturbances of the sleep-wake cycle are not routinely addressed during the initial rehabilitation and may persist for many years post injury if they remain untreated. Sleep disorders associated with TBI tend to exacerbate trauma-related cognitive, communication, and mood impairments [31]. Hence, timely identification and treatment of sleep disorders is essential to optimize recovery and outcomes, particularly to maximize the effectiveness of cognitive rehabilitation interventions.

Interventions for improvements in sleep quality and hygiene. Establishing a consistent daily schedule for individuals undergoing acute rehabilitation is critical for supporting the sleep-wake cycle that is often disrupted as a result of the injury. There is strong evidence for establishing a consistent sleep-wake schedule during very early stages of recovery and inpatient rehabilitation with the implementation of brain injury treatment protocols [32]. Initial sleep interventions rely on environmental modifications (e.g., reducing night-time stimuli, providing a quiet and dark sleep environment, minimizing nursing disruptions, waking the patient at a consistent time in the morning, providing natural morning light and orientation cues, minimizing daytime napping).

Education with patients and family about sleep hygiene can be helpful in early stages of brain injury rehabilitation as well as during post-acute recovery. Rehabilitation psychologists may also help with the implementation of these behavioural recommendations as part of health and behaviour interventions. Key components of sleep hygiene include:

– Maintaining a regular sleep schedule of going to bed and awakening around the same time every day, including holidays and weekends
– Using the bed only for sleep, and not eating, drinking, watching television, or using electronic devices in bed (or in the bedroom, if possible)
– Avoiding daytime naps or limiting naps to 20–30 minutes at most
– Getting out of bed if unable to fall asleep within 30 minutes of lying in bed and doing something relaxing, returning to bed when feeling sleepy
– Avoiding caffeine and alcohol in the afternoon
– Exercising earlier in the day and avoiding strenuous exercise late in the day
– Keeping the bedroom quiet and dark at night
– Reducing night-time stimuli and using relaxation techniques prior to bedtime.

For patients with more pronounced sleep disturbance (i.e., insomnia), the efficacy of cognitive behavioural therapy for insomnia (CBT-I) has been widely established [33]. It has been suggested that CBT-I reduces symptoms of insomnia and hence helps alleviate symptoms of depression, anxiety, fatigue, and pain. In the application for patients with TBI, it has been shown to reduce total wake time, improve sleep efficiency, reduce fatigue [34], and result in significant reductions in anxiety, depression, fatigue, and pain severity [35].

CBT-I is a manualized treatment [33] that provides education about sleep, circadian rhythms, impact of substances, and sleep restriction and offers instructions for stimulus control, stress management, cognitive restructuring, and suggestions for continued adjustment and relapse prevention. The treatment is usually delivered in a course of four sessions of 60 minutes each, generally at a pace of one session per week, according to the manual guidelines. Modifications of CBT-I protocol for individuals with brain injury were proposed to facilitate learning and retention of the information [35]. In session 1, a sleep diary is used to chart the daily sleep/wake patterns and is reviewed in order to address the existing sleep habits to tailor the intervention. This session focuses on psychoeducation on 'sleep rules' (e.g., avoiding daytime naps) and developing consistent times for going to bed and getting up. A useful modification for the neurorehabilitation population is the incorporation of preset alarms and reminders for digital calendars or writing in a traditional calendar to facilitate compliance, as well as the provision of summary handouts to aid learning, given diminished learning capacity secondary to TBI. In session 2, along with review of the sleep log, feedback is offered on optimizing sleep habits and further psychoeducation is provided. Patients are taught the 'constructive worry' technique in which the participant learns to manage pre-sleep worry, and instructed on the use of thought records for maladaptive thoughts and beliefs about insomnia. Sessions 3 and 4 are focused on making necessary adjustments to recommendations and reinforcing treatment adherence.

2.3.3 Fatigue

Fatigue is a prevalent complaint of patients with an acquired brain injury or neurological illness, regardless of its aetiology or severity. It is often reported as the most debilitating factor in movement disorders [36], multiple sclerosis [37], TBI [38], and stroke [39]. Cognitive and physical fatigue is the most commonly reported symptom of TBI irrespective of brain injury severity, with even more prevalence among individuals with mild TBI [40]. Studies estimated that 30% of persons with acquired brain injury experience severe fatigue six months after the injury, with limited improvement during the first year. Up to 70% of those with acquired brain injury reported fatigue five years after TBI, and some continued to experience fatigue even 10 years after the trauma, regardless of the severity of the injury, age, or time since insult [41]. Yet the subjective nature of fatigue complaints and the lack of strong evidence for specific interventions may often result in lack of treatment. Contributing factors include premorbid mental health, concurrent depression, pain, and sleep disturbance. Among suggested non-pharmacological treatments are physical activity, bright blue light, biofeedback, electrical stimulation, and CBT, but with insufficient evidence of efficacy for fatigue management [41].

Intervention for fatigue management. One of the promising approaches for mental fatigue management after acquired brain injury is the mindfulness-based stress reduction (MBSR) protocol. A systematic literature review and meta-analysis of mindfulness training in neurorehabilitation population indicated mindfulness-based interventions help with some relief of fatigue symptoms [39]. The formal practices in MBSR include sitting meditations, gentle yoga, and the body scan. Beginning with the awareness of the breath, the programme incorporates strategies for expanding awareness to include the body, mental states, and mental contents [42]. In an exploratory study, Johansson and colleagues found a statistically significant reduction in self-reported fatigue (as measured by self-assessment of mental fatigue, MFS) and improvements in processing speed after participation in an eight-week MBSR programme, regardless of age, gender, type of injury, or time since injury or stroke [43]. Another study by Johansson and colleagues [44] found that participation in an online MBSR programme also lad to significantly reduced mental fatigue after acquired brain injury.

Among other behavioural strategies for fatigue management are: proactive scheduling and structuring a day in advance; alternating high and low mental energy activities throughout the day; matching high-energy times with more demanding tasks; taking frequent short breaks with a motor activity or a relaxing activity (e.g., a brief walk or a few deep breaths); ensuring variation of pace and/or stimulation; maintaining a healthy diet with small, frequent meals to support steady glucose levels; and engaging in regular exercise. Primary goals for fatigue management in cognitive rehabilitation are to help minimize the impact of fatigue on available cognitive resources, as fatigue symptoms tend to exacerbate cognitive, emotional, and behavioural manifestations of brain injury.

2.3.4 Pain

Pain is a common complaint for neurorehabilitation patients and is often multifactorial in its aetiology and presentation. Pain suffering can be caused by polytrauma, weakness, spasticity, neuropathy, central pain, and/or headaches. It is estimated that between 22% and 95% of TBI survivors experience a chronic pain condition [45]. Pain also is prevalent after both ischemic and haemorrhagic strokes and may present as central neuropathic pain and/or pain due to peripheral mechanisms, such as shoulder pain, spasticity, persistent headache, and musculoskeletal pain [46]. The prevalence of pain condition after cerebrovascular accident ranges from 8% to 12% for central post-stroke pain up to 79% for overall post-stroke pain suffering [47].

In TBI, headaches are commonly the primary pain condition for many and are often accompanied by fatigue, sensory disturbances, increased photo- and phono-sensitivity, cognitive deficits, and emotional distress [48]. In addition, musculoskeletal, neuropathic, and central pain are frequently reported and may occur as a consequence of other injuries suffered during the traumatic event, or as a component of a persistent post-concussive syndrome [49]. Studies reported an inverse relationship between post-traumatic headache and the severity of the TBI, with the rates of headache ranging between 30% and 90% among those with a mild TBI, in contrast to the approximately 33% prevalence found among those with moderate to severe injuries [45, 50].

Intervention for behavioural pain management. Gironda and colleagues [49] reviewed existing treatment modalities and outcome studies and concluded that post-traumatic headaches may be resistant to treatment with medication alone, and better pain relief is achieved when medication is coupled with other treatment modalities, including CBT for pain with relaxation training and biofeedback, trigger identification, and stress-management strategies. Engagement in physical therapy and exercises for neck muscles may also reduce the frequency and intensity of tension headaches.

Tailoring CBT for pain to the neurological population facilitates engagement in rehabilitation and may enhance pain-coping skills, reduce associated disability and distress, and decrease pain intensity and frequency. As part of the interventions, it is important to address pain-related fear and activity avoidance, distinction between pain and harm, and potential for opioid analgesics addiction. It has been shown that education regarding behavioural pain management for patients and family tends to enhance compliance and reduce distress [51]. Mindfulness-based cognitive therapy (MBCT) has also been found to be beneficial for treatment of chronic headaches, in terms of reducing negative pain attributions, decreased pain interference, and catastrophizing [52].

2.4 Summary

The BI-ISIG Cognitive Rehabilitation Task Force of the ACRM has established evidence-based clinical recommendations for cognitive rehabilitation interventions through systematic review and analysis of the cognitive rehabilitation literature [1, 2, 3]. Furthermore, comprehensive clinical guidance for evidence-based cognitive rehabilitation protocols based on these reviews are provided in the *Cognitive Rehabilitation Manual: Translating Evidence-Based Recommendations into Practice* [4].

Domain-specific Practice Standard recommendations are based on substantive evidence of effectiveness in existing cognitive rehabilitation literature and involve: (1) metacognitive training for executive functioning deficits after TBI to help with emotional dysregulation and to bolster interventions for neglect, attention, and memory; (2) direct attention training and metacognitive training in post-acute neurorehabilitation for remediation of attention deficits; (3) memory strategy training using both internal and external memory strategies for remediation and compensation of mild memory deficits; (4) visual scanning training for left visual neglect after right hemisphere stroke; and (5) traditional cognitive-linguistic therapies for language deficits in left hemisphere stroke and development of social communication skills to help with functional communication deficits following TBI [3].

Practice Standard recommendations for cognitive rehabilitation also include comprehensive-holistic neuropsychological rehabilitation in post-acute settings given recognition that emotional, behavioural, and physical difficulties further exacerbate cognitive and functional impairments [3]. Individual psychotherapy, particularly CBT and MI modalities, help with positive coping strategies, reduction of emotional distress, and improved engagement in rehabilitation efforts. Sleep disturbance is common in brain injury and improvements are shown with behavioural and environmental interventions to help with sleep hygiene and CBT-I for issues with insomnia. Fatigue is prevalent in neurorehabilitation populations and associated with perceived disability. Neuropsychological rehabilitation interventions utilizing mindfulness and relaxation strategies help with improved fatigue management. Furthermore, cognitive behavioural neuropsychological rehabilitation interventions are effective in behavioural pain management neurorehabilitation populations. Neuropsychological interventions help with cognitive functioning by reducing the impact of emotional, behavioural, and physical factors that compete with already depleted cognitive resources. Interventions are also associated with improved rehabilitation engagement, functional independence, quality of life, and community reintegration. In addition to individual interventions, family therapy is recommended to help establish therapeutic goals within the external (e.g., home) environment to help with generalization of cognitive strategies to everyday life.

References

1. Cicerone KD, Dahlberg C, Kalmar, K, et al. Evidence-based cognitive rehabilitation: Recommendations for clinical practice. *Arch. Phys. Med. Rehabil.* 2000; 81: 1596–1615.

2. Cicerone KD, Dahlberg C, Malec, JF, et al. Evidence-based cognitive rehabilitation: Recommendations for clinical practice: Updated review of the literature from 1998 through 2002. *Arch. Phys. Med. Rehabil.* 2005; 86: 1681–92.

3. Cicerone KD, Langenbahn DM, Braden C, et al. Evidence-based cognitive rehabilitation: Updated review of the literature from 2003 through 2008. *Arch. Phys. Med. Rehabil.* 2011; 92: 519–30.

4. Haskins EC, Cicerone K, Dams-O'Connor K, et al. *Cognitive rehabilitation manual: Translating evidence-based recommendations into practice.* Reston, VA: ACRM Publishing, 2012.

5. Sohlberg M, Mateer C. *Cognitive rehabilitation: An integrative neuropsychological approach.* New York, NY: Guilford Press, 2001.

6. Fleming J, Ownsworth T. A review of awareness interventions in brain injury rehabilitation. *Neuropsychol. Rehabil.* 2006, 16: 474–500.

7. Kennedy MRT, Coelho C, Turkstra L, et al. Intervention for executive functions after traumatic brain injury: A systematic review, meta-analysis and clinical recommendations. *Neuropsychol. Rehabil.* 2008, 12: 257–99.

8. Sohlberg M, Turkstra L. *Optimizing cognitive rehabilitation: Effective instructional methods.* New York, NY: Guilford Press, 2011.

9. Sohlberg M, Mateer C. *Attention process training assessment.* Washington, DC: Association for Neuropsychological Research and Development, 1987.

10. Sohlberg M, McLaughlin KA, Pavese A, et al. Evaluation of attention process training and brain injury education in persons with acquired brain injury. *J. Clin. Exp. Neuropsychol.* 2000; 22: 656–76.

11. Fasotti L, Kovacs F, Eling P, et al. Time pressure management as a compensatory strategy training after closed head injury. *Neuropsychol. Rehabil.* 2000; 10: 47–65.

12. Cicerone K. Remediation of working attention in mild traumatic brain injury. *Brain Inj.* 2002; 16: 185–95.

13. Winkens I, Van Heugten C, Wade D, et al. Training patients in time pressure management: A cognitive strategy for mental slowness. *Clin. Rehabil.* 2009; 23: 79–90.

14. Caplan B. Rehabilitation psychology and neuropsychology with stroke survivors. In Frank RG, Rosenthal M, Caplan, B. eds. *Handbook of rehabilitation psychology.* Washington, DC: American Psychological Association, 2010; 63–94.

15. Hawley L, Newman J. Group Interactive Structured Treatment (GIST): A social competence intervention for individuals with brain injury. *Brain Inj.* 2010; 24: 1292–7.

16. McDonald S, Tate R, Togher L, et al. Social skills treatment for people with severe, chronic acquired brain injuries: A multicenter trial. *Arch. Phys. Med. Rehabil.* 2008; 89: 1648–59.

17. Coleman RD, Rapport LJ, Ergh TC, et al. Predictors of driving outcomes after traumatic brain injury. *Arch. Phys. Med. Rehabil.* 2002; 83: 1415–22.

18. Sherer M, Novack TA, Sander AM, et al. Neuropsychological assessment and employment outcome after traumatic brain injury: A review. *Clin. Neuropsychol.* 2002; 16: 157–78.

19. Zgaljardic D, Seale G, Schaefer L, Temple R, Foreman J, Elliott T. Psychiatric disease and post-acute traumatic brain injury. *J. Neurotrauma* 2015; 32: 1911–25.

20. Fann J, Katon W, Uomoto J, et al. Psychiatric disorders and functional disability in outpatients with traumatic brain injuries. *Am. J. Psychiatry* 1995; 152: 1493–9.

21. Lequerica AH, Kortte, K.Therapeutic engagement: A proposed model of engagement in medical rehabilitation. *Am. J. Phys. Med. and Rehabil.* 2010; 89: 415–22.

22. Potter S, Brown R, Fleminger S. Randomized, waiting list controlled trial of cognitive-behavioral therapy for persistent postconcussional symptoms after predominantly mild-moderate traumatic brain injury. *J. Neurol., Neurosurg. Psychiatry* 2016; 87: 1075–83.

23. Waldron B, Casserly L, O'Sullivan C. Cognitive behavioral therapy for depression and anxiety in adults with acquired brain injury. What works for whom? *Neuropsychol. Rehabil.* 2013; 23: 64–101.

24. Miller WR, Rollnick S. *Motivational interviewing: Helping people change* (3rd edn.). New York: Guilford Press, 2013.

25. Medley A, Powell T. Motivational interviewing to promote self-awareness and engagement in rehabilitation following acquired brain injury: A conceptual review. *Neuropsychol. Rehabil.* 2010; 20: 481–508.

26. Cicerone KD, Mott T, Azulay J, et al. A randomized controlled trial of holistic neuropsychological rehabilitation after traumatic brain injury. *Arch. Phys. Med. Rehabil.* 2008; 89: 2239–49.

27. Hsieh M, Ponsford J, Wong D, et al. Motivational interviewing and cognitive behavior therapy for anxiety following traumatic brain injury: A pilot

randomized controlled trial. *Neuropsychol. Rehabil.* 2012; 22: 585–608.

28. Makley MJ, English SB, Drubach DA, et al. Prevalence of sleep disturbances in closed head injury patients in a rehabilitation unit. *Neurorehabil. Neural Repair* 2008; 22: 341–7.

29. Baumann CR. Traumatic brain injury and disturbed sleep and wakefulness. *Neuromolecular Med.* 2012; 14: 205–12.

30. Wiseman-Hakes C, Colantonio A, Gargaro J. Sleep and wake disorders following traumatic brain injury: A systematic review. *Crit. Rev. Phys. and Rehabil. Med.* 2009; 21: 317–74.

31. Wiseman-Hakes C, Murray B, Colantonio A, et al. Evaluating the impact of treatment for sleep/wake disorders on recovery of cognition and communication in adults with chronic TBI. *Brain Inj.* 2013; 27: 1364–77.

32. Nakase-Richardson R, Sherer M, Barnett SD, et al. Prospective evaluation of the nature, course, and impact of acute sleep abnormality after traumatic brain injury. *Arch. Phys. Med. Rehabil.* 2013; 94: 875–82.

33. Edinger J, Carney C. *Overcoming insomnia: A cognitive-behavioral therapy approach, workbook* (2nd edn. [e-book]). New York, NY: Oxford University Press, 2015.

34. Oullet MC, Morin CM. Efficacy of cognitive-behavioral therapy for insomnia associated with traumatic brain injury: A single-case experimental design. *Arch. Phys. Med. Rehabil.* 2007; 88: 1581–92.

35. Lu W, Krellman J, Dijkers M. Can cognitive behavioral therapy for insomnia also treat fatigue, pain, and mood symptoms in individuals with traumatic brain injury? A multiple case report. *NeuroRehabilitation* 2016; 38: 59–69.

36. Herlofson K, Kluger B. Fatigue in Parkinson's disease. *J. Neurol. Sci.* 2017; 374: 38–41.

37. Wijenberg M, Stapert S, Köhler S, et al. Explaining fatigue in multiple sclerosis: Cross-validation of a biopsychosocial model. *J. Beh. Med.* 2016; 39: 815–22.

38. Ponsford J, Schönberger M, Rajaratnam S. A model of fatigue following traumatic brain injury. *J. Head Trauma Rehabil.* 2015; 30: 277–82.

39. Ulrichsen K, Kaufmann T, Nordvick J, et al. Clinical utility of mindfulness training in the treatment of fatigue after stroke, traumatic brain injury and multiple sclerosis: A systematic literature review and meta-analysis. *Frontiers in Psychol.* 2016; 7: 912.

40. Borgaro S, Baker J, Wethe J, et al. Subjective reports of fatigue during early recovery from traumatic brain injury. *J. Head Trauma Rehabil.* 2005; 20: 416–25.

41. Cantor J, Ashman T, Dijkers M, et al. Systematic review of interventions for fatigue after traumatic brain injury: A NIDRR traumatic brain injury model systems study. *J. Head Trauma Rehabil.* 2014; 29: 490–7.

42. Kabat ZJ. *Full catastrophe living: How to cope with stress, pain and illness using mindfulness meditation* (15th edn.). London, UK: Piatkus Books, 2001.

43. Johansson B, Bjuhr H, Rönnbäck L. Mindfulness-based stress reduction (MBSR) improves long-term mental fatigue after stroke or traumatic brain injury. *Brain Inj.* 2012; 26: 1621–8.

44. Johansson B, Bjuhr H, Karlsson M, et al. Mindfulness-based stress reduction (MBSR) delivered live on the Internet to individuals suffering from mental fatigue after an acquired brain injury. *Mindfulness* 2015; 6: 1356–65.

45. Uomoto JM, Esselman PC. Traumatic brain injury and chronic pain: Differential types and rates by head injury severity. *Arch. Phys. Med. Rehabil.* 1993; 74: 61–4.

46. Seifert CL, Chakravarty M, Sprenger T. The complexities of pain after stroke: A review with a focus on central post-stroke pain. *Paminerva Med.* 2013; 55: 1–10.

47. Oh H, Seo W. A comprehensive review of central post-stroke pain. *Pain Manag. Nurs.* 2015; 16: 804–18.

48. Nicholson K, Martelli MF. The problem of pain. *J. Head Trauma Rehabil.* 2004; 19: 2–9.

49. Gironda R, Clark M, Scholten J, et al. Traumatic brain injury, polytrauma, and pain: Challenges and treatment strategies for the polytrauma rehabilitation. *Rehabil. Psychol.* 2009; 54: 247–58.

50. Couch JR, Bearss C. Chronic daily headache in the posttrauma syndrome: Relation to extent of head injury. *Headache* 2001; 41: 559–64.

51. Sherer M, Evans CC, Leverenz J, et al. Therapeutic alliance in post-acute brain injury rehabilitation: Predictors of strength of alliance and impact of alliance on outcome. *Brain Inj.* 2007; 21: 663–72.

52. Day M, Thorn B, Kilgo G, et al. Mindfulness-based cognitive therapy for the treatment of headache pain: A pilot study. *Clin. J. Pain.* 2014; 30: 152–61.

Chapter 3

Management of Mood and Behaviour in Neurorehabilitation

Lewys Morgan and Abhijeeth Shetty

3.1 Introduction

The association between physical illness and emotional distress is well known [1]. People make adjustments to their lifestyle throughout the course of their illness in order to allow them to deal with the stressful consequences of being unwell. This process of adjustment has to be repeated many times in patients with chronic physical illnesses as the disease progresses, disability increases, or new complications arise [2]. Around a quarter of all those with a physical illness will go on to develop diagnosable psychiatric illnesses, of which mood and behavioural disorders are the most common [2]. Patients with neurological diseases can be particularly vulnerable to develop psychiatric disorders due to the impact of their illnesses on their physical and social functioning as well as the direct psychological consequence of the neurological disease process or brain lesions [3]. Disorders of mood and behaviour can impact an individual's ability to engage in rehabilitative activities and if untreated can negatively impact rehabilitation outcomes. Poor coping with the physical illness can be associated with self-harm and increased suicide risk, particularly in rehabilitation and neurology settings, which is traumatic to the patient, their family, and healthcare professionals looking after them [4]. It is therefore important that healthcare professionals have an understanding of the common mood and behavioural problems that occur in the neurorehabilitation setting and the management options available to them.

3.2 Adjustment Disorders

The emotional impact of a neurological illness can manifest itself in a manner that interferes with an individual's social, occupational, or other areas of functioning to a degree that it is categorized as a mental disorder. The International Statistical Classification of Diseases and Related Health Problems (ICD-10) [5] and the Diagnostic and Statistical Manual of Mental Disorders (DSM-V) [6]

are the two most frequently used resources containing descriptions of mental disorders. Both of these resources describe a condition known as an adjustment disorder where a stressor, which can be due to any cause including a neurological illness, has affected an individual's identity, values, social network, or social support, or has precipitated a major transition or crisis to such a degree as to cause a significant impact on that person's functioning [5,6].

Symptoms may manifest themselves as low mood, anxiety and worry, irritability and anger, social withdrawal or aggression, along with subjective feelings of an inability to cope or plan for the future in their current state. In order to diagnose an adjustment disorder, it is assumed that the condition would not have arisen if it were not for the occurrence of the stressor and is out of proportion to the severity of the stressor.

The aforementioned symptoms are a part of the normal adjustment process and tend to resolve within a few weeks of the onset of the stressor; however, in some the related emotional and behavioural disturbances do not. This may be in the context of the persistence of the stressor, persistence of the symptoms in spite of resolution of the stressor, or the individual finding it difficult to adapt to the stressor [7]. If symptoms persist, psychiatric intervention is often required. The prevalence of adjustment disorder in neurorehabilitation has not been systematically investigated.

Table 3.1 shows examples of factors that can affect psychological adjustment [8]. If clinicians are able to ensure that they acknowledge and attempt to address these factors early in the care of a neurorehabilitation patient, they will have the best opportunity to promote adaptive emotional recovery.

If an individual does develop an adjustment disorder with persistent symptoms, then treatment options include social, psychological, and/or pharmacological support. There is no consensus on optimal treatment options for adjustment disorders in general

Table 3.1 Modified from [8]

Factors that can affect psychological adjustment	
Lack of privacy	Chronic fatigue
Loss of independence	Medication side effects
Changes to social role and lifestyle	Isolation
Uncertainty regarding the future	Boredom
Sense of helplessness	Medical complications
Separation from family and friends	Cognitive problems
Inability to control basic bodily functions	Lack of family, friends, and social supports
Changes in physical health and functional ability	Chronic pain
Changes in body image	Premorbid personality

let alone in relation to neurorehabilitation settings [7]. By definition adjustment disorders are time limited and hence brief therapies should be considered initially. Addressing the factors which affect psychological adjustment as detailed in Table 3.1 should be the first step. The limited evidence in this field supports brief psychological interventions [7].

The goals of such therapy include: (a) identify the stressor and determine if it can be eliminated or minimized (problem solving); (b) understand the meaning of the stressor for the patient and reframe it positively; (c) normalize emotions related to the grief reaction and enable acceptance, distress tolerance, and emotional self-regulation; (d) bring to awareness and reduce maladaptive coping including avoidance and substance misuse; (e) mobilize sources of support, e.g., family, friends, peer support groups, and statutory and voluntary agencies.

These interventions can take the form of psycho-educational, supportive, family, peer, cognitive, behavioural, interpersonal, mindfulness-based, or psychodynamic therapies. Crisis and contingency planning should be considered. The role of the rehabilitation clinician would be to identify adjustment difficulties including risk to the patient and others, provide psycho-education, signpost to self-management options, and refer to psychology or psychiatry for specialist assessment and management.

In terms of pharmacological management of adjustment disorder, the most frequently prescribed

medications are antidepressants to improve low mood and anxiety symptoms. Both hypnotic and anxiolytic medications such as benzodiazepines are often prescribed for those experiencing an adjustment disorder with predominant anxiety features. There is no firm evidence to suggest whether outcomes are better for those treated with antidepressants or anxiolytics; however, it is often the case that their quick onset of action and perceived effectiveness make benzodiazepine anxiolytics appealing for control of symptoms along with psychological therapies [7]. Benzodiazepines can be a useful adjunctive in the management of severe emotional distress; however, they should be used sparingly and as a short-term remedy due to the high risk of dependence and oversedation, as well as the difficulties in cessation due to withdrawal effects [9]. If antidepressants are effective, then it is recommended that they are gradually withdrawn after at least six months of stable mental state.

3.3 Mood Disorders

Mood disorders found commonly in neurorehabilitation patients tend to be those highly prevalent in the general population such as depression and anxiety and hence frequently described in the literature. However, less common mood disorders such as bipolar disorder and emotional incontinence have been identified and studied in some specific conditions.

3.3.1 Depressive Disorders

Depressive disorder, often known simply as depression, is a syndrome characterized by low mood, poor energy, and a lack of interest or pleasure in activities. Identifying depression within neurorehabilitation populations can be challenging due to the fact that many of its symptoms, such as poor sleep, poor appetite, fatigue, poor concentration, and reduced libido, may be the sequelae of the neurological illness itself. Hence, psychological symptoms of depression are more useful in diagnosis; these include feelings of guilt, worthlessness, helplessness, hopelessness, and suicidal thoughts.

Depression can be diagnosed and measured either by using clinical assessment incorporating ICD-10 or DSM-V criteria, or by utilizing evidence-based rating scales. In clinical practice useful and widely used rating scales include the Public Health Questionnaire (PHQ-9), the Hamilton Depression Rating Scale, and the Beck Depression Inventory; in older people the Geriatric Depression Scale can also be valuable [10].

Rates of depression in the general population are estimated to range from 7% to 21% [11]. The rates are significantly higher in those with chronic physical ill health. The highest rates of clinically significant depressive symptoms (30% to 50%) are found in certain neurological conditions like epilepsy, Huntington's disease, Parkinson's disease, multiple sclerosis (MS), and stroke [2, 11, 12, 13, 14].

Depending on the number of symptoms and their functional impact, depression is divided into mild, moderate, and severe categories. The National Institute for Health and Care Excellence (NICE) guidelines suggest that mild depression is initially treated with psychosocial support, which is often delivered in primary care settings. Moderate or severe depression requires more specialist interventions; this usually takes the form of a combination of high-intensity psychological therapy and an antidepressant. Cognitive behavioural therapy (CBT) and interpersonal therapy (IPT) are favoured by NICE due to the more robust research evidence supporting their use in treating depression in otherwise healthy populations [15].

CBT is a psychological therapy designed to focus on modifying how an individual thinks, feels, and behaves in relation to themselves and/or others in order to feel better. CBT is focused on tasks and steered by a therapeutic alliance between the patient and the therapist. An example of a vicious circle of negative thoughts and related feelings and behaviours is shown in what follows; the intention of CBT would be to try and move the patient from unhelpful to helpful patterns. A person may have a series of unhelpful negative

thoughts, feelings, and behaviours that need careful unravelling during the sessions [16].

CBT is delivered over up to 20 sessions which are each around an hour long. Group and online or computer-aided CBT have also proven effective in the treatment of depression [17].

IPT is based on an individual's interactions with others and how these impact the individual's emotions. IPT focuses on four problem areas – grief, interpersonal disputes, role transitions, and interpersonal deficits. A number of techniques are used to address these areas and help the patient to address their depressive symptoms [18].

Whilst both of these psychological therapies have robust evidence for their use in the general population, their efficacy amongst neurorehabilitation populations has not been widely studied and results of the few published studies are mixed. A Cochrane review into the treatment of post-stroke depression completed in 2008 found that only four psychotherapy trials were available and there was no overall evidence of any benefit from the intervention [19]. A more recent review into depression in Parkinson's disease found that CBT and psychodynamic therapy are both effective compared to control groups [13].

Antidepressants are indicated for treatment of moderate to severe depression or mild depression which is unresponsive to psychosocial interventions [15]. Antidepressants increase the levels of extracellular synaptic neurotransmitters such as serotonin, noradrenaline, and dopamine [9]. A Cochrane review included 13 trials of patients with post-stroke depression; the review concluded that antidepressant medication produced improvements in depressive symptoms compared to placebo [19]. A review of antidepressant use in Parkinson's disease highlighted

Table 3.2 A model of cognitive behavioural therapy

	Unhelpful	Helpful
Thoughts	Since my stroke all my friends have left me; they must think I'm not fun or interesting any more.	Since my stroke my friends have not been in touch; I wonder if they know how I am/they must be finding it difficult to deal with.
Emotional Feelings	Upset, low in mood, guilty, anxious	Empathize with friends, positive and curious
Physical Feeling	Low energy, headache, palpitations, sweating, nausea	Comfortable
Action	Avoid friends, don't make contact with them, isolate self.	Talk to friends, send messages. Make sure they are doing okay and let them know how you are.

Table 3.3 A model of interpersonal therapy

Grief	Grief for loss of physical abilities or altered self-image
Interpersonal Disputes	Inability to meet expected roles at home or work, anger at own or partner's illness or disability
Role Transitions	Loss of job, marriage difficulties, adaptation to pain or physical illness, post-traumatic symptoms
Interpersonal Deficits	Difficulty forming new relationships, loss of social functioning

the variable efficacy of selective serotonin reuptake inhibitors (SSRIs), serotonin-noradrenaline reuptake inhibitors (SNRIs), and tricyclic antidepressants compared to placebo [13]. Both psychotherapy and antidepressant trials in neurorehabilitation suffer from significant methodological issues, which makes evidence-based recommendation difficult.

The choice of the antidepressant should be driven by the tolerability and side-effect profile of the drug. The presence of co-morbid illnesses and drug interaction should be borne in mind. The first-line antidepressant is an SSRI, although the risk of side effects, in particular gastrointestinal problems including bleeding and hyponatremia, need careful monitoring, especially in the elderly. Patients should be warned about the risk of anxiety and restlessness in the first two weeks of starting an antidepressant as well as the risk of increased suicidal thoughts in some patients. If well supported during this period, the therapeutic effect can be expected in two to four weeks at an adequate tolerated dose. Any antidepressant must be continued for at least six months (12 months in the elderly) following the resolution of all depressive symptoms in order to prevent relapse. A combination of antidepressants and psychosocial treatments is likely to be more effective than antidepressants alone [15].

3.3.2 Anxiety Disorders

Anxiety is a broad title for a group of disorders including phobias, panic disorder, and generalized anxiety disorder. Anxiety disorders can be diagnosed clinically or by utilizing evidence-based rating scales. Commonly used rating scales include the Generalized Anxiety Disorder 7 (GAD-7), the Beck Anxiety Inventory, and the Hospital Anxiety and Depression Scale (HADS) [20]. Within the general population the prevalence of phobias and panic disorder is reported as 0.6% and 2.4%, respectively, with generalized anxiety being more prevalent at 5.9% [9].

A brief description of generalized anxiety disorder and its treatment approaches follows as a guide to anxiety disorders in general. ICD-10 criteria for generalized anxiety disorder include persistent nervousness, trembling, muscular tensions, sweating, lightheadedness, palpitations, dizziness, and epigastric discomfort. The patient may also have one or more overwhelming fears, e.g., fear of dying, and fear of hospitals. The generalized nature refers to the fact that these symptoms are persistent and independent of the environmental situation that the sufferer is in [5].

Meta-analysis of studies into anxiety in patients with stroke, MS, and Parkinson's disease estimated prevalence rates of clinically significant anxiety symptoms in about 24%, 34%, and 40% of all patients, respectively [20, 14, 13].

At present, most published studies into the treatment of anxiety in neurorehabilitation populations have included small numbers of participants; however, these studies suggest promising results from utilizing psychological and pharmacological treatments recommended for anxiety in the general population.

NICE recommends that initial treatment for uncomplicated generalized anxiety involves low-intensity psychological therapies such as individual self-help or psycho-educational groups. If there is no improvement after use of these interventions, then the recommendation is that high-intensity psychological interventions such as CBT or applied relaxation are utilized, along with the use of an antidepressant medication [21]. CBT used in anxiety follows the same structure and principles as those used in depression. Applied relaxation is a coping skill that can be applied in any situation to reduce the anxiety response and introduce relaxation responses. The technique utilized is progressive muscle relaxation, which involves tensing and releasing various muscle groups to relax the body. The aim is to coach the patient into developing these relaxation skills as a habit that is automatically enacted when in an anxiety-provoking situation [22].

Pharmacological management of anxiety is indicated if psychological input has not been successful or if the patient has expressed a preference for this option. As with depression, SSRIs are considered the most effective and acceptable medications to trial first line. In the case of anxiety, NICE recommends sertraline as the first-line SSRI for cost-effectiveness reasons [21]. The choice, cautions, monitoring arrangement, and maintenance treatment with antidepressants as described in the section on depressive disorders apply to anxiety disorders as well.

Anxiety disorders by definition last six months or longer and hence benzodiazepines, such as lorazepam and diazepam, should usually be avoided except as a short-term measure to manage severe anxiety, agitation, or panic symptoms [21]. As described in the section on adjustment disorders, benzodiazepines carry a high risk of dependence, over-sedation, and withdrawal symptoms after long-term use.

3.3.3 Emotional Incontinence

Lesions in the lenticulo-capsular and brainstem areas have been associated with emotional incontinence, a condition characterized by excessive and inappropriate crying or laughing without the expected stimuli to motivate such behaviour [23]. Emotional incontinence can occur in a variety of neurological conditions, but is often seen post stroke, post traumatic brain injury (TBI), and in MS. The condition can often be mistaken for depression or mania, but a clinician should be able to differentiate between the two by examining the patient's affect, i.e. identifying the immediate expressed emotion, whether that corresponds with the patient's mood, frequency of changes in affect, and identifying whether there is an appropriate stimulus for the emotion. The mainstay of treatment is antidepressants, particularly SSRIs, which have been shown to be an effective first option to alleviate emotional incontinence [23].

3.3.4 Other Mood Disorders

Bipolar disorder is characterized by patterns of manic and depressive mood episodes. Evidence suggests that patients with MS are at a higher lifetime risk of developing any type of bipolar disorder, particularly type 2

(characterized by hypomania and depressive episodes) when compared with the general population (7.5% versus 1%) [24]. There is little research into the treatment of bipolar disorder in MS populations, so by default, treatment options are the same as in the general population. For patients presenting in the manic or hypomanic phase, treatment consists of withdrawal of any antidepressant and commencement of an antipsychotic medication. If the presentation is that of bipolar depression, then commencement of an antidepressant alongside an antipsychotic or a mood stabilizer is indicated. Longer-term mood management will often utilize a mood stabilizer such as sodium valproate or lithium as prophylaxis [25]. Diagnosis and initial management of bipolar disorders will require specialist psychiatric input.

If the neurological illness develops after a traumatic incident, such as in some cases of TBI, post-traumatic stress disorder (PTSD) has been identified as a potential complication [26]. PTSD is characterized by flashbacks and nightmares about the traumatic event, avoidance of situations that are reminiscent of the trauma, and hypervigilance. These symptoms are present against a background of a feeling of emotional numbness and detachment [5]. The recommended treatment of PTSD is CBT or other psychological therapies; currently there are no clinical trials of treatments specifically in TBI populations. It is also important to ensure any co-morbid depression and anxiety disorders are well managed [26].

3.4 Suicide

Suicide is the cause of more than 6,000 deaths per year in the United Kingdom and currently ranks as the leading cause of death in those aged between 20 and 34 [27]. These statistics highlight the importance of being aware of groups vulnerable to suicidal thoughts and intent. Neurorehabilitation populations can be particularly at risk of developing suicidal thoughts and acting upon them. This is secondary not only to the high prevalence of mood disorders but also to factors such as the stress of the trauma and potential increase in impulsivity and disinhibition that may come with neurological injuries and disorders [28].

Studies have suggested that those who have suffered a TBI have a fourfold increase in risk of death by suicide compared to the general population [28]. Studies of post-stroke populations have identified an increased risk of suicidality especially in women and young adults. Risks of suicidal thoughts, plans, and acts are all increased after stroke compared to the general population [29]. Progressive degenerative neurological conditions appear to significantly increase suicide risk. Huntington's disease has been reported as having up to an eightfold increase in completed suicide, and suicide in MS populations is 1.6- to 14-fold higher than in the general population [30, 31].

It is important therefore to assess the risk of suicide in neurorehabilitation populations routinely. All clinicians should have an understanding of how to undertake a risk assessment, although complex risk assessments will require specialist mental health input.

It is often advisable for those with little experience of conducting risk assessments to use a risk assessment tool such as the 'tool for assessment of suicide risk' (TASR) [32]. Using the TASR allows the clinician to ensure that pertinent questions are asked sensitively. It lets the clinician make an informed decision on how to manage the risk and provides easy documentation of a risk assessment [33].

Managing patients with suicidal thoughts and intent can be complex and challenging. If the clinician has concerns that the patient is experiencing suicidal thoughts, then psychiatric advice should be sought. Identifying and managing mood and behavioural problems described in this chapter can contribute to reducing and preventing suicide risk.

3.5 Challenging Behaviour

All of the disorders outlined earlier can lead to behavioural challenges that may prohibit effective neurorehabilitation and create difficulties for family and healthcare professionals. Accurate diagnosis and satisfactory management of the condition should help to alleviate some of these challenges: however, there are times when behavioural problems may occur in the absence of any diagnosable mental disorder, or persist in spite of optimal treatment of such a disorder.

The physical and psychosocial difficulties faced by those who have suffered from an illness requiring neurorehabilitation can lead to a variety of unpleasant emotional responses. These may manifest themselves as irritability, anger, agitation, and aggression. Clinicians find these behaviours the most challenging to deal with. It is therefore useful for the healthcare professional to have the skills to deal with such behaviours.

The way the clinician responds to challenging behaviour is important to prevent them from antagonizing a distressed patient further, which can escalate into violence. Richmond et al. outline some important rules (highlighted in the paragraphs that follow in italics) to consider when engaging in verbal de-escalation of challenging behaviour in patients [34].

The clinician should check that it is **safe to approach** the patient and **respect personal space** by always remaining two arm's lengths away, thus reducing risk of harm to them and reducing the patient's perception of threat from the clinician. There should be easy access to the exit for both. The clinician should **avoid being provocative** by ensuring that hands are visible and open, stand at an angle to the patient, and keep a calm demeanour and facial expression.

The clinician should ensure that only one person interacts with the patient at any one time, although it is helpful for other staff members to be nearby for support. They should **initiate verbal contact** by introducing themselves, provide reassurance, and orientate the patient. The clinician should **be concise** by utilizing short sentences, simple language, and repetition to ensure understanding. Attempts should be made to **identify the wants and feelings** of the patient. If the patient is not communicative, body language and past knowledge of the patient may be of use. In order to really understand the patient, the clinician must **listen closely to what the patient is saying** through active listening such as receptive body language, clarifying, and summarizing. They should imagine what the patient is saying as true even if they know it is not, to get an idea of how the patient is feeling.

Wherever possible the clinician should **agree or agree to disagree.** The clinician may agree with the truth of events, agree with the patient's version of events, or just agree to disagree. Whilst agreeing with the patient avoids conflict and allows for collaboration, it is important that the consequences of unacceptable behaviour are clear. The clinician should **establish clear boundaries** in a matter-of-fact and non-threatening manner. The clinician should **offer realistic choices** about alternative behaviours which can empower the patient and provide **hope.**

In order to restore the therapeutic relationship between staff and patients, there must be a *debrief of the patient and staff*. The patient and staff should be able to explain their version of events and explore alternatives for managing similar situations. By following these simple but powerful rules, the healthcare professional can increase the chances of a successful and conflict-free de-escalation [34].

In addition to verbal de-escalation, environmental conditions must be taken into account. It may be vital to remove the patient from a certain situation or for the staff to remove themselves for safety reasons. It may be necessary to ensure that objects that could be a risk to the patient, professional, or others are removed and that the patient's environment is altered to prevent them being overstimulated [34].

If verbal de-escalation and environmental modification have been unsuccessful, consideration must be made for the use of chemical sedation or, in some circumstances, physical restraint and seclusion. All healthcare facilities, where challenging behaviours are likely to occur, should have their own guidelines with regard to sedation, restraint, and seclusion. If the aim is rapid tranquilization, then the first-line drug of choice is a short-acting benzodiazepine like lorazepam or an antipsychotic medication, typically haloperidol with promethazine intramuscularly [35].

In situations where challenging behaviour has become a longer-term issue, specialist help from a psychiatrist should be called for. Underlying causes of challenging behaviours need reassessment and appropriate management. For long-term use, alternative medications must be considered due to the unfavourable side-effect profiles of both benzodiazepines and antipsychotics. A Cochrane review into the management of agitation post TBI found that the most promising medications were beta-blockers such as propranolol [36]. A more recent systematic review suggests that whilst beta-blockers show good results in managing agitation in TBI, the expert consensus recommendation is the use of mood stabilizers such as carbamazepine and sodium valproate as first-line drugs [37]. In addition, the review found little evidence of a beneficial effect with the use of antipsychotic agents in the absence of psychotic symptoms [37]. The Maudsley *Prescribing Guidelines in Psychiatry* is a useful resource for pharmacological management of mood and behavioural disorders [38].

3.6 Conclusion

Mood and behavioural problems are common within all types of neurorehabilitation patient groups. They cause distress to patients, affect patients' ability to engage in rehabilitation, and result in poorer outcomes without treatment. Neurorehabilitation professionals find these challenging to identify and treat. Whilst literature exists to illustrate the high prevalence of these disorders, there is little in the way of high-quality trials into their management. Unless contraindicated, evidence-based treatment guidelines for mood and behavioural disorders in the general population should be followed. The authors recommend that the multidisciplinary team in neurorehabilitation is supported by health psychologists and liaison psychiatrists for appropriate management of mood and behavioural problems.

References

1. Naylor C, Parsonage M, McDaid D et al. *Long-term conditions and mental health: The cost of co-morbidities.* London, UK: The King's Fund and Centre for Mental Health, 2012.

2. Guthrie E, Nayak A. Psychological reaction to physical illness. In Guthrie E, Temple M. eds. *Seminars in liaison psychiatry.* London, UK: Royal College of Psychiatrists, 2012; 51–65.

3. Jorge R, Robinson R. Mood disorders following traumatic brain injury. *International Review of Psychiatry* 2003; 15(4).

4. Hung CI, Liu CY, Liao MN, et al. Self-destructive acts occurring during medical general hospitalization. *General Hospital Psychiatry* 2000; 22(2): 115–21.

5. World Health Organization. *The ICD-10 classification of mental and behavioural disorders: Clinical descriptions and diagnostic guidelines.* Geneva, Switzerland: World Health Organization, 1992.

6. American Psychiatric Association. *Diagnostic and statistical manual of mental disorders* (5th edn.). Washington, DC: American Psychiatric Association, 2013.

7. Casey P. Adjustment disorder: New developments. *Current Psychiatry Reports* 2014; 16: 451.

8. Dezarnaulds A, Ilchef R. *Psychological adjustment after spinal cord injury: Useful strategies for health professionals* (2nd edn.). New South Wales, Australia: New South Wales Agency for Clinical Innovation, 2014.

9. Joint Formulary Committee. *British national formulary.* Vol. **74**. London, UK: BMJ Group and Pharmaceutical Press, 2017.

10. Bienenfeld D. Medscape. Screening Tests for Depression. 2016. http://emedicine.medscape.com/article/1859039-overview. (Accessed 3 September 2017).

11. Bromet E, Andrade LH, Hwang I, Sampson NA, Alonso J, de Girolamo G, et al. Cross-national epidemiology of DSM-IV major depressive episode. *BMC Med.* 2011; 9(90).

12. Paolucci S. Role, indications and controversies of antidepressant therapy in chronic stroke patients. *European Journal of Physical and Rehabilitation Medicine* 2013; 49: 233–41.

13. Renfroe J, Turner JH, Hinson VK. Prevalence, impact, and management of depression and anxiety in patients with Parkinson's disease. *Journal of Parkinsonism and Restless Legs Syndrome* 2016; 6: 15–22.

14. Boeschoten RE, Braamse AMJ, Beekman ATF, et al. Prevalence of depression and anxiety in multiple sclerosis: A systematic review and meta-analysis. *Journal of Neurological Sciences* 2017; 372: 331–41.

15. National Institute of Clinical Excellence (NICE). *Depression in adults with a chronic physical health problem: Recognition and management. NICE guideline 2009. (CG91).* London, UK: National Institute of Clinical Excellence, 2009.

16. Royal College of Psychiatrists. *Cognitive behavioural therapy.* 2013. [Patient Information Leaflet].

17. Andersson G, Cuijpers P. Pros and cons of online cognitive-behavioural therapy. *British Journal of Psychiatry* 2008; 193(4): 270–1.

18. Lipsitz J, Markowitz J. Mechanisms of change in interpersonal therapy (IPT). *Clinical Psychology Review* 2013; 33(8): 1134–47.

19. Hackett M, Anderson C, House AO, Xia J. Interventions for treating depression after stroke. *Cochrane Database of Systematic Review* 2008; 4: 1–95.

20. Burton C, Murray J, Holmes J et al. Frequency of anxiety after stroke: A systematic review and meta-analysis of observational studies. *International Journal of Stroke* 2013; 8: 545–59.

21. National Institute of Clinical Excellence (NICE). *Generalised anxiety disorder and panic disorder in adults: Management. NICE guidelines 2011. (CG113).* London, UK: National Institute of Clinical Excellence.

22. Hayes-Skelton SA, Roemer L, Orsillo SM, Borovec TDA Contemporary view of applied relaxation for generalised anxiety disorder. *Cognitive Behavioural Therapy* 2013; 42(4): 292–302.

23. Kim JS. Post-stroke mood and emotional disturbances: Pharmacological therapy based on mechanisms. *Journal of Stroke* 2016; 18(3): 244–55.

24. Carta MG, Moro MF, Lorefice L et al. Multiple sclerosis and bipolar disorders: The burden of comorbidity and its consequences on quality of life. *Journal of Affective Disorders* 2014; 167: 192–7.

25. National Institute of Clinical Excellence (NICE). *Bipolar disorder: Assessment and management. NICE guidelines 2016. (CG185).* London, UK: National Institute of Clinical Excellence.

26. Schwartzbold M, Diaz A, Martins ET. Psychiatric disorders and traumatic brain injury. *Neuropsychiatric Disease and Treatment* 2008; 4(4): 797–816.

27. Mental Health Foundation. *Suicide.* 2017. www.mentalhealth.org.uk/a-to-z/s/suicide. (Accessed 2 October 2017).

28. Wasserman L, Shaw T, Vu M, et al. An overview of traumatic brain injury and suicide. *Brain Injury* 2008; 22(11): 811–19.

29. Pompili M, Venturini P, Lamis DA et al. Suicide in stroke survivors: Epidemiology and prevention. *Drugs and Aging* 2015; 32: 21–9.

30. Hubers A, Duijn E, Roos R. Suicidal ideation in a European Huntington's disease population. *Journal of Affective Disorders* 2013; 151(1): 248–58.

31. Marrie RA. What is the risk of suicide in multiple sclerosis? *Multiple Sclerosis Journal* 2017; 23(6): 755–6.

32. Chehil S, Kutcher SP. *Suicide risk management: A manual for health professionals* (2nd edn.). Chichester, UK: Wiley-Blackwell, 2012.

33. BMJ Best Practice. *Suicide Risk Management.* 2016. http://bestpractice.bmj.com/best-practice/monograph/1016/diagnosis/step-by-step.html. (Accessed 5 October 2017).

34. Richmond JS et al. Verbal de-escalation of the agitated patient: Consensus statement of the American Association for Emergency Psychiatry Project BETA De-escalation Workgroup. *Western Journal of Emergency Medicine* 2012; 13(1): 17–25.

35. National Institute of Clinical Excellence (NICE). *Violence and aggression: Short-term management in mental health, health and community settings. NICE guidelines (NG10).* 2015. London, UK: National Institute of Clinical Excellence.

36. Fleminger S, Greenwood RJ, Oliver DL. Pharmacological management for agitation and aggression in people with acquired brain injury. *Cochrane Database of Systematic Reviews* 2006; 18(4).

37. Plantier D, Luaute J. Drugs for behaviour disorders after traumatic brain injury: Systematic review and expert consensus leading to French recommendations for good practice. *Annals of Physical and Rehabilitation Medicine* 2016; 59(1): 42–57.

38. Taylor D, Paton C, Kapur S. *Prescribing guidelines in psychiatry* (Maudsley 11th edn.). Chichester, UK: Wiley-Blackwell, 2012.

Chapter 4

Management of Disorders of Consciousness in Neurorehabilitation

Andreas Bender

4.1 Introduction

Long-term management of patients with disorders of consciousness (DOC) following severe brain injury is a demanding task. Challenges include diagnosis, prognostication, complications, and relative lack of evidence-based treatments, as well as end-of-life decisions with medico-legal implications. The Royal College of Physicians has recently updated its national clinical guidelines for such patients, which is an excellent source for more detailed information [1].

4.1.1 The Clinical Spectrum of Disorders of Consciousness (DOC)

There is no commonly accepted definition for consciousness, but most attempts agree that it refers to a state of reflected awareness of the self and the environment [2]. In order to fully comprehend the distinctions between different types of disorders of consciousness (DOC), it is important to acknowledge that two components are mandatory for 'normal'

consciousness: arousal (being awake) and awareness. These two aspects of consciousness can dissociate as a consequence of brain injury, e.g., leading to a state with sufficient arousal and alertness (eyes open) but lack of apparent awareness, the so-called unresponsive wakefulness syndrome (UWS).

The term DOC usually comprises four different consciousness states, but it is important to note that this has to be considered as a DOC continuum rather than completely distinct entities (Table 4.1).

The most obvious clinical distinction lies between coma and the UWS, when wakefulness with open eyes starts to occur. It is suggested to use the term UWS rather than its predecessors 'vegetative state' or 'apallic syndrome', because of the negative associations with them [6]. In contrast to the patients with UWS, Minimally conscious syndrome (MCS) patients typically can respond to some simple commands or do visual pursuit. As soon as patients regain functional communication or functional object use abilities, they emerge from the MCS. This state with regained but typically far from 'normal' consciousness lacks its own

Table 4.1 Clinical characteristics of disorders of consciousness

Type of DOC	Definition/clinical criteria	Reference
Coma	• Typically occurs immediately following severe brain injury, lasting approx. two weeks (without sedation) • Complete lack of arousal with eyes constantly closed • Inability to follow commands	[3]
Unresponsive wakefulness syndrome (UWS)	• Alternating phases of opened and closed eyes • No purposeful behavioural responses to the environment and commands • Spontaneous and reflex movements can occur	[4]
Minimally conscious state (MCS)	• Reproducible evidence of simple command following (termed MCS+) OR • Non-reflex, purposeful behaviour, such as visual pursuit or adequate emotional response (termed MCS−)	[5]
Emergence from MCS/ confusional state (CS)	• Ability for functional communication OR • Ability for functional object use • Confusion and disorientation	[5]

terminology, but is often referred to as a confusional state (CS) with disorientation.

4.1.2 The Challenge of the Correct Clinical Diagnosis

It is challenging to correctly diagnose the level of consciousness in brain-injured patients. It is estimated that the rate of misdiagnosis is close to 40% [7]. In most cases, MCS patients are mistaken to be in the UWS. There are several explanations for the lack of diagnostic precision: (1) examiners do not use standardized and well-operationalized clinical scales; (2) patients transition back and forth between UWS and MCS so that repeated clinical evaluations are warranted; (3) patients may be severely aphasic or completely locked in so that commands are either not understood or motor output in response to command is not possible despite consciousness.

Several neurobehavioral clinical rating scales have been developed to differentiate UWS, MCS, and CS, as well as to provide a measure for clinical progress. Currently, the JFK Coma Recovery Scale – Revised (CRS-R) is probably the internationally most widely used scale [8]. While it is not perfect, it has recently been recommended as the assessment method with the least limitations [9]. It ranges from 0 (deep coma) to a maximum of 23 points and clearly operationalizes features identifying MCS and emergence therefrom (Table 4.2).

Visual pursuit often is the first sign of emergence from UWS to MCS. It can best be elicited by using a mirror (or possibly the selfie side of a smartphone camera) and slowly moving it in front of the patient's eyes [10]. Yet lack of visual pursuit may not be taken as proof of UWS because many patients may suffer from cortical blindness as the occipital lobe seems to be especially prone to hypoxic-ischemic brain damage.

Even the most experienced clinician may miss signs of consciousness despite repeated examinations. This is due to a fundamental problem within the area of the evaluation of consciousness. Patients can only overcome the thresholds for conscious behaviour in the various clinical rating scales, if they retain the ability for movement control, and be it only for occulomotor responses. Patients may be conscious, but may be unable to show it due to complete loss of motor control. It is often a challenge to identify patients in a locked-in syndrome (LIS), but they at

Table 4.2 JFK Coma Recovery Scale – Revised (CRS-R)

Subscale/Items	If present, defining:
Auditory Function Scale	
4 – Consistent Movement to Command	MCS
3 – Reproducible Movement to Command	MCS
2 – Localization to Sound	
1 – Auditory Startle	
0 – None	
Visual Function Scale	
5 – Object Recognition	MCS
4 – Object Localization: Reaching	MCS
3 – Visual Pursuit	MCS
2 – Fixation	MCS
1 – Visual Startle	
0 – None	
Motor Function Scale	
6 – Functional Object Use	emMCS
5 – Automatic Motor Response	MCS
4 – Object Manipulation	MCS
3 – Localization to Noxious Stimulation	MCS
2 – Flexion Withdrawal	
1 – Abnormal Posturing	
0 – None/Flaccid	
Oromotor/Verbal Function Scale	
3 – Intelligible Verbalization	MCS
2 – Vocalization/Oral Movement	
1 – Oral Reflexive Movement	
0 – None	
Communication Scale	
2 – Functional: Accurate	emMCS
1 – Non-Functional: Intentional	MCS
0 – None	
Arousal Scale	
3 – Attention	
2 – Eye Opening w/o Stimulation	
1 – Eye Opening with Stimulation	
0 – Unarousable	

Note that for definition of MCS or emMCS, only one corresponding item needs to be present.
MCS = Minimally Conscious State; emMCS = emergence from MCS; UWS = Unresponsive Wakefulness Syndrome

least typically have volitional vertical eye movements. There seems to be a population of patients with severe brain injury, though, who lack even this minimal motor output despite being conscious or at least minimally conscious. There has been a strong scientific interest in developing methods that can detect such 'hidden consciousness'. Electrophysiological methods (mainly EEG) analyse event-related potentials (ERP) or other specific bioelectrical signals following stimuli or commands. Imaging methods, such as functional MRI or FDG-PET, focus on identifying brain networks that are necessary for consciousness or on eliciting responses in specific brain areas, which are typical for conscious awareness [11]. Several such studies have suggested that 10–20% of UWS patients may indeed be conscious and in rare instances, communication by means of the MRI signal seemed to be possible in the scanner [12]. Identifying patients with preserved yet concealed consciousness may not only be scientifically interesting but also of clinical and prognostic relevance because they may have a more favourable long-term outcome [13].

It has to be stressed, though, that all of these methods are still mainly in the research realm and have hardly entered clinical routine.

4.1.3 Neuroanatomy and Pathophysiology

DOC can arise from strategic lesions in areas, which are believed to be critical components of arousal and consciousness networks, such as the brainstem containing the ascending reticular activating system (ARAS) or the central thalamus bilaterally [14]. In contrast, diffuse brain injury due to anoxic-ischemic encephalopathy (AIE) or traumatic brain injury (TBI) may cause DOC by disrupting thalamo-cortical or cortico-cortical (especially frontoparietal) projections. Anterior and posterior midline neuronal hubs of the so-called default mode network (DMN) seem to be especially important for awareness of the self and the environment [15].

It is important to critically evaluate standard neuroimaging and electrophysiology findings in a given DOC patient and to correlate these findings with the clinical syndrome. Anterior brainstem lesions in the corticospinal tract along with preserved EEG activity in the alpha range should be a red flag in an unresponsive patient and should trigger careful examination of volitional eye movements in order not to mistake an LIS for a UWS.

4.2 Introduction to Treatment

Treatment of patients with DOC can be divided into measures to avoid or treat common complications and strategies aimed at enhancing the recovery process, i.e. stimulation approaches to increase the level of consciousness. Overall, evidence and quality of evidence for clinical efficacy of treatments for DOC patients are low [16, 17]. For the purpose of this chapter, we focus on treatments to further recovery of consciousness.

The brain injuries underlying DOC are often so severe and diffuse that they may be beyond the reach of current treatment strategies. The clinical studies have been limited by lack of standardized consciousness assessment protocols and heterogeneous nature of the study populations (traumatic versus non-traumatic, coma versus UWS versus MCS, acute versus chronic).

4.2.1 Non-Pharmacological Treatments

4.2.1.1 Verticalization to Near-Standing Position
Rationale and Indication:

Changing posture and body position is a frequent feature of normal behaviour which is lacking in patients with severe DOC. Clinical experience, as well as limited evidence from smaller clinical trials, suggests that DOC patients benefit from repeated mobilization to near-standing position, in terms of improved arousal and alertness as well as a stabilization of the cardiovascular and respiratory system [18]. Being transferred from a supine to a standing position provides additional multisensory stimulation for patients, which can often be directly observed as patients begin to open their eyes and explore their environment once verticalized. Also, positive effects can clinically be seen with regard to the level of spasticity. On the other hand, there are also concerns that early mobilization might have a negative impact on cerebral autoregulation and brain perfusion.

Main indications for DOC patients are:

- Additional sensory stimulation to further arousal and attention
- Stabilization and training of the cardiovascular and respiratory system
- Prophylaxis for spastic equinovarus foot
- Normalization of generalized increased muscle tone

Main contraindications for DOC patients are:

- Severe cardiovascular instability (i.e., need for inotropic drugs)
- Unstable intracranial pressure (e.g., first week after acute brain injury with increased intracranial pressure)
- Fractures of lower limbs (e.g., as part of polytrauma injury in TBI patients)
- Severe spastic equinovarus foot

Description of Technique:

There are various ways to mobilize patients to a near-standing position, each having distinct advantages or disadvantages:

- *Stabilizing the joints of the legs by means of casts or splints and transferring patients to a standing table to lean against and rest the arms on:*
  This method is time-consuming and often requires two or three therapists to support the patient's head and trunk and carry weight while transferring. Another disadvantage is that patients may experience a cardiovascular syncope because of postural hypotension. This often limits the actual time in standing position.
  The advantage of this method is that it doesn't involve costly equipment and that it provides a sensation of near-normal standing on one's own feet to the patients.
- *Use of a standard tilt table:*
  Patients are transferred in supine position from their bed to a tilt table and then the table is gradually tilted up to a near-standing position. While this method is faster than the casting/splinting technique, it carries the same limitations with regard to cardiovascular instability. It is easier, though, to stabilize the head and neck as they can rest on the surface of the table.
- *Use of a tilt table with integrated robotic leg training:*
  This is the most recent development and has the advantage of activating the cardiovascular system by means of stimulating the muscles of the leg, thereby increasing the return of venous blood to the heart. Robotic stepping can be accompanied by functional electrical stimulation (FES) of thigh and calf muscles, synchronized with the corresponding stepping pattern and providing even more sensorimotor stimulation. Transfer from bed to device is as quick as with standard tilt

tables, but preparation for robotic training or even FES requires significant additional time. Other disadvantages are high investment costs and difficulties in cleaning and disinfecting the robotic mechanical parts. Also, patients with pacemakers or other implanted electrical devices, as well as patients with poorly controlled seizures, cannot be treated by FES.

If verticalization techniques are employed, it is necessary to monitor cardiac and respiratory functions, in order not to exceed the cardiorespiratory capacity.

Review of Evidence:

Two recent randomized controlled clinical trials have addressed the question whether tilt table verticalization with robotic stepping leg movements has benefits for DOC patients.

In the first, 44 patients in UWS or MCS were randomized to receive either tilt table therapy with robotic stepping training (ERIGO® device from Hocoma, Switzerland) or conventional tilt table therapy for a total of 10 sessions over a three-week period [19]. Both the ERIGO® and the conventional groups improved over time in their scores of the CRS-R scale. There seemed to be a small statistical superiority of the conventional tilt table group, even though sample size and power were low. Overall, there was no statistical difference between groups. Net therapy times were greater in the robotic therapy group compared to the conventional group. The robotic treatment was less prone to cause hypotension, presyncope, or syncope than standard tilt table. Standard tilt table treatment seemed to have a slightly greater impact on recovery of consciousness than the more sophisticated device, when measured by the CRS-R. Unfortunately, the study did not have a control group without sham intervention.

An Italian trial randomized 40 DOC patients in UWS or MCS to receive either ERIGO® treatment or conventional in-bed physiotherapy, five times a week for three weeks [18]. As in the previous study, both groups improved in all outcome measures at the end of the study compared to clinical status at enrolment. Levels of consciousness measured by the CRS-R seemed to improve statistically more in the robotic tilt table than in the control group. These findings are in accordance with smaller previous series that suggested improved arousal and consciousness levels when tilt tables were used for verticalization [20].

Recommendations for verticalization strategies:

- Rehabilitation units that treat DOC patients should have verticalization protocols and standards.
- DOC patients should regularly be mobilized to near-standing vertical positioning to increase the likelihood of recovery of consciousness.
- Tilt tables with robotic leg movements are more efficient in delivering effective verticalization time than standard tilt tables, especially in patients who are prone to hypotension or syncope.

4.2.1.2 Sensory Stimulation and Music Therapy

Rationale and Indication:

It has long been suggested that sensory stimulation as a means of enriched environment and prevention of sensory deprivation could increase neuronal plasticity in DOC patients. Sensory stimulation programmes have long been used as treatments in UWS or MCS patients following acute brain injury [21]. Depending on the types and number of senses that are targeted, unimodal or multimodal stimulation programmes have been developed. It has been cautioned that non-specific overstimulation lead to habituation and might hinder recovery of consciousness and cognition.

The various sensory stimulation programmes differ in the stimuli provided to the patients. For example for auditory senses, they range from simple but repetitive sounds to emotionally more complex stimuli, such as familiar (family) voices repetitively saying the patient's own name or reading stories [22]. Sensory stimulation may address one or a combination of senses: olfactory, visual, auditory, gustatory, tactile, kinaesthetic.

Music therapy is also a form of sensory stimulation, where specialized music therapists use music to elicit reactions from DOC patients [23, 24]. These reactions can be very subtle, such as a slight change in breathing or facial expression. Music therapists are trained to detect these changes and vary their music depending on these reactions. Special musical instruments have been developed to incorporate patients into the body of the instrument in order for them to be exposed not only to the sound but also to the vibrations for example of a harp. It was suggested that music therapy is capable of stimulating areas, which are important hubs in consciousness networks [25]. It was shown that music therapy with preferred songs can promote arousal and attention in DOC patients, in contrast to noise or disliked music [26].

Review of Evidence:

In 2002, a Cochrane review compared three different multimodal sensory stimulation programmes [27]. Altogether, 68 patients had been enrolled in three studies. The authors concluded that the quality of the evidence was low and insufficient to draw firm conclusions.

An evidence-based review of interventions to promote arousal from coma identified eight different sensory stimulation studies [16]. Again, the quality of the evidence was low and no clear recommendations could be given.

Recently, a small trial randomized 15 TBI patients with DOC to receive either 40 minutes per day of familiar auditory sensory training (FAST) or a control condition with silence during the same time for a total of six weeks [28]. The FAST intervention consisted of playing customized recordings of meaningful stories told by people well known to the patient. Patients in the intervention group had significantly improved scores in a coma scale compared to the control group. In addition, in an fMRI paradigm, they had greater activation in the brain language network than patients without FAST therapy.

In another study, 30 comatose TBI patients were randomly assigned to two different multimodal sensory stimulation protocols or a conventional physiotherapy session for two weeks [29]. At the end of follow-up, patients in the intervention groups had higher scores in coma and consciousness scales compared to the control group. The stimulation protocol consisting of 20-minute sessions five times per day seemed to be most effective.

Music therapy has been shown to have direct effects on arousal and attention in DOC patients [26, 30]. Neurobehavioral responses depended on whether music was salient or disliked or just white noise. Despite these obvious direct effects, randomized clinical trials on the effects of music therapy on outcome in DOC patients have not yet been published.

In our clinical experience, though, music therapy may also be useful in calming down severely affected DOC patients in a sympathetic hyperactivity state, i.e.

sweating, tachycardic, tachypnoeic, hyperthermic. There is no evidence, however, to support this clinical impression.

Recommendations for sensory stimulation programmes:

- Sensory stimulation programmes may be useful in increasing arousal and awareness in DOC patients.
- Auditory sensory stimulation may be more effective than addressing other senses.
- While evidence for positive effects of music therapy on outcome is lacking, it has obvious direct effects on arousal and behaviour in DOC patients.

4.2.1.3 Electric/Electromagnetic Stimulation Techniques

Rationale and Indication:

Electric or electromagnetic stimulation of specific brain areas in DOC patients has attracted considerable interest in the research community. In DOC, parts of the neuronal consciousness network are hypoactive, possibly because of disruption of thalamocortical, thalamostriatal, and corticocortical excitatory projections. The general rationale behind electrical stimulation of the brain is to specifically target these hypoactive hubs of the consciousness network, thereby promoting arousal and awareness. Stimulation can be done by means of transcranial direct current stimulation (tDCS) or transcranial magnetic stimulation (TMS). As an alternative, continuous electric stimulation of the median nerve is intended to deliver somatosensory input to the thalamus and its respective projection areas, thereby enhancing plasticity and reorganization of the consciousness network. Finally, direct application of electricity to deep grey matter brain areas – deep brain stimulation (DBS) – is also an option but is discussed in the section on surgical treatment.

Description of Technique:

tDCS is a form of non-invasive modulation of electrical cortical activity by means of weak polarizing currents. Depending on the placement of the surface electrodes, it can either be used to increase excitability in the cortex adjacent to the anode ('anodal tDCS') or to decrease it by placing the cathode over the target area ('cathodal tDCS'). In DOC patients, usually anodal tDCS is performed to stimulate frontal cortical

areas. The cathode is placed at the other side of the skull above the eye so that the current will be directed from the anode through frontal brain areas towards the cathode. A typical treatment session would consist of 20 minutes of stimulation with 2 mA [31].

Review of Evidence:

In the only randomized controlled trial, a single 20-minute session of anodal tDCS over the left dorsolateral prefrontal cortex (DLPFC) was used in 55 UWS or MCS patients [31]. It was a randomized crossover study, where all patients received anodal tDCS as well as sham stimulation, but in different treatment sequences. Repeated CRS-R scoring was performed before and after true and sham stimulation as well as at final follow-up after 12 months. While there were direct positive treatment effects of anodal tDCS with an increase in the CRS-R in the MCS subgroup of patients, scores in the UWS subgroup did not change significantly. The long-term outcome at 12 months did not differ between treatment responders and non-responders. From a safety aspect, no treatment-related side effects were observed. This is in line with previous studies, where no major adverse events were noted in healthy subjects [32].

Several lines of evidence suggest that tDCS responders and non-responders might be identifiable pre-treatment by means of fMRI, MRI, or FDG-PET to identify and target the intact and metabolic active brain areas [31, 33].Currently, several trials are being conducted, where repeated tDCS is applied to DOC patients over a longer treatment period in order to evaluate its effect on outcome.

So far, there are no published data about randomized controlled trials on the efficacy of TMS in DOC patients. An evidence-based review concluded that there was conflicting evidence whether median nerve stimulation could promote faster recovery from DOC [16]. A large single-centre controlled trial from China randomized a total of 437 TBI patients with GCS ≤ 8 at two weeks post injury to receive either right median nerve electric stimulation (RMNS) or 'standard neurosurgical treatment' [34]. RMNS was conducted with surface electrodes applying 15–20 mA biphasic pulses at 40 Hz for 20 seconds per minute. This protocol was applied eight hours per day for two weeks. At the end of the two-week daily stimulation protocol, patients in the RMNS group showed better improvement in GCS than patients in the control group. At six months follow-up, significantly more patients from the

RMNS group had regained consciousness and fewer were in UWS than in the control group. Unfortunately, there was no sham stimulation group in this trial, so it remains questionable whether the observed outcome differences were attributable to the stimulation as such or other biasing factors unrelated to stimulation. No safety issues were associated with continuous RMNS.

Recommendations for electric/electromagnetic stimulation:

- tDCS to the left DLPFC promotes short-term arousal in DOC patients. Whether repeated application has long-term positive effects is currently unclear.
- A treatment protocol with two weeks of RMNS may promote recovery of consciousness in TBI patients with GCS < 8. Yet evidence to support this effect is limited by poor study design.
- Given the very good safety profile of tDCS and RMNS, an individual treatment trial may be considered.

4.2.2 Pharmacological Treatment

4.2.2.1 Amantadine

Rationale and Indication:

Amantadine is the only drug with good evidence to support its routine use for promoting recovery of consciousness. Its exact mechanism of action is not fully understood, but antagonism at N-methyl-D-aspartate receptors, as well as indirect dopamine agonist activity, is considered to play an important role [35]. Amantadine may enhance dopaminergic neurotransmission in nigrostriatal, mesolimbic, and frontostriatal neuronal circuits that play an important role in arousal and consciousness networks. Its modulation effect on dopaminergic neurotransmission has led to its use in patients with Parkinson's disease. Administration of amantadine to promote awakening in DOC patients has been part of neurocritical and neurorehabilitative care for many years, despite the paucity of substantial scientific evidence at the time.

Pharmacology and Side Effects:

Amantadine is available as oral formulation (typically 100 mg and 200 mg tablets) or as IV infusion solution, where 200 mg are dissolved in 500 ml 0.9% NaCl. It is 67% bound to plasma proteins and has a satiable transport system across the blood–brain barrier.

Maximum concentrations in plasma occur two and eight hours after application of a single dose (depending on the formulation). Steady-state plasma concentrations are achieved after four to seven days. Elimination half-life is between 10 and 30 hours (and approx. six days in brain tissue), whereby increasing age as well as impaired renal function lead to increased elimination times, as 90% of amantadine is excreted in urine.

Typical daily effective doses for treatment of coma range from 200 to 400 mg/day. Usually, treatment is started with 100 mg amantadine twice daily. Applications in the evenings (past 4 PM) should be avoided as amantadine may lead to agitation and restlessness. Amantadine doses have to be reduced in cases of impaired kidney function, depending on the GFR (refer to product information for details).

Special care has to be taken with intravenous application of amantadine. Infusions should be administered very slowly over a time period of at least three hours.

Amantadine is contraindicated in cases of severe heart failure (NYHA IV), cardiomyopathy, myocarditis, heart block (AV block > °II), bradycardia with heart rate < 55 bpm, ventricular arrhythmias, hypokalaemia, hypomagnesaemia, and long QT-interval (QTc > 420 ms; U-waves). ECG has to be performed before the first dose of amantadine as well as at one and three weeks into therapy to rule out long QT syndrome.

Main side effects are insomnia, confusion, agitation, urinary retention in patients with prostate hyperplasia, and livedo reticularis. For treatment of coma, amantadine is often started intravenously and then later switched to oral application.

Evidence:

Amantadine is the only intervention for treatment of DOC with good clinical evidence so far. This evidence stems from a multicentre, multinational, randomized controlled trial in 184 patients who had suffered severe TBI either in UWS or MCS [36]. The amantadine group started with 100 mg twice daily for two weeks. The dose was then increased to 300 mg per day and, if necessary, i.e. lack of clinical improvement, to a final dose of 400 mg per day. Total treatment time was four weeks and final assessments took place after six weeks. The amantadine group improved significantly faster in clinical consciousness ratings than the control group, while study medication was given. Both UWS and MCS patients benefited from the active study medication.

After tapering study medication at four weeks, improvement rates of the amantadine group slowed while those of the placebo group remained constant so that at the end of the six weeks follow-up, the extent of functional recovery had begun to converge again. From a safety aspect, both groups had comparable frequencies of adverse events, the most frequent ones being hypertonia/spasticity, agitation, insomnia, and vomiting.

It is unclear whether there are equally positive effects of amantadine in patients with DOC of non-traumatic origin. From clinical experience, though, there are several non-traumatic patients who show immediate positive effects upon initiation of an individual trial of amantadine.

Recommendation:

- Eligible patients (i.e., no contraindications) in UWS/MCS within four months of TBI should receive a four-week trial of amantadine in doses starting at 200 mg per day and increased to 400 mg per day, if necessary.
- A similar amantadine trial may be considered in DOC patients with non-traumatic aetiology.

4.2.2.2 Zolpidem

Rationale and Indication:

Several case reports have suggested that single doses of zolpidem could lead to transient recovery of consciousness and functional communication skills in chronic DOC patients [37]. This seems paradoxical because zolpidem is a hypnotic drug. It is a short-acting selective gamma-aminobutyric acid (GABA) agonist but not of the benzodiazepine type [38]. Based on the mesocircuit hypothesis of DOC, under normal conditions, the striatum inhibits the globus pallidus internus (GPi), thereby preventing its inhibitory function on the thalamus and its important excitatory thalamocortical projections [39]. According to this hypothesis, severe brain injury leads to disruption of this circuit, leaving the GPi disinhibited, resulting in increased inhibition of the thalamus. Zolpidem has a high affinity to inhibitory GABAergic receptors on the GPi and could thereby release the thalamus from its excessive inhibition and thus indirectly activating frontal cortical areas [40].

Pharmacology and Side Effects:

Zolpidem comes in tablets of 5 mg or 10 mg. The maximum daily dose is 10 mg. Maximum plasma levels are reached between 0.5 and 3 hours, and its elimination half-life is 2–4 hours. It is metabolized in the liver by the CYP3A4 system into inactive metabolites. Its clearance is reduced in older patients, as well as in patients with impaired liver function, so smaller doses should be used.

Expected side effects include diarrhoea, vomiting, hallucinations, agitation, and respiratory tract infections.

Evidence:

Apart from several case reports, two controlled trials randomized DOC patients in UWS or MCS to receive either 10 mg of zolpidem or placebo in a single dose. The first was a crossover trial with 84 patients [41]. Five per cent of patients were rated as responders with improved behavioural responses. There was no obvious clinical pattern permitting prediction of responder status.

In the second study, 60 DOC patients of traumatic and non-traumatic aetiology received 10 mg of Zolpidem in an open label screening trial [42]. Twelve patients were found to be responders (20%) with a change in total CRS-R scores or improved behavioural responses within one hour after administration of zolpidem. Yet, in only 1 of these 12 patients did the consciousness diagnosis change post study medication, i.e. before zolpidem the patient was diagnosed as MCS and post zolpidem as emerged from MCS. In this patient, in a second study phase, a placebo-controlled trial (crossover) was initiated but failed to confirm a clear zolpidem response. In the other 11 responders, improvements did not cross a clinical threshold necessary for a change in diagnosis.

A small case series with three known zolpidem responders who were in chronic MCS showed that only zolpidem, but not placebo, led to brief emergence from MCS, which was paralleled by an increased glucose metabolism in prefrontal cortical areas [40].

Recommendation:

- Given the uncritical safety profile in a controlled environment, a single therapeutic trial of 5–10 mg zolpidem may be performed in DOC patients, even though responder rates are expected to be less than 10%.

4.2.2.3 Other Pharmacological Agents

Intrathecal Baclofen:

The intrathecal baclofen given for control of severe spasticity may lead to pronounced improvement of arousal and consciousness. Several small case series have been published supporting this hypothesis [43, 44]. These findings mirror our own clinical experience. Yet the mechanisms behind this obvious effect are not understood. The reduction of oral baclofen because of a new intrathecal delivery system may be part of this effect.

Dopaminergic Drugs (Other Than Amantadine):

Levodopa and bromocriptine have also been used in therapeutic trials for disorders of consciousness [16]. While positive effects have been reported in small case series, no randomized controlled trials have been published so far.

Modafinil:

Modafinil is indicated for treating excessive sleepiness in cases of narcolepsy, obstructive sleep apnoea, and shift work sleep disorders. It increases cortical catecholamine levels, upregulates serotonin and glutamate, and decreases GABA [45]. One retrospective analysis identified 17 of 24 DOC patients who responded to a therapeutic trial of modafinil with improvements in arousal and awareness [46]. No results of randomized controlled trials have been reported so far.

4.2.3 Surgical Treatment

4.2.3.1 Deep Brain Stimulation (DBS)

There are no established and evidence-based surgical treatment options to promote recovery of consciousness in DOC patients. Deep brain stimulation (DBS) has been tried and evaluated for more than 30 years in these conditions [47]. While immediate positive effects on arousal were noted in UWS patients with electrodes implanted in the mesencephalic reticular formation or thalamus, lack of control conditions did not permit for an analysis of long-term effects on outcome. More recently, a more scientific approach on a single-case basis provided a better understanding of effects attributable to thalamic DBS [48]. In this multiple crossover study, a patient who had been in MCS for several years received bilateral DBS with repeated stimulation in the on and off phases and intensive behavioural testing. Stimulation was associated with behavioural improvements with regard to motor control, oral feeding abilities, and arousal when compared with the off phases. Just recently, another case series with three DOC patients with bilateral thalamic stimulation was published [49]. They had been in chronic UWS or MCS for between two and eight years prior to surgery. CRS-R scores improved by an average of two or three points during the course of active high-frequency DBS of at least 18 months, but no patient emerged from MCS. Interestingly, a significant reduction of spasticity and myoclonus was noted in all patients during stimulation phases. It is unclear whether a CRS-R increase of two or three points crosses the threshold of a meaningful real-life improvement.

While DBS remains a very interesting and promising therapeutic option, current data are not providing enough evidence to consider this method outside of carefully planned and conducted clinical trials. Recently, as a basis for future steps into this direction, inclusion and exclusion criteria as well as ethical and medico-legal implications and issues have been proposed and discussed [50].

References

1. Royal College of Physicians. *Prolonged disorders of consciousness: National clinical guidelines.* London, UK: Royal College of Physicians, 2013.

2. Giacino JT, Fins JJ, Laureys S, et al. Disorders of consciousness after acquired brain injury: The state of the science. *Nat. Rev. Neurol.* 2014; **10**: 99–114.

3. Jennett B, Teasdale G. Aspects of coma after severe head injury. *Lancet* 1977; **1**: 878–81.

4. Laureys S, Celesia GG, Cohadon F, et al. Unresponsive wakefulness syndrome: A new name for the vegetative state or apallic syndrome. *BMC Med* 2010; **8**: 68.

5. Giacino JT, Ashwal S, Childs N, et al. The minimally conscious state: Definition and diagnostic criteria. *Neurology* 2002; **58**: 349–53.

6. Gosseries O, Bruno MA, Chatelle C, et al. Disorders of consciousness: What's in a name? *NeuroRehabilitation* 2011; **28**: 3–14.

7. Van Erp WS, Lavrijsen JC, Vos PE, et al. The vegetative state: Prevalence, misdiagnosis, and treatment limitations. *J. Am. Med. Dir. Assoc.* 2015; **16**: 85 e9–85 e14.

8. Giacino JT, Schnakers C, Rodriguez-Moreno D, et al. Behavioral assessment in patients with disorders of

consciousness: Gold standard or fool's gold? *Prog. Brain Res.* 2009; **177**: 33–48.

9. Seel RT, Sherer M, Whyte, J, et al. Assessment scales for disorders of consciousness: Evidence-based recommendations for clinical practice and research. *Archives of Physical Medicine and Rehabilitation* 2010; **91**: 1795–813.

10. Di H, Nie Y, Hu X, et al. Assessment of visual fixation in vegetative and minimally conscious states. *BMC Neurol.* 2014; **14**: 147.

11. Bender A, Jox RJ, Grill E, et al. Persistent vegetative state and minimally conscious state: A systematic review and meta-analysis of diagnostic procedures. *Dtsch. Arztebl. Int.* 2015; **112**: 235–42.

12. Monti MM, Vanhaudenhuyse A, Coleman MR, et al. Willful modulation of brain activity in disorders of consciousness. *New England Journal of Medicine* 2010; **362**: 579–89.

13. Stender J, Gosseries O, Bruno MA, et al. Diagnostic precision of PET imaging and functional MRI in disorders of consciousness: A clinical validation study. *Lancet* 2014; **384**: 514–22.

14. Young GB. Coma. *Ann. N. Y. Acad. Sci.* 2009; **1157**: 32–47.

15. Di Perri C, Bahri MA, Amico E, et al. Neural correlates of consciousness in patients who have emerged from a minimally conscious state: A cross-sectional multimodal imaging study. *Lancet Neurol.* 2016; **15**: 830–42.

16. Meyer MJ, Megyesi J, Meythaler J, et al. Acute management of acquired brain injury Part III: An evidence-based review of interventions used to promote arousal from coma. *Brain Injury* 2010; **24**: 722–9.

17. Oliveira L, Fregni,F. Pharmacological and electrical stimulation in chronic disorders of consciousness: New insights and future directions. *Brain Injury* 2011; **25**: 315–27.

18. Frazzitta G, Zivi I, Valsecchi R, et al. Effectiveness of a very early stepping verticalization protocol in severe acquired brain injured patients: A randomized pilot study in ICU. *PLoS One* 2016; **11**: e0158030.

19. Krewer C, Luther M, Koenig E, et al. Tilt table therapies for patients with severe disorders of consciousness: A randomized, controlled trial. *PLoS One* 2015; **10**: e0143180.

20. Riberholt CG, Thorlund JB, Mehlsen J, et al. Patients with severe acquired brain injury show increased arousal in tilt-table training. *Dan. Med. J.* 2013; **60**: A4739.

21. Tolle P, Reimer M. Do we need stimulation programs as a part of nursing care for patients in 'persistent vegetative state'? A conceptual analysis. *Axone* 2003; **25**: 20–6.

22. Padilla R, Domina A. Effectiveness of sensory stimulation to improve arousal and alertness of people in a coma or persistent vegetative state after traumatic brain injury: A systematic review. *Am. J. Occup. Ther.* 2016; **70**: 7003180030: pp. 1–8.

23. Schnakers C, Magee WL, Harris B. Sensory stimulation and music therapy programs for treating disorders of consciousness. *Front Psychol.* 2016; **7**: 297.

24. Magee WL, O'Kelly J. Music therapy with disorders of consciousness: Current evidence and emergent evidence-based practice. *Ann. N. Y. Acad. Sci.* 2015; **1337**: 256–62.

25. Vanhaudenhuyse A, Noirhomme Q, Tshibanda LT, et al. Default network connectivity reflects the level of consciousness in non-communicative brain-damaged patients. *Brain* 2010; **133**: 161–71.

26. O'Kelly J, James L, Palaniappan R, et al. Neurophysiological and behavioral responses to music therapy in vegetative and minimally conscious states. *Front. Hum. Neurosci.* 2013; **7**: 884.

27. Lombardi F, Taricco M, De Tanti A, et al. Sensory stimulation of brain-injured individuals in coma or vegetative state: Results of a Cochrane systematic review. *Clin. Rehabil.* 2002; **16**: 464–72.

28. Pape TL, Rosenow JM, Steiner M, et al. Placebo-controlled trial of familiar auditory sensory training for acute severe traumatic brain injury: A preliminary report. *Neurorehabil. Neural. Repair* 2015; **29**: 537–47.

29. Megha M, Harpreet S, Nayeem Z. Effect of frequency of multimodal coma stimulation on the consciousness levels of traumatic brain injury comatose patients. *Brain Injury* 2013; **27**: 570–7.

30. Binzer I, Schmidt HU, Timmermann T, et al. Immediate responses to individual dialogic music therapy in patients in low awareness states. *Brain Injury* 2016; **30**(7): 1–7.

31. Thibaut A, Bruno MA, Ledoux D, et al. tDCS in patients with disorders of consciousness: Sham-controlled randomized double-blind study. *Neurology* 2014; **82**: 1112–18.

32. Kessler SK, Turkeltaub PE, Benson JG, et al. Differences in the experience of active and sham transcranial direct current stimulation. *Brain Stimul.* 2012; **5**: 155–62.

33. Cavaliere C, Aiello M, Di Perri C, et al. Functional connectivity substrates for tDCS response in minimally conscious state patients. *Front Cell Neurosci.* 2016; **10**: 257.

34. Lei J, Wang L, Gao G, et al. Right median nerve electrical stimulation for acute traumatic coma patients. *J. Neurotrauma* 2015; **32**: 1584–9.

35. Peeters M, Page G, Maloteaux JM, et al. Hypersensitivity of dopamine transmission in the rat

striatum after treatment with the NMDA receptor antagonist amantadine. *Brain Res.* 2002; **949**: 32–41.

36. Giacino JT, Whyte J, Bagiella E, et al. Placebo-controlled trial of amantadine for severe traumatic brain injury. *N. Engl. J. Med.* 2012; **366**: 819–26.

37. Gosseries O, Charland-Verville V, Thonnard M, et al. Amantadine, apomorphine and zolpidem in the treatment of disorders of consciousness. *Curr. Pharm. Des.* 2014; **20**: 4167–84.

38. Kovacic P, Somanathan R. Zolpidem, a clinical hypnotic that affects electronic transfer, alters synaptic activity through potential GABA receptors in the nervous system without significant free radical generation. *Oxid. Med. Cell. Longev.* 2009; **2**: 52–7.

39. Schiff ND. Recovery of consciousness after brain injury: A mesocircuit hypothesis. *Trends in Neurosciences* 2010; **33**: 1–9.

40. Chatelle C, Thibaut A, Gosseries O, et al. Changes in cerebral metabolism in patients with a minimally conscious state responding to zolpidem. *Front. Hum. Neurosci.* 2014; **8**: 917.

41. Whyte J, Rajan R, Rosenbaum A, et al. Zolpidem and restoration of consciousness. *Am. J. Phys. Med. Rehabil.* 2014; **93**: 101–13.

42. Thonnard M, Gosseries O, Demertzi A, et al. Effect of zolpidem in chronic disorders of consciousness: A prospective open-label study. *Funct. Neurol.* 2013; **28**: 259–64.

43. Margetis K, Korfias SI, Gatzonis S, et al. Intrathecal baclofen associated with improvement of

consciousness disorders in spasticity patients. *Neuromodulation* 2014; **17**: 699–704: discussion 704.

44. Al-Khodairy AT, Wicky G, Nicolo D, et al. Influence of intrathecal baclofen on the level of consciousness and mental functions after extremely severe traumatic brain injury: Brief report. *Brain Injury* 2015; **29**: 527–32.

45. Battleday RM, Brem AK, Modafinil for cognitive neuroenhancement in healthy non-sleep-deprived subjects: A systematic review. *Eur. Neuropsychopharmacol.* 2015; **25**: 1865–81.

46. Dhamapurkar SK, Wilson BA, Rose A, et al. Does modafinil improve the level of consciousness for people with a prolonged disorder of consciousness? A retrospective pilot study. *Disabil. Rehabil.* 2016; 1–7.

47. Yamamoto T, Katayama Y, Obuchi, T, et al. Deep brain stimulation and spinal cord stimulation for vegetative state and minimally conscious state. *World Neurosurg.* 2013; **80**: S30 e1–9.

48. Schiff ND, Giacino JT, Kalmar K, et al. Behavioural improvements with thalamic stimulation after severe traumatic brain injury. *Nature* 2007; **448**: 600–3.

49. Magrassi L, Maggioni G, Pistarini C, et al. Results of a prospective study (CATS) on the effects of thalamic stimulation in minimally conscious and vegetative state patients. *J. Neurosurg.* 2016; **125**: 972–81.

50. Giacino J, Fins JJ, Machado A, et al. Central thalamic deep brain stimulation to promote recovery from chronic posttraumatic minimally conscious state: Challenges and opportunities. *Neuromodulation* 2012; **15**: 339–49.

Management of Communication Disorders in Neurorehabilitation

Rajani Sebastian and Donna C. Tippett

5.1 Introduction

Acquired communication disorders, particularly aphasia, dysarthria, and apraxia of speech (AOS), are common socially and functionally limiting problems in patients with stroke and other neurologic diseases. The term 'aphasia' is used to describe an acquired loss or impairment of the language system following brain damage [1]. The most common cause of aphasia is a cerebrovascular accident or stroke, mainly to the left hemisphere. About one-third of all people who experience a stroke develop aphasia [2, 3]. More than 2 million people in the United States have acquired aphasia [4]. Dysarthria has been defined as a 'neurologic motor speech impairment that is characterized by slow, weak, imprecise, and/or uncoordinated movements of the speech musculature and may involve respiration, phonation, resonance, and/or oral articulation' [5]. Estimates of the prevalence of dysarthria following stroke vary from 20% to 30% [6, 7]. AOS is a disruption in spatial and temporal planning and/or programming of movements for speech production and is characterized by slowed speech rate with distorted phonemes, distorted phoneme substitutions, and a tendency to segregate speech into individual syllables and equalize stress across adjacent syllables [8, 9]. Although AOS can involve all speech subsystems, it is predominantly a disorder of articulation and prosody.

In this chapter, we discuss the approaches underlying rehabilitation of communication disorders following a stroke, including speech-language pathology intervention, adjunctive approaches, and medical/pharmacological intervention. Some degree of recovery of speech and language skills is typical after a stroke, mostly occurring within the first few months; however, severe and debilitating speech and language deficits frequently persist. Given the public health and personal implications of communication disorders, treatment is a compelling topic.

Speech-language pathology intervention or behavioural intervention is the mainstay treatment for acquired communication disorders after stroke [10]. Increasingly, speech-language pathology intervention is evidence-based and person-centred [11]. Recent advances in neuroimaging contribute new understandings of the structural and functional correlates of speech and language processing and the neurobiology of recovery. Speech and language treatments are informed by these advances, and adjuncts to traditional behavioural therapy are being investigated. Transcranial direct current stimulation (tDCS) is one method that has been proposed to boost behavioural language treatment in post-stroke aphasia [12, 13]. Emerging research points to the promise of acetylcholinesterase inhibitors and memantine for aphasia [14]. In addition, there are expanded indications for medical and surgical interventions to ameliorate the impact of stroke through reperfusion [15, 16, 17]. Furthermore, there is an increased interest in using technology to improve treatment delivery for communication disorders.

5.2 Behavioural Treatment: Speech-Language Pathology

Speech and language therapy is both restorative and compensatory. Therapy may vary in intervention regimen, theoretical approach, or delivery model. Principles of neuroplasticity support early and intense therapy; however, questions remain regarding specific intervention strategies given the variable nature of aphasia, dysarthria, and AOS. The rationale for early intervention is also based on the principles of neuroplasticity such that therapy capitalizes on spontaneous recovery in the immediate post-stroke period [18]. For example, in aphasia rehabilitation, research has shown that speech therapy is beneficial over spontaneous recovery; treated individuals have almost twice the degree of recovery of untreated individuals when therapy is commenced within the first three months post stroke [10].

Historically, clinicians base therapy largely on assessment data. Therapy tasks are developed to target specific domains, such as word retrieval at a single word level for aphasia rehabilitation. This follows a traditional medical model which emphasizes impairment of function, and is therapist-centred. Clinicians currently use many behavioural treatment techniques in the clinical setting to treat acquired communication disorders. For example, for AOS rehabilitation, therapy approaches may focus on improving accuracy of articulation by imitation, phonetic approaches, integral stimulation, and key word techniques [19]. However, the medical model of treatment has limitations. For example, in aphasia rehabilitation therapy may focus on word retrieval by increased ability to name pictured objects in a treatment task that does not necessarily translate to a relevant outcome, such as improvement in functional communication [20].

Given the limitations of medical-centred models of speech therapy, a social model of therapy has emerged which encompasses equalizing the social relations of service delivery, the authentic involvement of users (patients), the creation of engaging experiences, user control, and accountability [11]. This practice is consistent with the conceptual framework for contemporary models of healthcare of the International Classification of Functioning, Disability, and Health (ICF) of the World Health Organization [21]. This approach encourages patient-centred care, focusing on development of goals which address individual needs and circumstances. Therapy is a collaborative process. Patients, families, and caregivers identify goals which are important to them. Clinicians conduct formal assessment, and then negotiation occurs between patients and therapists to define a treatment plan. This is in contrast to therapist-controlled approaches; a genuine patient-centred approach allows patients, their families, and their caregivers, rather than the clinician, to lead the goal-setting process [22].

A specific example of a patient-centred approach is the Life Participation Approach to Aphasia (LPAA) [23]. This approach places the life concerns of those affected by aphasia at the centre of all decision-making. It empowers the consumer to select and participate in the recovery process and to collaborate on the design of interventions that aim for a more rapid return to active life. Therefore, this intervention has the potential to reduce the consequences of disease and injury that contribute to long-term health costs [23]. Specific tasks can also be adapted to conform to a patient-centred approach. For example, the Activity Card Sort [24] can be tailored to elicit information from individuals with aphasia about their level of engagement in meaningful activities as well as hindrances to participation, allowing clinicians to obtain qualitative information about interests, level of involvement, and priorities which could then be used to shape the direction of therapy [25].

Current speech-language pathology practice standards dictate that therapy must be evidence-based and person-centred. Evidence-based practice refers to an approach in which current, high-quality research evidence is integrated with practitioner expertise and client preferences and values [26]. A growing literature documents the evidence base for treatment of acquired communication disorders [27, 28, 29], although a more cautious interpretation is offered for treatment of AOS [30].

The efficacy of speech and language therapy applied in aphasia treatment has been reported in two Cochrane analyses [10, 31]. The Cochrane analyses indicate that speech and language therapy benefits functional use of language, language comprehension, and language production, when compared with no access to therapy, but it was unclear how long these benefits might last. Furthermore, the review also found that many hours of therapy over a short period of time (high intensity) appeared to help participants' language use in daily life and reduced the severity of their aphasia problems. However, the time when speech and language therapy should start [32] and its duration and intensity [33] are still controversial. Similarly, a Cochrane review of the research effort targeting treatment efficacy and effectiveness of speech therapy in dysarthria found no evidence to support or refute the effectiveness of speech and language therapy interventions for dysarthria following non-progressive brain damage. The authors found that most of the studies have been small-scale and often favoured single-case or small N design [34].

Applications of the principles governing brain organization and reorganization may contribute to the development of more meaningful therapy approaches. Neuroscience research has now provided clear evidence that behavioural training can induce plasticity and reorganization [35, 36]. One promising training approach is the development of constraint-induced language therapy, which has demonstrated positive clinical outcomes for stroke patients with aphasia. Constraint-induced principles, known also as 'use dependent learning' principles, were derived from basic neuroscience investigations [37]. Approaches for treating post-stroke language impairments based upon constraint-induced principles were introduced in 2001 [38]. A relatively large number of studies have used constraint-induced language therapy, a technique in which massed practice is an integral part of the intervention [39, 40, 41]. Overall, beneficial effects on language functions using standardized tests, connected speech measures, and functional communication have been reported in most studies that used constraint-induced language therapy in patients with chronic aphasia.

Advances in structural and functional brain mapping have greatly expanded our knowledge regarding the relationship between brain connectivity, neural network integrity, and speech and language recovery. Several neuroimaging measures have shown promise as biomarkers and predictors for treatment-related language improvement, including measures of structure and function, in gray matter and white matter. For example, Fridriksson and colleagues [42] examined the relationship between regional and global structural white matter neural network architecture and the ability to improve naming performance after naming treatment in patients with chronic aphasia. All patients underwent naming treatment using semantic and phonological cueing hierarchies [43]. They found that preserved global white matter neural network architecture, with maintenance of the left temporal lobe influence in the configuration of the brain neural networks, is crucial to support naming recovery in individuals with chronic aphasia. Their finding has the potential to encourage the translation of brain connectivity studies into real-life clinical contexts, by providing health practitioners with a tool to assess the potential for recovery.

In summary, there is a strong consensus that speech and language therapy is beneficial for recovery of function after a stroke; however, several challenges limit the implementation of evidence-based, patient-centred care. In addition, the optimal intervention intensity has not yet been established [44], clinical effectiveness for several therapy strategies remains unknown, and no reports from randomized trials have mentioned cost-effectiveness [45]. Despite an increase in randomized controlled trials of optimized speech and language therapy for communication difficulties after stroke, an urgent need remains for good-quality research in this area, especially for dysarthria and AOS. Speech and language treatment is progressively more informed by advances in understanding of the neurobiology of recovery. The use of neuroimaging techniques may further increase our understanding of the underlying mechanisms of spontaneous and treatment-induced recovery. This in turn may prompt changes to existing approaches and/or the development of new treatment paradigms that may contribute to the efficacy of rehabilitation efforts.

5.3 Non-Invasive Brain Stimulation

Non-invasive brain stimulation is a recent adjunct to the field of communication disorders. There has been a growing interest in the use of non-invasive brain stimulation techniques such as transcranial direct current stimulation (tDCS) and transcranial magnetic stimulation (TMS) to enhance recovery of communication disorders in acquired brain injury. Please see [46, 47] for detailed reviews. This interest stems from the growing body of evidence indicating that non-invasive brain stimulation techniques can induce long-lasting changes in neural excitability resulting in functional reorganization and improved speech and language performance. According to Cotelli et al. [48], there are three possible mechanisms by which TMS or tDCS may trigger adaptive neuroplasticity in people with neurological conditions, including: (1) the reactivation of canonical networks, partly damaged or made dysfunctional by the cerebral lesion; (2) the recruitment of compensatory networks, mostly contralateral homologue cortical regions; and (3) the additional recruitment of peri-lesional brain regions.

TMS is thought to modify cortical excitability by increasing or decreasing activity in targeted areas of the cortex by using a rapid time-varying magnetic field [49, 50]. The application of TMS in the treatment of communication disorders is mostly limited to post-stroke aphasia. The majority of studies that have investigated the use of repetitive TMS (rTMS) as a treatment for aphasia have utilized an inhibitory rTMS paradigm for the stimulation of the non-lesioned right inferior frontal gyrus (pars triangularis, BA45) aimed at reducing overactivity. A series of studies by Naeser and colleagues has shown that the application of low-frequency (1 Hz) rTMS, suppressing the activation of the right Broca's homologue, improved the performance of chronic, non-fluent participants with aphasia in naming [51, 52, 53]. Note that TMS has also been applied to the lesioned left hemisphere to reactivate brain regions ipsilateral to the lesion. For example, Cotelli et al. [48] examined the effects of TMS to the left dorsolateral prefrontal cortex along with speech and language therapy. All participants showed an improvement in object naming up to 48 weeks post stimulation.

tDCS is a non-invasive brain stimulation technique that can promote neuroplasticity by modulation of spontaneous cortical activity in the brain. Unlike TMS, which elicits action potentials in neurons, tDCS does not. tDCS involves application of low-amplitude direct current to the scalp via two surface electrodes which modulate the excitability of cortical neurons without directly inducing neuronal action potentials [54]. The effects of the stimulation depend on the polarity of the current flow, with brain excitability being usually increased by anodal tDCS and decreased by cathodal tDCS [55].

Recent years have seen increasing interest in the use of tDCS as a treatment for aphasia [12, 56, 57, 13]. Some studies have examined the effect of anodal or excitatory tDCS applied to the lesioned left hemisphere to improve language recovery via enhancement of neuronal activity in the peri-lesional cortical area [12, 56, 13]. For example, Baker et al. [12] applied either anodal tDCS or sham tDCS over peri-lesional brain regions along with a computerized anomia treatment for five days to individuals with chronic aphasia. The findings indicated a significant improvement in naming accuracy for treated items after anodal tDCS compared with sham tDCS, with the treatment effect persisting for one week post treatment. Similarly, Marangolo et al. [58] examined the effects of tDCS to the left Broca's area along with concomitant intensive articulatory therapy for five days in patients with severe AOS, using anodal and sham stimulations. The results indicated that anodal stimulation had a beneficial effect on the recovery of apraxia. Further, the follow-up testing revealed retention of the achieved improvement only for the anodal condition.

Other studies have examined the effect of cathodal or inhibitory tDCS applied to the contralateral hemisphere to decrease activity in the right hemisphere to improve language function [59, 57]. For example, Jung et al. [59] applied cathodal stimulation

(1mA for 20 min) to the right homologue of Broca's area in individuals with subacute and chronic aphasia. tDCS stimulation was combined with speech-language therapy for 10 sessions and all participants showed significant improvement in aphasia quotients based on the Korean version of the Western Aphasia Battery.

In summary, these studies offer promise that non-invasive brain stimulation may be a tool that could augment the treatment of communication disorders following brain damage. To date, the data supporting the benefits of TMS are more consistent than that reported for tDCS. Several research groups have shown the benefits of inhibitory rTMS applied to the right Broca's area to improve language outcomes in chronic non-fluent patients with aphasia. In contrast, the findings of tDCS studies are less consistent. A recent Cochrane review on the use of tDCS in post-stroke aphasia, based on 12 randomized controlled cross-over trials with 136 participants, concluded that there was no evidence for the effectiveness of tDCS in improving functional communication, language impairment, and cognition [60]. Several questions remain, ranging from the mechanism of tDCS action, anodal versus cathodal stimulation, duration and timing of intervention, effect of stimulation on brain networks, and long-term benefits. More research is needed to determine the selection of the most appropriate therapeutic approach (i.e., excitation of the perilesional area of the left hemisphere versus inhibition of the overactive right hemisphere) that will maximize the effectiveness of TMS and tDCS. In addition, further research is indicated to establish if neuromodulation combined with language therapy affects functional communication in ways which are meaningful to individual circumstances and needs, central to the concept of patient-centred care [61].

5.4 Pharmacological Treatment

There has been a recent emphasis on augmenting rehabilitation with medical treatments that may hasten recovery of speech and language skills. Pharmacotherapy has been recognized as a potential adjunct to behavioural therapy for the treatment of communication disorders due to stroke [62, 63, 64, 65]. Please see [14, 66, 67] for reviews on this topic. Pharmacological interventions for aphasia are mainly designed to strengthen networks subserving language and language-related cognitive functions such as attention and memory [66]. The theoretical rationale for pharmacological intervention in aphasia is based on the notion that re-establishing the activity of specific neurotransmitters in dysfunctional, but not irretrievably damaged, brain regions may strengthen neural activity in networks mediating attention, word learning, and memory [68, 69]. Many different pharmacological agents have been tried with roughly half of the studies pairing a drug with behavioural therapy in an attempt to boost language recovery. We briefly cover the main pharmacological treatment drugs that have been used in aphasia recovery. Most studies have examined the efficacy of drugs acting on noradrenergic, dopaminergic, cholinergic, and glutamatergic neurotransmitter systems.

Dopaminergic- and noradrenergic-based drugs. The most widely investigated class of drugs so far has been the catecholamines such as bromocriptine, levodopa, dextroamphetamine, and amantadine, which are involved in neuromodulation of the dopaminergic and noradrenergic systems [62, 70, 71, 65, 72, 73]. Albert et al. [62] were the first researchers who evaluated the role of bromocriptine in a stroke patient with chronic, transcortical motor aphasia. Beneficial changes were noted in speech initiation, pause in conversation, paraphasias, and naming, with these attributed to enhanced dopaminergic tone in the mesocortical pathway [62]. Positive effects of bromocriptine have been found in other single cases, cases series and open-label trials mainly on non-fluent patients with aphasia [62]. Similarly, levodopa had positive effects in chronic patients when combined with language therapy on naming and repetition especially in patients with frontal lobe damage [65]. However, pharmacotherapeutic interventions using catecholamines have shown only varying degrees of success. The language gains reported were partial, especially among patients with moderate to severe impairment, in whom certain language problems (e.g., non-fluency) persisted even after treatment, showing limited to no long-term effects [66]. Furthermore, many of the studies did not combine drug therapy with concomitant language therapy.

Cholinergic- and glutamatergic-based drugs. Drugs targeting the cholinergic and glutamatergic neurotransmitter systems in aphasia recovery include ameridin, bifemelane, aniracetam, galantamine, piracetam, donepezil, and memantine. The use of donepezil and memantine in aphasia treatment was inspired, in part, by their positive effects on language and communication in patients with Alzheimer's disease and vascular dementia [66]. In several studies, cholinergic- or glutamatergic-based interventions have been found to improve performance on naming and comprehension tasks among aphasic patients with posterior lesions and patients with fluent aphasia [74, 75, 76, 63, 68]. For example, a pilot case control study of donepezil in patients with acute aphasia showed that cholinergic augmentation improved the rate and the amount of recovery in spontaneous speech, comprehension, repetition, and naming functions relative to a non-treated group [76]. Other studies also found improvement in language skills by combining donepezil with speech and language therapy in patients with chronic aphasia [74]. Similarly, memantine used in combination with intensive language-action therapy revealed significant gains in language and communication deficits in patients with chronic aphasia [38, 75]. Piracetam is another drug that is commonly used in the treatment of aphasia [63, 68, 77]. A randomized placebo-controlled trial of piracetam combined with intensive speech and language therapy in acute aphasia found significant improvements in several language tests (spontaneous speech, comprehension, naming, written language, and Token test) and verbal communication [68].

In addition to these, there are other pharmacological treatment drugs aimed at improving language deficits in aphasia, including serotonin, norepinephrine, and γ-aminobutyric acid. For example, the selective serotonin reuptake inhibitor fluvoxamine improved naming abilities in a small sample of fluent aphasic patients [78].

In summary, based on the current evidence, there is some beneficial effect of drug therapy when combined with language therapy in augmenting language and communication deficits post stroke. However, the benefits are not evident for all drugs and data on long-term benefits are limited. For example, dopaminergic- and noradrenergic-based drugs are mostly beneficial for patients with a frontal lesion with mild to moderate deficits but not moderate to severe deficits. Further, the neuroplastic changes that are taking place as a result of pharmacotherapy are still unclear.

Therefore, in future trials of drug therapies targeting aphasia recovery, efforts should be directed to identify appropriate candidates using well-defined clinical criteria and combining structural and functional neuroimaging techniques to understand the mechanism of neural recovery.

5.5 Medical and Surgical Treatment

Surgical and neurovascular approaches to the treatment of communication disorders are mainly limited to the field of acute post-stroke aphasia. A variety of surgical and interventional neuroradiology procedures have been developed that can complement rehabilitation in the first days after stroke by restoring blood flow to dysfunctional but salvageable brain tissue [79]. The focus of acute stroke interventions, such as thrombolysis, embolectomy, and stenting, is to restore blood flow to ischemic tissue that is receiving enough blood to survive, but not enough to function ('ischemic penumbra'). Many of these interventions have been shown to augment aphasia recovery, by allowing recovery of tissue function before there is permanent damage to the entire affected area. Increasing blood pressure is one approach that investigators have used to improve stroke symptoms. Several studies have shown that increasing blood pressure by intravenous phenylephrine can augment acute aphasia recovery [80, 16]. Carotid stenting, with or without angioplasty, is another common procedure to restore blood flow, prevent stroke, and/or improve tissue function. For example, Hillis et al. have shown that acute aphasia resolved after left carotid stenting associated with reperfusion of the language cortex [81]. In another study, complete resolution of aphasia was observed after intra-arterial or intravenous thrombolysis that resulted in improved perfusion [82]. Intravenous thrombolysis has been shown to be effective in improving long-term language after acute ischemic stroke in the left hemisphere, but this intervention is generally limited to the small subset of patients who get to the hospital within three hours of onset of symptoms. In a series of studies, Hillis et al. evaluated the hypothesis that restoring blood flow to specific cortical regions in the left hemisphere after acute stroke results in improvement in language performance [15, 17].

5.6 Music Therapy

Music therapy has been used in rehabilitation of communication disorders to stimulate brain functions involved in speech and language. The most common intervention using melody and rhythm is the Melodic Intonation Therapy (MIT) [83]. MIT consists of speaking with a simplified and exaggerated prosody, characterized by a melodic component (two notes, high and low) and a rhythmic component (two durations, long and short). This treatment program combines several facilitation techniques, including intoned speech, Sprechgesang (i.e., rhythmically emphasized prosody), unison production with the clinician, and lip-reading. The goal of MIT is to restore propositional speech. The rationale is that patients can learn a new way to speak through singing by using language-capable regions of the right hemisphere. Although MIT is regarded as a language treatment for Broca's aphasia, it has also been used in the treatment of AOS. Several music therapy variations have been developed mostly based on MIT principles such as the Modified Melodic Intonation Therapy, MMIT [84], and Singing Intonation, Prosody, breathing (German: *Atmung*), and Rhythm and Improvisation, SIPARI [85].

Over the years, several studies have shown the beneficial effects of MIT on language production in individuals with severe aphasia [86, 87, 88]. A recent review examined the efficacy of MIT in recovery of speech and language skills [89]. Results of the review indicated that treatment outcomes were positive in most of the studies; however, most studies were case studies, focusing on the effect of MIT in the chronic phase after stroke. Furthermore, the mechanisms of recovery pertaining to music therapy remain unclear. Some studies via neuroimaging techniques supported the role of the right hemisphere [90], whereas some reports are contradictory [91]. In summary, music therapy appears to have a promising role in speech and language recovery. Future studies should focus on the understanding of the working mechanisms, and thus a better implementation and timing of MIT in speech and language rehabilitation.

5.7 Computer Technology

There has been tremendous increase in attention in research regarding the use and application of technology to improve treatment delivery of communication disorders. There is an emerging consensus for the need to enhance treatment intensity in chronic aphasia [10]. However, given the limited financial resources of the healthcare system and the limited number of clinicians available to provide such services, alternative ways to enhance treatment intensity need to be explored. One approach to increase the availability of treatment hours is by utilizing computerized treatment. Rehabilitation of communication disorders, especially aphasia rehabilitation, is particularly suited for remote/telerehabilitation due to the emphasis on speech/visual and auditory communication. Individuals with aphasia have reported benefits from the increased autonomy, the ability to type rather than write, and the flexibility in scheduling therapy times [92].

Several efforts have been made to apply various forms of computer technology to rehabilitation of communication disorders resulting from stroke. These include communication aids such as Sentence-Shaper (Psycholinguistic Technologies, Jenkintown, PA), Lingraphica (Lingraphica Inc., Princeton, NJ), and Touchspeak (Touchspeak, London, England). In addition, Internet-based software treatment programs have been increasingly available for individuals with brain damage, and most of these software programs specifically target aphasia therapy. These include Sentactics (Sentactics Corporation, Concord, CA [93]), ORLA-VT (Oral Reading for Language in Aphasia (ORLA [94]), and Constant Therapy [95].

A recent review by Zheng, Lynch, and Taylor [95] indicated that computer therapy is effective when compared to no therapy. Computer therapy appears to deliver equivalent results to clinician-delivered therapy in individuals with chronic aphasia. This is a promising result, particularly in light of recent literature indicating the need for intensive therapy for optimal outcomes [96]. As researchers implement treatments from the computer and through mobile devices, it is essential to incorporate evidence-based treatment programs in computer therapy. For example, Constant Therapy is a mobile rehabilitation application designed for brain rehabilitation that incorporates evidence-based therapy in aphasia recovery. In this software program, therapy tasks are divided into language and cognitive tasks and are personalized for each patient, based on standardized tests and baseline performance.

In summary, recent technological advances, especially smart tablets, provide a unique way for stroke patients to take control of their rehabilitation, by giving them access to treatment technologies. These technologies allow patients to continue therapy outside the traditional clinical setting and stay connected with their clinician to manage their rehabilitation program. These advances in technology have the potential to reshape the way rehabilitation is conducted for individuals who require ongoing communication therapy but struggle to find practical and financially viable options to continue their rehabilitation.

5.8 Conclusion

Major advances have occurred in the past two decades in the development of interventions for communication disorders in stroke rehabilitation. There is a strong consensus that speech and language therapy is beneficial after stroke; however, there is still no clear evidence regarding the optimal timing, intensity, and type of therapy. Along with routine management of aphasia, there is a need for the development of interdisciplinary protocols to address the associated negative outcomes of aphasia over the long term [3]. Early intervention by speech-language pathologists may improve functional communication and quality of life for survivors and caregivers; however, the mechanisms that drive recovery of impairments need to be better understood. Given the prolonged course of behavioural speech and language therapy, the prospect of augmenting the effectiveness of this therapy is attractive to clinicians, patients, and patients' families and caregivers. Several approaches have been used as adjuvants to traditional speech and language therapy such as pharmacotherapy and non-invasive brain stimulation. Advances in technology are also important, and computer therapy can offer new opportunities for intensive, tailored and personalized language treatment at whatever time point a patient wishes to engage with therapy after stroke. Greater insight into biomarkers and predictors of the effects of speech and language therapy may be key to maximizing the impact of this emerging class of therapies for stroke patients. For example, knowing where the lesion is and what peri-lesional tissue is anatomically intact is critical to identify which brain region to stimulate using non-invasive brain stimulation to augment speech and language therapy. Future research should place greater emphasis on randomized controlled trials and evidence-based research.

5.9 Acknowledgement

This research was supported by NIDCD K99 DC015554 and P50 DC014664. The content is solely the responsibility of the authors and does not necessarily represent the views of the National Institutes of Health.

References

1. Benson DF, Ardila A. *Aphasia: A clinical perspective.* London, UK: Oxford University Press, 1996.

2. Engelter ST, Gostynski M, Papa S, et al. Epidemiology of aphasia attributable to first ischemic stroke incidence, severity, fluency, etiology, and thrombolysis. *Stroke* 2006; **37**(6): 1379–84.

3. Flowers HL, Skoretz SA, Silver FL, et al. Poststroke aphasia frequency, recovery, and outcomes: A systematic review and meta-analysis. *Archives of Physical Medicine and Rehabilitation* 2016; **97**(12): 2188–201.

4. National Aphasia Association. *Aphasia.* New York, NY: National Aphasia Association, 2016.

5. Yorkston KM. Treatment efficacy: Dysarthria. *Journal of Speech, Language, and Hearing Research* 1996; **39**(5): S46–7.

6. Arboix A, Marti-Vilalta JL. Lacunar infarctions and dysarthria. *Archives of Neurology* 1990; **47**(2): 127–7.

7. Melo TP, Bogousslavsky J, van Melle G, Regli F. Pure motor stroke: A reappraisal. *Neurology* 1992; **42**(4): 789–9.

8. Duffy JR. *Motor speech disorders: Substrates, differential diagnosis, and management.* St. Louis, MO: Elsevier Mosby, 2013.

9. McNeil MR, Robin DA, Schmidt RA. Apraxia of speech: Definition, differentiation, and treatment. In McNeil MR. ed. *Clinical management of sensorimotor speech disorders.* New York, NY: Thieme, 2009; 249–68.

10. Brady MC, Kelly H, Godwin J, Enderby P. Speech and language therapy for aphasia following stroke. *Cochrane Database of Systematic Reviews* 2012; Issue 5. Art. No.: CD000425.

11. Byng S, Duchan JF. Social model philosophies and principles: Their applications to therapies for aphasia. *Aphasiology* 2005; **19**(10–11): 906–22.

12. Baker J, Rorden C, Fridriksson J. Using transcranial direct current stimulation (tDCS) to treat stroke patients with aphasia. *Stroke: A Journal of Cerebral Circulation* 2010; **41**(6): 1229–36.

13. Vestito L, Rosellini S, Mantero M, Bandini F. Long-term effects of transcranial direct-current stimulation in chronic post-stroke aphasia: A pilot study. *Frontiers in Human Neuroscience* 2014; **8**: 1–7.

14. Beristain X, Golombievski E. Pharmacotherapy to enhance cognitive and motor recovery following stroke. *Drugs & Aging* 2015; **32**(10): 765–72.

15. Hillis AE, Barker PB, Beauchamp NJ, Winters BD, Mirski M, Wityk RJ. Restoring blood pressure reperfused Wernicke's area and improved language. *Neurology* 2001; **56**(5): 670–2.

16. Hillis AE, Ulatowski JA, Barker PB. A pilot randomized trial of induced blood pressure elevation: Effects on function and focal perfusion in acute and subacute stroke. *Cerebrovascular Diseases* 2003; **16**(3): 236–46.

17. Hillis AE, Kleinman JT, Newhart M, et al. Restoring cerebral blood flow reveals neural regions critical for naming. *Journal of Neuroscience* 2006; **26**(31): 8069–73.

18. Raymer AM, Beeson P, Holland A, et al. Translational research in aphasia: From neuroscience to neurorehabilitation. *Journal of Speech, Language, and Hearing Research* 2008; **51**(1): S259–75.

19. Peach RK. Acquired apraxia of speech: Features, accounts, and treatment. *Topics in Stroke Rehabilitation* 2004; **11**(1): 49–58.

20. Hersh, D. Ten things our clients might say about their aphasia therapy ... if we only asked. *ACQ: Issues in Language, Speech and Hearing* 2004; **6**(2): 102–5.

21. World Health Organization. *ICF: International classification of functioning, disability and health-report.* Geneva, Switzerland: World Health Organization, 2001.

22. Leach E, Cornwell P, Fleming J, Haines T. Patient centered goal-setting in a subacute rehabilitation setting. *Disability and Rehabilitation* 2010; **32**(2): 159–72.

23. Chapey R, Duchan RJ, Garcia LJ, Kagan A, Lyon JG, Simmons-Mackie N. Life-participation approach to aphasia: A statement of values for the future. In Chapey R. ed. *Language interventions strategies in aphasia and related neurogenic communication disorders.* Philadelphia, PA: Lippincott Williams & Wilkins, 2001; 279–89.

24. Baum CM, Edwards D. *ACS: Activity card sort.* St. Louis, MO: Washington University School of Medicine, 2001.

25. Haley K, Jenkins K, Hadden C, Womack J, Hall J, Schweiker C. Sorting pictures to assess participation in life activities. *SIG 2 Perspectives on Neurophysiology and Neurogenic Speech and Language Disorders* 2005; **15**(4): 11–15.

26. American Speech-Language-Hearing Association. *Evidence-based practice in communication disorders: Position statement.* Rockville, MD: American Speech-Language-Hearing Association, 2005.

27. Cherney LR, Patterson JP, Raymer AM. Intensity of aphasia therapy: Evidence and efficacy. *Current*

Neurology and Neuroscience Reports 2011; **11**(6): 560–9.

28. Persad C, Wozniak L, Kostopoulos E. Retrospective analysis of outcomes from two intensive comprehensive aphasia programs. *Topics in Stroke Rehabilitation* 2013; **20**(5): 388–97.

29. Yorkston KM, Spencer KA, Duffy JR, et al. Evidence-based practice guidelines for dysarthria: Management of velopharyngeal function. *Journal of Medical Speech-Language Pathology* 2001; **9**(4): 257–74.

30. Wambaugh JL, Nessler C, Cameron R, Mauszycki SC. Treatment for acquired apraxia of speech: Examination of treatment intensity and practice schedule. *American Journal of Speech-Language Pathology* 2013; **22**(1): 84–102.

31. Brady MC, Kelly H, Godwin J, Enderby P, Campbell P. Speech and language therapy for aphasia following stroke (Review). *Cochrane Database of Systematic Reviews* 2016; Issue 6. Art. No.: CD000425.

32. Allen L, Mehta S, McClure JA, Teasell, R. Therapeutic interventions for aphasia initiated more than six months post stroke: A review of the evidence. *Topics in Stroke Rehabilitation* 2014; **19**(6): 523–35.

33. Dignam J, Copland D, McKinnon E, Burfein P, O'Brien K, Farrell A, Rodriguez AD. Intensive versus distributed aphasia therapy: A nonrandomized, parallel-group, dosage-controlled study. *Stroke* 2015; **46**(8): 2206–11.

34. Sellars C, Hughes T, Langhorne P. Speech and language therapy for dysarthria due to non-progressive brain damage. *Cochrane Database of Systematic Reviews* 2005; Issue 3, Art. No.: CD002088.

35. Crinion JT, Leff AP. Using functional imaging to understand therapeutic effects in poststroke aphasia. *Current Opinion in Neurology* 2015;**28**(4): 330–7.

36. Meinzer M, Breitenstein C. Functional imaging studies of treatment-induced recovery in chronic aphasia. *Aphasiology* 2008; **22**(12): 1251–68.

37. Taub E, Uswatte G, Elbert T. New treatments in neurorehabilitation founded on basic research. *Nature Reviews Neuroscience* 2002; **3**(3): 228–36.

38. Pulvermüller F, Neininger B, Elbert T, Mohr B, Rockstroh B, Koebbel P, Taub E. Constraint-induced therapy of chronic aphasia after stroke. *Stroke* 2001; **32**(7): 1621–6.

39. Maher LM, Kendall D, Swearengin JA, Rodriguez A, Leon SA, Pingel K ... Rothi LJG. A pilot study of use-dependent learning in the context of constraint induced language therapy. *Journal of the International Neuropsychological Society* 2006; **12**(06): 843–52.

40. Meinzer M, Djundja D, Barthel G, Elbert T, Rockstroh B. Long-term stability of improved language

functions in chronic aphasia after constraint-induced aphasia therapy. *Stroke* 2005; **36**(7): 1462–6.

41. Szaflarski JP, Ball AL, Grether S, Al-fwaress F, Griffith NM, Neils-Strunjas J ... Reichhardt R. Constraint-induced aphasia therapy stimulates language recovery in patients with chronic aphasia after ischemic stroke. *Medical Science Monitor: International Medical Journal of Experimental and Clinical Research* 2008; **14**(5): CR243.

42. Bonilha L, Gleichgerrcht E, Nesland T, Rorden C, Fridriksson J. Success of anomia treatment in aphasia is associated with preserved architecture of global and left temporal lobe structural networks. *Neurorehabilitation and Neural Repair* 2016; **30**(3): 266–79.

43. Linebaugh CW. Cueing hierarchies and word retrieval. In Brookshire RH. ed. *Clinical aphasiology*. Minneapolis, MN: BRK Publishers, 1997; 19–31.

44. Cherney LR. Aphasia treatment: Intensity, dose parameters, and script training. *International Journal of Speech-Language Pathology* 2012; **14**(5): 424–31.

45. Marsh K, Bertranou E, Suominen H, Venkatachalam M. An economic evaluation of speech and language therapy. *Matrix Evidence* 2010.

46. Sebastian R, Tsapkini K, Tippett DC. Transcranial direct current stimulation in post stroke aphasia and primary progressive aphasia: Current knowledge and future clinical applications. *NeuroRehabilitation* 2016; **39**: 141–52.

47. Naeser MA, Martin PI, Ho M, Treglia E, Kaplan E, Bashir S, Pascual-Leone A. Transcranial magnetic stimulation and aphasia rehabilitation. *Archives of Physical Medicine and Rehabilitation* 2012; **93**(1): S26–S34.

48. Cotelli M, Fertonani A, Miozzo A, Rosini S, Manenti R, Padovani A ... Miniussi C. Anomia training and brain stimulation in chronic aphasia. *Neuropsychological Rehabilitation* 2011; **21**(5): 717–41.

49. Hallett M. Transcranial magnetic stimulation and the human brain. *Nature* 2000; **406**(6792): 147–50.

50. Walsh V, Pascual-Leone A. *Neurochronometrics of mind: TMS in cognitive science.* Cambridge, MA: MIT Press, 2003.

51. Martin PI, Naeser MA, Ho M, Doron KW, Kurland J, Kaplan J ... Pascual-Leone A. Overt naming fMRI pre-and post-TMS: Two nonfluent aphasia patients, with and without improved naming post-TMS. *Brain and Language* 2009; **111**(1): 20–35.

52. Naeser MA, Martin PI, Nicholas M, Baker EH, Seekins H, Kobayashi M ... Doron KW. Improved picture naming in chronic aphasia after TMS to part of right Broca's area: An open-protocol study. *Brain and Language* 2005; **93**(1): 95–105.

53. Naeser MA, Martin PI, Theoret H, Kobayashi M, Fregni F, Nicholas M ... Pascual-Leone A. TMS suppression of right pars triangularis, but not pars opercularis, improves naming in aphasia. *Brain and Language* 2011, **119**(3): 206–13.

54. Nitsche MA, Paulus W. Excitability changes induced in the human motor cortex by weak transcranial direct current stimulation. *Journal of Physiology* 2000; **527**(3): 633–9.

55. Liebetanz D, Nitsche MA, Tergau F, Paulus W. Pharmacological approach to the mechanisms of transcranial DC-stimulation-induced after-effects of human motor cortex excitability. *Brain* 2002; **125**(10): 2238–47.

56. Fridriksson J, Richardson JD, Baker JM, Rorden C. Transcranial direct current stimulation improves naming reaction time in fluent aphasia: A double-blind, sham-controlled study. *Stroke* 2011; **42**(3): 819–21.

57. Kang EK, Kim YK, Sohn HM, Cohen LG, Paik NJ. Improved picture naming in aphasia patients treated with cathodal tDCS to inhibit the right Broca's homologue area. *Restorative Neurology and Neuroscience* 2011; **29**(3): 141–52.

58. Marangolo P, Marinelli CV, Bonifazi S, Fiori V, Ceravolo MG, Provinciali L, Tomaiuolo F. Electrical stimulation over the left inferior frontal gyrus (IFG) determines long-term effects in the recovery of speech apraxia in three chronic aphasics. *Behavioural Brain Research* 2011; **225**(2): 498–504.

59. Jung I-Y, Lim JY, Kang EK, Sohn HM, Paik N-J. The factors associated with good responses to speech therapy combined with transcranial direct current stimulation in post-stroke aphasic patients. *Annals of Rehabilitation Medicine* 2011; **35**(4): 460–9.

60. Elsner B, Kugler J, Pohl M, Mehrholz J. Transcranial direct current stimulation (tDCS) for improving aphasia in patients with aphasia after stroke. *Cochrane Database of Systematic Reviews* 2015; Issue 5. Art. No.: CD009760.

61. Byng S, Cairns D, Duchan J. Values in practice and practising values. *Journal of Communication Disorders* 2002; **35**(2): 89–106.

62. Albert ML, Bachman D, Morgan A, Helm-Estabrooks N. Pharmacotherapy of aphasia. *Neurology* 1988; **38**: 877–9.

63. Güngör L, Terzi M, Onar MK. Does long term use of piracetam improve speech disturbances due to ischemic cerebrovascular diseases? *Brain and Language* 2011; **117**(1): 23–7.

64. McNamara P, Albert ML. Neuropharmacology of verbal perseveration. *Seminars in Speech and Language* 2004; **25**(4): 309–32.

65. Seniów J, Litwin M, Litwin T, Leśniak M, Członkowska A. New approach to the rehabilitation of post-stroke focal cognitive syndrome: Effect of levodopa combined with speech and language therapy on functional recovery from aphasia. *Journal of the Neurological Sciences* 2009; **283**(1), 214–18.

66. Berthier ML, Pulvermüller F, Dávila G, Casares NG, Gutiérrez A. Drug therapy of post-stroke aphasia: A review of current evidence. *Neuropsychology Review* 2011; **21**(3): 302–17.

67. Cahana-Amitay D, Albert ML, Oveis A. Psycholinguistics of aphasia pharmacotherapy: Asking the right questions. *Aphasiology* 2014; **28**(2): 133–54.

68. Kessler J, Thiel A, Karbe H, Heiss WD. Piracetam improves activated blood flow and facilitates rehabilitation of poststroke aphasic patients. *Stroke* 2000; **31**: 2112–16.

69. Berthier ML, Pulvermüller F. (2011). Neuroscience insights improve neurorehabilitation of poststroke aphasia. *Nature Reviews. Neurology* 2011; **7**: 86–97.

70. de Boissezon X, Peran P, de Boysson C, Démonet JF. Pharmacotherapy of aphasia: Myth or reality? *Brain and Language* 2007; **102**: 114–25.

71. Sabe L, Leiguarda R, Starkstein SE. An open-label trial of bromocriptine in nonfluent aphasia. *Neurology* 1992; **42**: 1637–8.

72. Walker-Batson D, Curtis S, Natarajan R, Ford J, Dronkers N, Salmeron E, et al. Double-blind, placebo-controlled study of the use of amphetamine in the treatment of aphasia. *Stroke* 2001; **32**: 2093–8.

73. Whiting E, Chenery HJ, Chalk J, Copland DA. Dexamphetamine boosts naming treatment effects in chronic aphasia. *Journal of International Neuropsychological Society* 2008; **13**: 972–9.

74. Berthier ML, Green C, Higueras C, Fernandez I, Hinojosa J, Martín MC. A randomized, placebo-controlled study of donepezil in poststroke aphasia. *Neurology* 2006; **67**: 1687–9.

75. Berthier ML, Green C, Lara JP, Higueras C, Barbancho MA, Dávila G, Pulvermüller F. Memantine and constraint-induced aphasia therapy in chronic poststroke aphasia. *Annals of Neurology* 2009; **65**(5): 577–85.

76. Chen Y, Li Y-S, Wang Z-Y, Xu Q, Shi G-W, Lin Y. The efficacy of donepezil for post-stroke aphasia: A pilot case control study. *Zhonghua Nei Ke Za Zhi (Chinese Journal of Internal Medicine)* 2010; **49**(2): 115–18.

77. Orgogozo JM. Piracetam in the treatment of acute stroke. *Pharmacopsychiatry* 1999; **32**(1): 25–32.

78. Tanaka Y, Bachman DL. Pharmacotherapy of aphasia. In Connor LS, Obler LK. eds. *Neurobehavior of*

language and cognition studies of normal aging and brain damage. Berlin: SpringerLink, 2007; 159–62.

79. Hillis AE. Pharmacological, surgical, and neurovascular interventions to augment acute aphasia recovery. *American Journal of Physical Medicine & Rehabilitation* 2007; **86**(6): 426–34.

80. Rordorf G, Cramer SC, Efird JT, Schwamm LH, Buonanno F, Koroshetz WJ. Pharmacological elevation of blood pressure in acute stroke clinical effects and safety. *Stroke* 1997; **28**(11): 2133–8.

81. Hillis AE, Wityk RJ, Barker PB, Beauchamp NJ, Gailloud P, Murphy K … Metter EJ. Subcortical aphasia and neglect in acute stroke: The role of cortical hypoperfusion. *Brain* 2002; **125**(5): 1094–104.

82. Perler BA, Murphy K, Sternbach Y, Gailloud P, Shake JG. Immediate postoperative thrombolytic therapy: An aggressive strategy for neurologic salvage when cerebral thromboembolism complicates carotid endarterectomy. *Journal of Vascular Surgery* 2000; **31**(5): 1033–7.

83. Albert ML, Sparks RW, Helm NA. Melodic intonation therapy for aphasia. *Archives of Neurology* 1973; **29**(2): 130–1.

84. Baker FA. Modifying the melodic intonation therapy program for adults with severe non-fluent aphasia. *Music Therapy Perspectives* 2000; **18**(2): 110–14.

85. Jungblut M. SIPARI1: A music therapy intervention for patients suffering with chronic, nonfluent aphasia. *Music and Medicine* 2009; **1**(2): 102–5.

86. Belin P, Zilbovicius M, Remy P, Francois C, Guillaume S, Chain F … Samson Y. Recovery from nonfluent aphasia after melodic intonation therapy: A PET study. *Neurology* 1996; **47**(6): 1504–11.

87. Bonakdarpour B, Eftekharzadeh A, Ashayeri H. Melodic intonation therapy in Persian aphasic patients. *Aphasiology*, 2003; **17**(1): 75–95.

88. Schlaug G, Marchina S, Norton, A. From singing to speaking: Why singing may lead to recovery of expressive language function in patients with Broca's aphasia. *Music Perception: An Interdisciplinary Journal* 2008; **25**(4): 315–23.

89. van der Meulen I, van de Sandt-Koenderman, ME, Ribbers GM. Melodic intonation therapy: Present controversies and future opportunities. *Archives of Physical Medicine and Rehabilitation* 2012; **93**(1): S46–S52.

90. Schlaug G, Marchina S, Norton A. Evidence for plasticity in white-matter tracts of patients with chronic Broca's aphasia undergoing intense intonation-based speech therapy. *Annals of the New York Academy of Sciences* 2009; **1169**(1): 385–94.

91. Breier JI, Randle S, Maher LM, Papanicolaou AC. Changes in maps of language activity activation following melodic intonation therapy using magnetoencephalography: Two case studies. *Journal of Clinical and Experimental Neuropsychology* 2010; **32**(3): 309–14.

92. Petheram B. The behaviour of stroke patients in unsupervised computer-administered aphasia therapy. *Disability and Rehabilitation* 1996; **18**(1): 21–6.

93. Thompson CK, Choy JJ, Holland A, Cole R. Sentactics®: Computer-automated treatment of underlying forms. *Aphasiology* 2010; **24**(10): 1242–66.

94. Cherney LR. Oral reading for language in aphasia (ORLA): Evaluating the efficacy of computer-delivered therapy in chronic nonfluent aphasia. *Topics in Stroke Rehabilitation* 2010; **17**(6): 423–31.

95. Zheng C, Lynch L, Taylor N. Effect of computer therapy in aphasia: A systematic review. *Aphasiology* 2016; **30**(2–3): 211–44.

96. Bhogal SK, Teasell RW, Foley NC, Speechley MR. Rehabilitation of aphasia: More is better. *Topics in Stroke Rehabilitation* 2015; **19**(6): 523–35.

97. Lee AW, Hillis AE. The pharmacological treatment of aphasia. In Stemmer B, Whitaker HA. eds. *Handbook of the neuroscience of language.* London, UK: Academic Press, 2008; 407–15.

98. Miltner WH. Plasticity and reorganization in the rehabilitation of stroke. *Zeitschrift für Psychologie* 2016; **224**: 91–101.

99. Nitsche MA, Liebetanz D, Tergau F, Paulus W. Modulation of cortical excitability by transcranial direct current stimulation. *Der Nervenarzt* 2002; **73**(4): 332–5.

Management of Disorders of Eating, Drinking, and Swallowing in Neurorehabilitation

Chapter 6

Rachel Mulheren, Alba Azola, and Marlís González-Fernández

6.1 Introduction

Nutrition and hydration are integral to health and quality of life. To initiate the process of eating or drinking, a substance must be recognized as nutritive and delivered to the oral cavity. Swallowing requires the coordination of neuromuscular events in the aerodigestive tract to deliver a bolus from the oral cavity through the pharynx and oesophagus to the stomach. Coordination of breathing and swallowing, including a brief moment of apnoea, prevents food from entering the airway and lungs. Swallowing has both a voluntary and involuntary or reflexive component. Food and drink are swallowed differently depending on sensory properties such as consistency, size, temperature, and taste [1–3]. These adjustments depend on a neural network including the cranial nerves,

brainstem swallowing pattern generators, cerebral cortex, thalamus, and cerebellum for motor planning, motor execution, and sensory processing [4–6].

Swallowing involves several structures of the head and neck (Figure 6.1). Liquid and solid boluses differ in how they are managed in the oral phase of swallowing [7, 8]. During the oral preparatory phase, liquids are positioned in the oral cavity with the posterior tongue and soft palate approximating to prevent premature spillage. Then, during the oral propulsive stage, liquids are transferred posteriorly to the oropharynx as the anterior tongue approximates the hard palate. Solids are first transferred to the lower teeth by the tongue and cheeks, mixed with saliva, and masticated during stage 1 transport. During stage 2 transport, the tongue tip touches the hard palate and transfers processed solids to the oropharynx.

During the pharyngeal phase, the soft palate retracts and contacts the posterior pharyngeal wall to seal the nasal cavity and generate pressure for bolus propulsion. The larynx moves anteriorly and superiorly as the true and false vocal folds approximate and the epiglottis inverts over the closed larynx. The tongue base contacts the posterior pharyngeal wall, which moves the bolus through the pharynx in muscular waves. The upper oesophageal sphincter relaxes, and the bolus passes into the oesophagus. Finally, during the oesophageal phase, the bolus is transported by peristalsis and gravity through the lower oesophageal sphincter to the stomach.

Disordered swallowing, or dysphagia, is reported in 16% of the general population [9], in up to 34% of the elderly population [10], and in 50% of stroke patients [11]. Dysphagia may arise from a breakdown at any point in the neuroanatomical swallowing system and may involve compromised strength, timing, range of motion, or coordination during any phase of swallowing. Aetiologies of dysphagia are numerous and include neurological disorder, brain injury, pharmacological side effects, degenerative disease, psychogenesis, and craniofacial

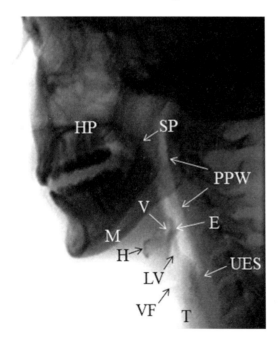

Figure 6.1 Anatomy of the head and neck involved in swallowing VF, vocal folds; H, hyoid bone; M, mandible; UES, upper oesophageal sphincter; T, trachea; V, valleculae; PPW, posterior pharyngeal wall; E, epiglottis; HP, hard palate; SP, soft palate; LV, laryngeal vestibule

trauma or abnormality. The natural aging process may result in changes to swallowing function [12]. Cognitive impairments may also impact deglutition. In some cases, swallowing function may improve over time with spontaneous recovery (as may be the case after stroke). On the other hand, dysphagia may never fully resolve or worsen.

Swallowing function is assessed by clinical and instrumental evaluation. Initially, risk of dysphagia/aspiration may be screened by a brief medical history review and observation of water swallows. A clinical swallowing evaluation is more thorough than the initial screen and determines whether a swallowing disorder is present and, if so, provides a breakdown of impairments and how they can be treated. First, the patient's history and pertinent physical exam is obtained, including a cranial nerve exam and an assessment of cough and hyolaryngeal elevation during a saliva swallow. Different sizes and consistencies of solids and liquids are trialled as the clinician observes for signs and symptoms of dysphagia (Table 6.1). Swallowing physiology is best assessed by instrumental techniques such as the videofluoroscopic swallowing study (VFSS) or fibre-optic endoscopic evaluation of swallowing (FEES). Both procedures provide video imaging of sequential swallowing events and allow the evaluation of penetration into the laryngeal vestibule and aspiration into the trachea. For most cases these tests are considered to provide complementary information although penetration or aspiration during the swallow cannot be observed using FEES. Exploration of other instrumental techniques such as high-resolution manometry, dynamic magnetic resonance imaging, high-resolution ultrasound, and multi-slice computed tomography is currently under way.

Table 6.1 Observable signs and symptoms of dysphagia during clinical swallow evaluation

Wet, gurgly vocal quality
Coughing
Choking
Throat clear
Watering eyes
Residue in oral cavity after swallowing
Anterior loss of bolus
Nasal regurgitation
Effortful, prolonged mastication
No swallow initiated

6.2 Treatment

Treatment of dysphagia is individualized based on medical history, patient goals, pathophysiology, and prognosis. The goal of dysphagia therapy is to facilitate oral intake to the greatest degree possible, with supplementation by non-oral routes of nutrition as necessary for achieving adequate nutrition and hydration. In addition to factors of quality of life, such as socialization and pleasure during mealtimes, oral intake prevents degradation of swallowing function, or disuse atrophy, as may occur during prolonged *nils per os* status. Speech-language pathologists design and conduct swallowing therapy with input from dieticians, physiatrists, radiologists, neuropsychologists, otorhinolaryngologists, respiratory therapists, and other healthcare professionals.

Treatment can take place in any location, ranging from the bedside in the medically compromised patient to home, where the patient can perform an exercise regimen. The earlier treatment can be initiated, depending on medical status and patient willingness, the better. In fact, prophylactic swallowing exercises are recommended for head and neck cancer patients prior to chemoradiation or tumour resection [18, 19]. In cases of degenerative disorders where restoration of function may be limited, treatment of swallowing disorders may serve to maintain the current level of function.

Dysphagia treatment may compensate for lost function, facilitate restoration of function, or combine both. Compensatory strategies modify the environment and conditions in which swallowing occurs to promote safety and efficiency during swallowing. For example, postural changes such as the chin tuck or head turn manoeuvres optimize the direction of bolus flow; changes to bolus properties alter sensory input to the swallowing network to modulate how a bolus is swallowed. Alternative intake methods such as parenteral nutrition or tube feeding entirely bypass the oropharyngeal structures to deliver nutrition. These techniques allow the patient to maintain nutrition and hydration but do not restore compromised neurophysiology. Similar to assistive devices for ambulation, once compensatory strategies are removed, swallowing returns to baseline.

Restorative treatment strategies target the mechanisms underlying dysphagia to produce lasting improvement in function. Exercises may be introduced to strengthen swallowing musculature, to improve the timing of swallowing events, to increase range of motion, and to promote coordination of swallowing physiology.

Generally, treatment of dysphagia is non-pharmacological, and includes a customized programme of diet modifications, exercises, and sensorimotor stimulation. Pharmacological and surgical management are applicable to specific cases based on their ability to address particular causal mechanisms.

6.3 Treatment: Non-Pharmacological

The consistency of food can be altered to maximize swallowing safety and efficiency; however, all consistencies should be tested during an instrumental swallowing evaluation to ascertain the specific effects on patients' swallowing physiology. For example, thickened liquids may reduce penetration and aspiration if thin liquid spills from the oral cavity prior to swallow initiation or if airway closure is inadequate [13]. Conversely, thickened liquids may be more difficult to swallow in the case of weakness, which may result in a greater amount of pharyngeal residue that is at risk of being aspirated. Additionally, thickened liquids may affect hydration status due to thickening agents and reduced liquid intake associated with low palatability. In cases of penetration or minimal aspiration, patients may be prescribed thickened liquids during meals, with thin water allowed after oral care between meals, as aspiration of water may pose a lower risk of pneumonia than aspiration of food or residue [14, 15]. Solids may be mechanically altered to varying degrees to accommodate weakness or poor coordination during the oral phase of swallowing. Although consistency nomenclature may vary by country and facility, definitions of liquid and solid flow properties have been developed by the International Dysphagia Diet Standardization Initiative (iddsi.org/) (Figure 6.2). Modifying bolus size may improve swallowing function [16]. For example, in patients with risk of aspiration, smaller boluses may facilitate better coordination, whereas in patients with reduced sensation, a larger bolus may be needed to trigger the appropriate swallowing response.

Simple changes to the eating environment may facilitate swallowing function. The removal of external distractions such as television and noise promotes focus on the meal and following safe swallowing strategies. Although mealtimes are social in nature,

patients may benefit from refraining from speaking while food is in the oropharynx to prevent penetration, aspiration, or choking. Patients may have a more coordinated swallow if they feed themselves. An upright posture during intake reduces the risk of penetration and aspiration and allows for gravity to assist in the safe and efficient transfer of food to the stomach. For patients at risk of reflux, an upright posture should be maintained for at least one hour following eating or drinking [17]. A chin tuck may assist with airway protection in the case of premature spillage to the pharynx (Table 6.2); however, this posture may worsen penetration and aspiration in some patients, and should first be trialled during instrumental evaluation. In the case of significant unilateral residue due to weakness, turning the head to the weaker side closes the pyriform sinus on the weak side while directing the bolus to the stronger side of the pharynx. For patients with impaired oral transit, a backwards head tilt may be used to move the bolus to the pharynx (Table 6.2); however, this posture may cause or worsen penetration and aspiration if airway protection is not adequate.

The use of a straw allows for a bolus to bypass the anterior oral cavity, which may benefit patients with a weak or uncoordinated oral phase. However, if airway protection is delayed or incomplete, straws may be contraindicated due to the brisk bolus delivery directly to the pharynx. Special cups (e.g., Provale) and straws (e.g., SafeStraw™) can be used to limit the amount of liquid per bolus. Cut-out cups allow for complete tilting and extraction of liquid with little head movement. The angle and grip of utensils can be customized to improve manual delivery of food to the oral cavity. Plates may be fitted with dividers or barriers.

Due to the sensory-motor feedback loops in the swallowing network, oral stimulation with non-nutritive stimuli may improve swallowing function in patients with an intact peripheral nervous system. Thermal stimulation involves repeatedly rubbing the anterior faucial pillars with a cold stimulus to reduce the timing of swallowing [18]. Taste stimuli, particularly sour, may also improve the timing and coordination of swallowing in stroke patients and reduce aspiration in patients with other neurogenic aetiologies of dysphagia [19].

Certain swallowing exercises may be used in direct or indirect treatment (with or without food) (Table 6.2). The Mendelsohn manoeuvre, during

Table 6.2

Swallowing Manoeuvres and Exercises	Physiologic Target						
	Oral Bolus Transport	Initiation of Pharyngeal Swallow	Hyolaryngeal Excursion	Laryngeal Vestibule Closure	Pharyngeal Contraction	Tongue Base Retraction	UES Opening
Chin Tuck				X		X	
Head Turn				X			X
Chin Up	X						
Sensory Stimulation		X					
Mendelsohn Manoeuvre			X	X			X
Supraglottic Swallow		X	X	X		X	X
Super Supraglottic Swallow		X	X	X		X	X
Effortfull Swallow		X	X	X		X	X
Masako Manoeuvre					X	X	
Shaker Exercise			X	X			X
Expiratory Muscle Strength Training			X				
Surface Electrical Stimulation			X				

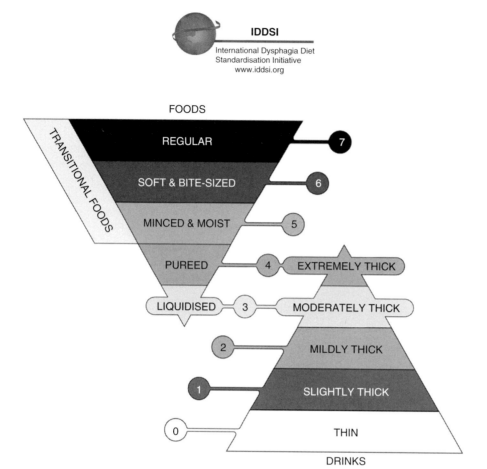

IDDSI
International Dysphagia Diet
Standardisation Initiative
www.iddsi.org

FOODS

TRANSITIONAL FOODS

REGULAR — 7
SOFT & BITE-SIZED — 6
MINCED & MOIST — 5
PUREED — 4 — EXTREMELY THICK
LIQUIDISED — 3 — MODERATELY THICK
2 — MILDLY THICK
1 — SLIGHTLY THICK
0 — THIN

DRINKS

Figure 6.2 The International Dysphagia Diet Standardization Initiative © The International Dysphagia Diet Standardization Initiative, 2016. iddsi.org/resources/framework/

which the patient is instructed to feel the thyroid notch and 'hold it up' for several seconds in the middle of swallow, facilitates and prolongs hyolaryngeal elevation, UES opening, pharyngeal contraction, and bolus transit [20, 21] (Figure 6.3). The supraglottic swallow involves holding the breath, swallowing, and immediately coughing to facilitate early and sustained glottic closure with prolonged UES opening; the super-supraglottic swallow adds a Valsalva manoeuvre, contributing to closure of the airway at the false vocal folds [22, 23]. Instructing patients to squeeze the muscles of the throat during swallowing, or an effortful swallow, promotes hyolaryngeal elevation, UES opening, and airway protection, and generates higher pressure in the oropharynx and oesophagus [24–26].

In contrast, some exercises are always completed without a food bolus (Table 6.2). The tongue hold exercise, or Masako manoeuvre, promotes anterior movement of the posterior pharyngeal wall by protruding the tongue and holding it between the teeth during a swallow [27]. The Shaker Exercise, completed in a supine position, involves multiple repetitions of nodding the head forward and holding for approximately one minute; this exercise targets hyolaryngeal excursion, UES opening, and strengthening of the suprahyoid muscles [28]. Strengthening and endurance exercises for the tongue may improve swallowing pressures and facilitate airway protection [29].

Biofeedback is especially useful in swallowing training, a task that naturally provides limited intrinsic feedback [30]. Additionally, most patients are not familiar with the regional anatomy. Surface electromyography of the submental musculature provides visual feedback as a waveform for every swallow relative to baseline for each session [31]. It is important to

A

B

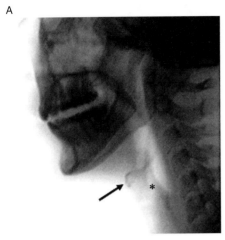

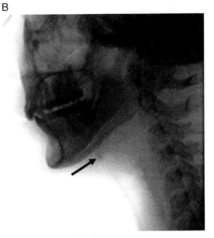

Figure 6.3 Mendelsohn manoeuvre performed under videofluoroscopy: (A) Structures at rest; note the open laryngeal vestibule (*) and the position of the hyoid. (B) Mendelsohn manoeuvre; hyoid elevation is sustained for at least two seconds.

STRUCTURES AT REST

HYOID ELEVATED,
LARYNGEAL VESTIBULE CLOSED

note that the submental muscles are also active during other co-occurring swallowing functions, including lingual movement and increases in the electromyographic signal do not necessarily represent swallowing. Pharyngeal and oesophageal manometry can provide visual biofeedback for generation of sequential pressures along the upper alimentary canal during swallowing [32, 33]. Training during and after instrumental evaluation (i.e., VFSS or FEES) allows patients to become familiar with their anatomy and physiology during swallowing and use that feedback to improve performance.

Surface electrical stimulation is often incorporated during direct and indirect treatment (Table 6.2). Electrode pairs are placed on the skin to deliver electrical currents to anterior neck. Placement of electrodes varies by manufacturer recommendation, though general regions include the submental and infrahyoid musculature. The current indiscriminately stimulates all areas within reach, with the highest intensity to the skin and with decreasing intensity to more distal muscles. At lower levels of current, only sensory afferents are stimulated, and at higher levels, the current may produce sensory stimulation as well as muscle contraction. A low, sensory stimulation may reduce aspiration and pooling of residue in patient with chronic dysphagia, whereas sensory and motor stimulation may interfere with airway protection by depressing the larynx during swallowing [34]. It is unclear if electrical stimulation provides benefit when combined with swallowing exercises [35]. The efficacy of

electrical stimulation for an individual patient can be assessed during instrumental evaluation and retested after a period of treatment.

As airway protection is crucial for swallowing safety, respiratory training may be incorporated in dysphagia treatment (Table 6.1). Expiratory muscle strength training (EMST) has been shown to improve swallowing outcomes for several patient populations. Recent studies indicate that EMST may increase expiratory pressure and improve reflex cough in stroke patients [36], increase pressure and swallowing kinematics in patients with amyotrophic lateral sclerosis (ALS) [37], and reduce penetration and aspiration in patients with Parkinson's disease (38). Initially, the target pressure is set at a fraction of baseline value; as performance improves, the target is adjusted to provide a challenging but appropriate load. The intensity and duration of respiratory training vary by patient.

Recent research suggests that transcranial magnetic stimulation and transcranial direct current stimulation may improve swallowing function of neurogenic aetiology by altering neuronal activity in the cortex. Although evidence is limited and results mixed, stimulation of either the damaged or intact hemisphere has been shown to improve swallowing outcomes in stroke patients [39].

When oral intake is not considered safe or the patient fails to meet nutritional demands alternate means of alimentation are considered. A short-term (< 30 days) alternative for providing enteric nutrition is the use of a nasogastric (NG) tube. There are risks associated to NG tubes feeding, including reflux aspiration, dislodgement, improper placement, and ulceration of pharyngeal or oesophageal tissues.

6.4 Pharmacological Treatment

The role of pharmacological agents in dysphagia management is limited, with a few medications such as anticholinergic drugs used to decrease sialorrhea and reduce aspiration of oral secretions [40] as described in Chapter 7. However, medical treatment of the underlying aetiologies resulting in dysphagia may improve swallowing function. For example, in patients with dermatomyositis responsive to medical treatment, swallowing function improves along with peripheral symptoms [41]. In the case of reflux-induced dysphagia the effect is limited. Wetscher et al. found that treatment with proton pump inhibitors and prokinetic agents improved dysphagia in only 27% of patients [42]. Despite mixed evidence, recent research suggests that dysphagia in Parkinson's disease may be ameliorated by dopaminergic medication [43]. In patients with Achalasia, the use of calcium channel blockers, nitrates, and anticholinergics to induce relaxation of the lower oesophageal sphincter offers little benefit and is limited by significant side effects. Botulin toxin injections are useful for temporary relief of trismus, lingual dystonia, cricopharyngeal hypertonia, and sialorrhea.

6.5 Surgical Treatment

If prolonged enteric nutrition is required, placement of a percutaneous gastrostomy or jujenostomy tube (PEG or PEJ) should be considered. Even though this does not eliminate the risk of aspiration, it decreases the risk when compared to continued oral feeding. The placement of the tube is a surgical procedure and it carries its own potential risk such as bleeding, infection, injury to adjacent organs, and leakage of gastric contents into the peritoneal cavity [44].

Referral for surgical management of dysphagia is appropriate in a few cases, for example structural abnormalities such as neuromuscular dysfunction of the cricopharyngeus muscles, oesophageal strictures, stenosis, and ventral cervical osteophytes. Botulinum toxin injections may improve symptoms in patients with hypertonicity of the upper oesophageal sphincter,

with a recent study showing symptomatic response in 47% of patients [45, 46]. However, this chemical myotomy is temporary, lasting between 3 and 12 months in most patients [47, 48]. Patients with milder impairments on videofluoroscopy and higher pressures in pharyngeal contraction had a better response to Botulinum injections. Management of oesophageal strictures is dictated by the aetiology and anatomy of the stricture, for example, benign versus malignant. Dilation of areas of narrowing in the aerodigestive tract with serial or pneumatic dilatation techniques is the primary treatment for benign strictures, albeit often offering temporary symptom relief and requiring multiple subsequent procedures [49]. Oesophageal stents and brachytherapy are typically used in palliative treatment of malignant strictures. In patients with crycopharyngeal dysfunction, endoscopic cricopharyngeal myotomy provides better long-term results than dilation with up to 95% of patients not experiencing dysphagia after the procedure [50]. Cervical ventral osteophytes are present in 20–30% of patients over the age of 65; the first line of therapy includes conservative treatments such as anti-inflammatory medications and diet modification [51]. Cervical osteophytectomy is reserved for those failing conservative management. Laryngeal diversion or laryngectomy, resulting in complete disassociation of the respiratory and digestive tract, may be contemplated in the setting of severe intractable aspiration caused by dysphagia. Although these measures eliminate aspiration, they result in loss of phonation, cough, and sense of smell, and there is potential for persistent pharyngeal dysphagia, and so these measures should only be considered in extreme cases.

6.6 Conclusion

Swallowing is a vital and intricate physiologic function that provides nutrition and hydration while preventing airway invasion. Proper function heavily relies on an intact central and peripheral nervous system, thus neurologic disorders can have a devastating impact on the patient's ability to swallow. Identification of the specific causal mechanisms contributing to the patient's dysphagia will guide the management. The effectiveness of strategies should be assessed with instrumental evaluation and periodic follow-up. Effective treatment of dysphagia requires a multidisciplinary approach and input from patients and caregiver.

References

1. Nagy A, Molfenter SM, Peladeau-Pigeon M, Stokely S, Steele CM. The effect of bolus consistency on hyoid velocity in healthy swallowing. *Dysphagia* 2015; **30**(4): 445–51.

2. Hamdy S, Jilani S, Price V, Parker C, Hall N, Power M. Modulation of human swallowing behaviour by thermal and chemical stimulation in health and after brain injury. *Neurogastroenterol. Motil.* 2003; **15**(1): 69–77.

3. Perlman AL, Schultz JG, VanDaele DJ. Effects of age, gender, bolus volume, and bolus viscosity on oropharyngeal pressure during swallowing. *J. Appl. Physiol.* (1985) 1993; **75**(1): 33–7.

4. Zald DH, Pardo JV. The functional neuroanatomy of voluntary swallowing. *Ann. Neurol.* 1999; **46**(3): 281–6.

5. Hamdy S, Aziz Q, Rothwell JC, Hobson A, Barlow J, Thompson DG. Cranial nerve modulation of human cortical swallowing motor pathways. *Am. J. Physiol.* 1997; **272**(4 Pt. 1): G802–8.

6. Jean A. Brain stem control of swallowing: Neuronal network and cellular mechanisms. *Physiol. Rev.* 2001; **81**(2): 929–69.

7. Palmer JB, Rudin NJ, Lara G, Crompton AW. Coordination of mastication and swallowing. *Dysphagia* 1992; **7**(4): 187–200.

8. Hiiemae KM, Palmer JB. Food transport and bolus formation during complete feeding sequences on foods of different initial consistency. *Dysphagia* 1999; **14**(1): 31–42.

9. Eslick GD, Talley N. Dysphagia: Epidemiology, risk factors and impact on quality of life – a population-based study. *Aliment. Pharmacol. Ther.* 2008; **27**(10): 971–9.

10. González-Fernández M, Humbert I, Winegrad H, Cappola AR, Fried LP. Dysphagia in old-old women: Prevalence as determined according to self-report and the 3-ounce water swallowing test. *J. Am. Geriatr. Soc.* 2014; **62**(4): 716–20.

11. Mann G, Hankey GJ, Cameron D. Swallowing function after stroke: Prognosis and prognostic factors at 6 months. *Stroke* 1999; **30**(4): 744–8.

12. Ekberg O, Feinberg MJ. Altered swallowing function in elderly patients without dysphagia: Radiologic findings in 56 cases. *AJR: Am. J. Roentgenol.* 1991; **156**(6): 1181–4.

13. Logemann JA, Gensler G, Robbins J, Lindblad AS, Brandt D, Hind JA, et al. A randomized study of three interventions for aspiration of thin liquids in patients with dementia or Parkinson's disease. *J. Speech Lang. Hear. Res.* 2008; **51**(1): 173–83.

14. Carlaw C, Finlayson H, Beggs K, Visser T, Marcoux C, Coney D, et al. Outcomes of a pilot water protocol project in a rehabilitation setting. *Dysphagia* 2012; **27**(3): 297–306.

15. Panther K. The Frazier free water protocol. *Persp. Swall. and Swall. Dis. (Dysphagia)* 2005; **14**(1): 4–9.

16. Ekberg O, Olsson R, Sundgren-Borgstrom P. Relation of bolus size and pharyngeal swallow. *Dysphagia* 1988; **3**(2): 69–72.

17. Kayser-Jones J, Pengilly K. Dysphagia among nursing home residents. *Geriatr. Nurs.* 1999; **20**(2): 77–84.

18. Rosenbek JC, Roecker EB, Wood JL, Robbins J. Thermal application reduces the duration of stage transition in dysphagia after stroke. *Dysphagia* 1996; **11**(4): 225–33.

19. Logemann JA, Pauloski BR, Colangelo L, Lazarus C, Fujiu M, Kahrilas PJ. Effects of a sour bolus on oropharyngeal swallowing measures in patients with neurogenic dysphagia. *J. Speech Hear. Res.* 1995; **38**(3): 556–63.

20. Lazarus C, Logemann JA, Gibbons P. Effects of maneuvers on swallowing function in a dysphagic oral cancer patient. *Head Neck* 1993; **15**(5): 419–24.

21. McCullough GH, Kamarunas E, Mann GC, Schmidley JW, Robbins JA, Crary MA. Effects of Mendelsohn maneuver on measures of swallowing duration post stroke. *Top. in Stroke Rehabil.* 2012; **19**(3): 234–43.

22. Ohmae Y, Logemann JA, Hanson DG, Kaiser P, Kahrilas PJ. Effects of two breath-holding maneuvers on oropharyngeal swallow. *Ann. Oto., Rhin. & Laryn.* 1996; **105**(2): 123–31.

23. Donzelli J, Brady S. The effects of breath-holding on vocal fold adduction: Implications for safe swallowing. *Arch. Oto.–Head & Neck Surg.* 2004; **130**(2): 208–10.

24. Pouderoux P, Kahrilas PJ. Deglutitive tongue force modulation by volition, volume, and viscosity in humans. *Gastroenterology* 1995; **108**(5): 1418–26.

25. Bülow M, Olsson R, Ekberg O. Videomanometric analysis of supraglottic swallow, effortful swallow, and chin tuck in patients with pharyngeal dysfunction. *Dysphagia* 2001; **16**(3): 190–5.

26. Hind JA, Nicosia MA, Roecker EB, Carnes ML, Robbins J. Comparison of effortful and noneffortful swallows in healthy middle-aged and older adults. *Arch. Phys. Med. Rehabil.* 2001; **82**(12): 1661–5.

27. Fujiu M, Logemann JA. Effect of a tongue-holding maneuver on posterior pharyngeal wall movement during deglutition. *Am. J. Sp.-Lang. Path.* 1996; **5**(1): 23–30.

28. Logemann JA, Rademaker A, Pauloski BR, Kelly A, Stangl-McBreen C, Antinoja J, et al. A randomized

study comparing the Shaker exercise with traditional therapy: A preliminary study. *Dysphagia* 2009; **24**(4): 403–11.

29. Robbins J, Kays SA, Gangnon RE, Hind JA, Hewitt AL, Gentry LR, et al. The effects of lingual exercise in stroke patients with dysphagia. *Arch. Phys. Med. Rehabil.* 2007; **88**(2): 150–8.

30. Azola AM, Sunday KL, Humbert IA. Kinematic visual biofeedback improves accuracy of learning a swallowing maneuver and accuracy of clinician cues during training. *Dysphagia* 2017; **32**(1): 115–22.

31. Crary MA, Carnaby GD, Groher ME, Helseth E. Functional benefits of dysphagia therapy using adjunctive sEMG biofeedback. *Dysphagia* 2004; **19**(3): 160–4.

32. Huckabee M, Lamvik K, Jones R. Pharyngeal mis-sequencing in dysphagia: Characteristics, rehabilitative response, and etiological speculation. *J. Neurol. Sci.* 2014; **343**(1): 153–8.

33. O'Rourke A, Humphries K. The use of high-resolution pharyngeal manometry as biofeedback in dysphagia therapy. *Ear, Nose & Throat Journal* 2017; **96**(2): 56.

34. Ludlow CL, Humbert I, Saxon K, Poletto C, Sonies B, Crujido L. Effects of surface electrical stimulation both at rest and during swallowing in chronic pharyngeal dysphagia. *Dysphagia* 2007; **22**(1): 1–10.

35. Langmore SE, McCulloch TM, Krisciunas GP, Lazarus CL, Van Daele DJ, Pauloski BR, et al. Efficacy of electrical stimulation and exercise for dysphagia in patients with head and neck cancer: A randomized clinical trial. *Head Neck* 2016; **38** Suppl. 1: E1221–31.

36. Hegland KW, Davenport PW, Brandimore AE, Singletary FF, Troche MS. Rehabilitation of swallowing and cough functions following stroke: An expiratory muscle strength training trial. *Arch. Phys. Med. Rehabil.* 2016; **97**(8): 1345–51.

37. Plowman EK, Watts SA, Tabor L, Robison R, Gaziano J, Domer AS, et al. Impact of expiratory strength training in amyotrophic lateral sclerosis. *Muscle Nerve* 2016; **54**(1): 48–53.

38. Troche MS, Okun MS, Rosenbek JC, Musson N, Fernandez HH, Rodriguez R, et al. Aspiration and swallowing in Parkinson disease and rehabilitation with EMST: A randomized trial. *Neurology* 2010; **75**(21): 1912–19.

39. Pisegna JM, Kaneoka A, Pearson WG, Jr, Kumar S, Langmore SE. Effects of non-invasive brain stimulation on post-stroke dysphagia: A systematic review and meta-analysis of randomized controlled trials. *Clin. Neurophysiol.* 2016; **127**(1): 956–68.

40. Hockstein NG, Samadi DS, Gendron K, Handler SD. Sialorrhea: A management challenge. *Am. Fam. Physician* 2004; **69**(11): 2628–34.

41. Mugii N, Hasegawa M, Matsushita T, Hamaguchi Y, Oohata S, Okita H, et al. Oropharyngeal dysphagia in dermatomyositis: Associations with clinical and laboratory features including autoantibodies. *PloS One* 2016; **11**(5): e0154746.

42. Wetscher GJ, Glaser K, Gadenstaetter M, Profanter C, Hinder RA. The effect of medical therapy and antireflux surgery on dysphagia in patients with gastroesophageal reflux disease without esophageal stricture. *Am. J. of Surg.* 1999; **177**(3): 189–92.

43. Warnecke T, Suttrup I, Schroder JB, Osada N, Oelenberg S, Hamacher C, et al. Levodopa responsiveness of dysphagia in advanced Parkinson's disease and reliability testing of the FEES-Levodopa-test. *Parkinsonism Relat. Disord.* 2016; **28**: 100–6.

44. Rahnemai-Azar AA, Rahnemaiazar AA, Naghshizadian R, Kurtz A, Farkas DT. Percutaneous endoscopic gastrostomy: Indications, technique, complications and management. *World J. Gastroenterol.* 2014; **20**(24): 7739–51.

45. Porter RF, Gyawali CP. Botulinum toxin injection in dysphagia syndromes with preserved esophageal peristalsis and incomplete lower esophageal sphincter relaxation. *Neurogastroenterol. Motil.* 2011; **23**(2): 139–44, e27–8.

46. Zaninotto G, Marchese Ragona R, Briani C, Costantini M, Rizzetto C, Portale G, et al. The role of botulinum toxin injection and upper esophageal sphincter myotomy in treating oropharyngeal dysphagia. *J. Gastrointest. Surg.* 2004; **8**(8): 997–1006.

47. Sharma S, Kumar G, Eweiss A, Chatrath P, Kaddour H. Endoscopic-guided injection of botulinum toxin into the cricopharyngeus muscle: Our experience. *J. Laryn. & Oto.* 2015; **129**(10): 990–5.

48. Terré R, Panadés A, Mearin F. Botulinum toxin treatment for oropharyngeal dysphagia in patients with stroke. *Neurogastroenterology & Motility* 2013; **25**(11): 896–e702.

49. Siersema PD. Treatment options for esophageal strictures. *Nature Clinical Practice Gastroenterology & Hepatology* 2008; **5**(3): 142–52.

50. Kocdor P, Siegel ER, Tulunay-Ugur OE. Cricopharyngeal dysfunction: A systematic review comparing outcomes of dilatation, botulinum toxin injection, and myotomy. *Laryngoscope* 2016; **126**(1): 135–41.

51. Chen Y, Sung K, Tharin S. Symptomatic anterior cervical osteophyte causing dysphagia: Case report, imaging, and review of the literature. *Cureus* 2016; **8**(2).

Management of Salivary Disorders in Neurorehabilitation

Nicole Rogus-Pulia, Joanne Yee, and Korey Kennelty

7.1 Introduction

7.1.1 The Basics of Saliva Production

Whole saliva (commonly referred to as saliva), or the mixture of specific salivary fluid as produced by individual glands, is composed primarily of water (~99.5%), with proteins (0.3%) and inorganic and trace substances (0.2%) comprising the remaining properties. Several factors influence the composition of saliva and its flow rate, including the type and size of the salivary glands producing saliva, stimulation, diet, age and sex of the individual, medications, circadian rhythm, and physiological status. As such, a large range of salivary flow rates is described to be within normal limits. Total daily whole saliva flow may be between 500 mL and 1.5 L depending upon the individual, with average values for pH and flow rate for healthy individuals as indicated in Table 7.1 [1]. Although wide variability exists in collection methods and stimuli used, evidence strongly suggests that a reduction in salivary flow is observed with aging [2].

Saliva is produced in major contralateral glands in the oral cavity, with the submandibular, sublingual, and parotid glands producing around 90–95% of resting saliva. The remaining 5–10% is produced by glands located throughout the oral mucosa, including the labial, buccal, lingual, and palatal mucosa. Each gland's secretions show variable composition and volume and are dictated by the cellular makeup of the gland [3].

Two different types of saliva assist in oropharyngeal health and function: stimulated saliva and unstimulated (resting) saliva. Stimulated saliva is produced before, during, and after eating due to various sensory inputs (e.g., mechanical, gustatory). Resting saliva is not produced in the presence of these apparent stimuli but has instead two components that affect its production – spontaneous and continuous secretion – as well as reflexive secretions to the sensation of dryness of the oral mucosa [4]. This complex process

serves in preserving the health of the oral cavity, while also maintaining adequate moisture (see Table 7.2 for the various functions of resting and stimulated saliva).

Each gland consists of a mixture of cell types, including acinar epithelial cells, of which there are two types: mucous and serous cells. Mucous cells produce secretions which are rich in mucin, a substance comprised mostly of proteins and amino acids. Serous cells secrete a watery fluid with comparatively few mucins. After being secreted by acinar cells, salivary fluid moves through the salivary ductal system, picking up electrolytes and other proteins, before finally arriving at the excretory surface of the gland. The variation in composition of each gland characterizes the fluid it produces, affecting viscosity and elasticity [4].

Saliva is largely controlled extrinsically by the autonomic nervous system, both sympathetic and parasympathetic divisions. Secretion is regulated via a reflex arch which has various influences. The afferent branch consists of chemoreceptors in taste buds and mechanoreceptors in the periodontal ligament. Afferent innervations of cranial nerves V, VII, IX, and X also play a role by carrying impulses to salivary nuclei in the medulla oblongata. Efferent influences are mainly parasympathetic via cranial nerve VII, which controls the submandibular, sublingual, and other minor glands, and cranial nerve IX, which influences the parotid gland.

7.1.2 Salivary Dysfunction

As mentioned earlier, typical salivary flow rates are difficult to establish without making a comparison to flow rates for individuals suffering from salivary dysfunction. Dysfunction comes in multiple forms and may be characterized by sialorrhea (i.e., hypersalivation or overproduction of saliva), hyposalivation (i.e., decreased production of salivary fluid), or xerostomia (the sensation of oral dryness that may or may not be accompanied by hyposalivation).

Table 7.1

	Unstimulated	Stimulated
Average whole saliva flow rate	0.3 mL per minute	7 mL per minute
pH (on a scale of 0–14)	6.2 (more acidic)	7.4 (more basic)

Table 7.2

Resting saliva functions	Stimulated saliva functions
Primarily secretions of submandibular, sublingual, and parotid glands	*Primarily secretions of submandibular and parotid glands*
• Maintains moisture	• Maintains taste receptor health
• Preventions dehydration	• Neutralizes food or bacterial acids
• Protects the surface of the teeth, via salivary pellicle and 'clumping' of microorganisms	• Lubricates oral cavity to protect teeth and mucosa during acts of deglutition
	• Prepares food for swallowing and digestion

7.1.2.1   What Are Hyposalivation and Xerostomia?

Hyposalivation can be described as an objective measurement of the decrease in typical salivary flow rate. Patients with hyposalivation may experience problems clearing food and bacteria from dental and oral surfaces; difficulty chewing, swallowing, and speaking; an increase in caries (tooth decay or cavities); and problems retaining dentures. A strong association has been observed between xerostomia and hyposalivation. Whereas hyposalivation is a measurable reduction in salivary flow from individual or all salivary glands, xerostomia is the subjective sensation of having dry mouth.

Interestingly, there are cases where xerostomia occurs without a documented decrease in salivary flow [5]. Reasons for this lack of association between xerostomia and hyposalivation are not clear, but lubrication and hydration functions of saliva are

hypothesized to relate to changes in the quality or composition of saliva rather than the quantity [6].

7.1.2.2   What Is Sialorrhea?

Sialorrhea, or hypersalivation, is a less-studied domain than hyposalivation and xerostomia [7]. Nevertheless, the presence of sialorrhea has a significant impact on the patients who suffer from it. Sialorrhea is defined as increased amount of accumulating saliva in the oral cavity, which may be caused by excessive production or by decreased clearance of saliva [8]. This build-up of saliva may result in drooling or ptyalis where this excess saliva in the mouth extends beyond the lip margin. The clinical and functional impact of sialorrhea may include impaired social functioning (particularly embarrassment or isolation), aspiration (entry of food/liquid into the airway), skin breakdown, odour, or infection.

7.1.2.3   Salivary Disorders in Patients with Long-Term Neurologic Conditions

As mentioned previously, sialorrhea occurs frequently in patients with long-term neurologic conditions, including Parkinson's disease (PD), motor neuron disease (most frequently amyotrophic lateral sclerosis [ALS]), and Wilson's disease [9–11]. Sialorrhea may be medication-induced through use of direct and indirect cholinergic agonists to treat dementia of the Alzheimer type and myasthenia gravis [12]. It may also be caused by failure of the systems which help to control, clear, and remove saliva from the oral cavity (e.g., muscle incoordination). Decreased neuromuscular control may result in impaired facial and oral motor control as well as dysphagia, or difficulty swallowing [10, 13, 14]. In fact, the existing literature on PD suggests that sialorrhea does not result from excessive saliva production but rather more often from impaired or infrequent swallowing [15, 16].

Interestingly, the opposite impairment, hyposalivation, can occur in patients with long-term neurologic conditions. The incidence of both PD and ALS increases with advancing age [11, 17], which may result in age- or medication-induced hyposalivation. Medications that most commonly induce dry mouth are tricyclic antidepressants, antipsychotics (particularly clozapine), anticholinergics, beta-blockers, and antihistamines [18]. Patients with neurologic disease often suffer from non-motor symptoms such as psychiatric and urinary disorders, which may require treatment by xerogenic medications. Cersosimo and colleagues found the prevalence of xerostomia in a group of 97 PD patients to be 61% [19]. In another study of patients with early-stage PD, it was suggested that hyposalivation is an early autonomic manifestation of PD [20]. The co-occurrence of sialorrhea and xerostomia in the same PD patient as documented by Cersosimo and colleagues reflects the different pathophysiological basis for these two symptoms [19]. Dry mouth is likely a manifestation of autonomic involvement of the salivary gland [21], while drooling is likely the consequence of impaired swallowing in the PD population.

7.2 Treatment Overview

7.2.1 Treatment for Hyposalivation and Xerostomia

A multitude of options exist for management of hyposalivation and xerostomia (Figure 7.1), although the strength of the evidence is variable. Behavioural management may include increasing consumption of water throughout the day to provide moisture to the oral cavity; avoiding mouth breathing; using a humidifier in the bedroom and during winter months; and avoiding caffeine or alcohol, which have drying and diuretic effects. Other strategies to alleviate xerostomia include utilizing sugar-free hard candies; frequently chewing sugar-free, xylitol-containing gum; or using various salivary substitutes. Acupuncture and electrical stimulation of the salivary glands have been described. Medication therapies, including cholinergic agonists such as pilocarpine or cevimeline, have been observed to be effective in relieving symptoms of xerostomia or hyposalivation [8].

7.2.2 Treatment for Sialorrhea

For individuals who suffer from sialorrhea, management ranges across a spectrum of conservative to more invasive approaches (Figure 7.1). Behavioural modification may involve myofunctional therapy to improve oromotor functionality or remind the patient to swallow, but these approaches have mostly been studied in paediatric populations. Where behavioural modification may not be an option, medical management in the form of medication therapy or injections may be considered. Anticholinergic agents, such as atropine, scopolamine (scopolamine), and glycopyrrolate, can be used to decrease salivation. In addition, botulinum toxin injections have been studied extensively and have demonstrated good success in patients with a variety of aetiologies [22, 23]. More permanent and invasive techniques include radiotherapy or surgery. Surgical interventions have mostly been carried out with paediatric patients with some success but also side effects [24].

7.3 Treatment Options for Hyposalivation/Xerostomia

7.3.1 Non-Pharmacological Treatments for Hyposalivation/Xerostomia

7.3.1.1 Topical Preparations

A variety of saliva-substitute sprays, gels, mouthwashes or mouth rinses, and special toothpastes are available for treatment of dry mouth and is commonly recommended for a variety of patients suffering with this condition. These saliva substitutes,

---

Hyposalivation and/or Xerostomia

- Topical preparations
- Acupuncture
- Electrical stimulation
- Cholinergic drugs (pilocarpine, cevimeline)

Hypersalivation and/or Sialorrhea

- Behavioural modifications (e.g., oral motor therapy, increasing swallowing frequency)
- Radiotherapy to salivary glands
- Botox injections into salivary glands
- Anti-cholinergic drugs (e.g., atropine, hyoscine, glycopyrrolate)
- Surgical interventions (e.g., Wilke's procedure)

Figure 7.1 Management of salivary disorders

whether in gel, spray, liquid, or toothpaste form, are intended to moisturize the oral and pharyngeal mucosa by retaining a coating as a replacement for inadequate natural saliva production [25, 26].

A multitude of saliva substitute products are being developed, with the majority based upon carboxymethylcellose (CMC), hydroxyethylcellulose (HEC), polyglycerylmethacrylate (PGM), hydroxypropylmethylcellulose (HPMC), or animal mucin [25]. Moisturizing gels require regular application to the oral mucosa. Sugar-free chewing gums sweetened with either sorbitol or xylitol may be used to stimulate saliva production through topical (gustatory) or mechanoreceptive/proprioceptive (masticatory) action. Toothpastes designed to treat dry mouth may be used as part of a full mouth care system (along with gels or mouthwashes) [25].

Despite the variety of products available, it does not appear, according to a recent Cochrane review, that the long-term impact of these products on oral and systemic health has been objectively established [25, 26]. Thirty-six trials were included in this review evaluating a range of different interventions or modes of delivery. The authors concluded there was not strong evidence to suggest that a specific topical therapy is effective for treating the symptom of dry mouth [26]. While moisturizing gels may lessen symptoms of mouth dryness, their use does not appear impact salivary gland function [25]. In contrast, while chewing gum was found to increase saliva production, there is no strong evidence that it relieves xerostomia [26].

Currently, there does not appear to be one type of topical agent that should be recommended over another. There is a clear need for well-designed, adequately powered studies with no risk of bias to address the effectiveness of these various products for treatment of dry mouth. Until then, while these products may continue to be recommended to patients, it is important to inform patients of the limitations of their use.

7.3.1.2 Acupuncture

Acupuncture has been used to stimulate the autonomic nervous system and increase peripheral blood flow, which may in turn stimulate saliva production [27, 28]. Electro-acupuncture includes the addition of a low-frequency current (2 Hz) being delivered to specific needles [25]. The exact mechanism of action is poorly understood, but could relate to sensory stimulation or placebo effect [25]. Many questions

remain regarding the ideal position and depth of the needles, as well as the intensity of treatment needed [27].

Acupuncture has been used most often for treatment of xerostomia following radiation therapy for head and neck cancer. A systematic review in 2010 analysed whether acupuncture resulted in improvement in dry mouth symptoms in this patient population [27]. Of 61 records screened, only 3 randomized controlled trials were selected for qualitative synthesis. All three studies reported a decrease in xerostomia following acupuncture, but, for two of the studies, there was an equivalent decrease for the control groups. This review highlighted the poor quality of the studies, lack of uniformity or consistency relative to the number of acupuncture points, duration of follow-up, and qualifications/experience of the acupuncturists [27]. Adverse effects of acupuncture include mild pain, bruising, or bleeding at the acupuncture sites, fatigue after treatment, and eye discomfort [28].

A Cochrane review conducted by Furness and colleagues in 2013 [28] examined effectiveness of nonpharmacological approaches to management of dry mouth, including acupuncture. Six acupuncture trials were included in the review. While small increases in unstimulated and stimulated whole saliva were observed, the carryover of this change to the symptom of dry mouth was not evaluated [28]. Given these limitations, there is a definite need for further well-designed double-blind trials with sufficient statistical power to determine the benefits of this treatment approach [28].

7.3.1.3 Electrostimulation

Electrostimulation can be used to apply electrical current to the skin covering the parotid gland area and on the oral mucosa in order to increase salivary secretion [25]. A recently developed device aims to increase saliva by delivering electrical stimulation in the area of the third molar along the oral mucosal surface 1–5 millimetres away from the lingual nerve [25]. Temporary side effects of these techniques may include twitching of facial musculature, anaesthesia of areas of skin next to the electrodes, or initial discomfort in the mucosal area in contract with electrodes [25, 29].

In the same Cochrane review of nonpharmacological treatments for xerostomia, Furness and colleagues included trials examining the effectiveness of electrostimulation in treating dry mouth [28]. Two trials of electrostimulation that compared a device with a placebo (sham device) were included. No significant differences in stimulated or unstimulated salivary flow rates were reported in either trial. A large trial of 114 patients with xerostomia over two months showed that a lingual nerve-stimulating device improved xerostomia severity and frequency, as well as swallowing difficulties over the sham [30]. This trial was not included in the Cochrane review as it employed a crossover design [30]. The same issues with bias risk and inadequate statistical power mentioned regarding the acupuncture trials are applicable to these electrostimulation trials as well. Given these limitations with the evidence supporting use of these devices, their use outside of the clinical trial setting remains difficult to justify [28].

7.3.2 Pharmacological Treatments for Hyposalivation/Xerostomia

Two medications, pilocarpine and cevimeline, are commonly used to treat xerostomia. Other less common medications that have been used clinically to treat xerostomia include anethole trithione, bethanechol, and nizatidine. Anethole trithione is a substituted dithiolethione and a bile secretion-stimulating medication; bethanechol is a choline ester with muscarinic agonist properties; and nizatidine is a histamine$_2$-receptor antagonist with the ability to inhibit acetylcholinesterase, resulting in an increased availability of acetylcholine [25]. While anethole trithione, bethanechol, and nizatidine have shown promise for increasing salivary flow, adequately powered and well-designed randomized clinical trials have yet to be conducted for an FDA-approved indication to treat xerostomia [25]. In what follows, we review pilocarpine and cevimeline, the two medications that have received FDA regulatory approval for this indication.

7.3.2.1 Pilocarpine

Pilocarpine hydrochloride (Salagan®) is indicated for the treatment of dry mouth in patients post-chemotherapy or radiation therapy for head and neck cancer and for patients with Sjogren's syndrome. In order for pilocarpine to be effective in increasing salivary flow, remaining functional salivary tissue must be present [25]. This medication increases salivary secretion by direct stimulation of salivary muscarinic receptors on the acinar cell surface, causing an increase in secretion of exocrine glands (e.g., salivary and sweat glands) and in the tone of smooth muscle in the gastrointestinal and urinary tracts.

Pilocarpine has been used most widely as a topical treatment for glaucoma [31]. An oral tablet formulation is available for the treatment of xerostomia. Pharmacokinetic properties of oral pilocarpine have not been well described in patients with xerostomia. Following two days of administration of oral pilocarpine 5 or 10 mg three times daily, mean peak plasma medication concentrations (C_{max}) of 15 and 41 μg/L in healthy adult males were reached in 1.25 and 0.85 hours (t_{max}), respectively [31, 32].

The recommended dosage for the initiation of treatment of xerostomia is 5 mg three times daily. Titration up to 10 mg three times daily can be used in patients who do not respond adequately to a lower dose [31]. According to current manufacturer labelling, dosing adjustment is not needed in patients with renal impairment, but adjustments should be made in patients with moderate hepatic impairment. Mild and often tolerable events are commonly reported with use of pilocarpine, and their occurrence has been shown to be dose related. This medication can also increase secretion by the other exocrine glands, including the sweat, lacrimal, gastric, pancreatic, and intestinal glands, and the mucous cells of the respiratory tract. Pilocarpine also increases smooth muscle tone and motility in the intestinal and urinary tracts, gallbladder, biliary ducts, and bronchi [31]. Given this, side effects can include sweating (most common), chills, nausea, dizziness, rhinitis, flushing, asthenia, urinary frequency, increased lacrimation, palpitations, and gastrointestinal tract disturbance [25, 31]. Also, since pilocarpine is a parasympathomimetic agent, there may be effects on the cardiovascular and pulmonary systems. No significant effects on heart rate, blood pressure, or cardiac conductivity have been reported, but studies were not conducted in patients with medical conditions like asthma or those taking beta-adrenergic antagonists [31]. Potential medication interactions for patients taking antidepressants who are experiencing impaired salivary function have not been studied either [31].

There are substantial efficacy data to support the use of pilocarpine for treatment of xerostomia. A number of well-designed randomized clinical trials have found pilocarpine to be effective in both patients with Sjogren's syndrome and those with head and neck cancer treated with radiation when administered at oral doses of 5–7.5 mg given three to four times daily [25]. Given these findings, this medication has regulatory approval for treatment of xerostomia in these patient populations in many countries [25]. Despite this, its effects in patients with long-term neurologic conditions have largely not been tested.

7.3.2.2 Cevimeline

Cevimeline (Evoxac®) is another FDA-approved medication for the treatment of xerostomia. Cevimeline is a cholinergic agonist that binds and activates muscarinic M_3 receptors on salivary and other exocrine glands. After administration of a single 30 mg capsule, Cevimeline was rapidly absorbed with a mean time to peak concentration of one and a half to two hours, with a half-life elimination of 5±1 hours. Cevimeline is largely metabolized by the liver and excreted in the urine. However, according to manufacturer labelling, no dosing adjustments are required for renal or hepatic impairment. When administered with food, there is a decrease in the rate of absorption and the peak concentration was reduced by 17.3%.

Cevimeline is generally well tolerated, but does have expected adverse events due to its parasympathomimetic effects resulting from its muscarinic agonist action. These can include sweating, cephalgia, visual disturbance, lacrimation, nausea, and dyspepsia, vomiting, diarrhoea, gastrointestinal spasm, sinusitis, infections of the upper respiratory system, rhinitis, atrioventricular block, tachycardia, bradycardia, hypotension, hypertension, shock, mental confusion, cardiac arrhythmia, and tremors [25].

Additionally, caution should be taken when administering cevimeline to patients taking beta-adrenergic antagonists due to a possibility of cardiac conduction disturbances. It is expected that, if another medication with parasympathomimetic effects were administered concurrently, there would be additive effects. Also, it is possible that cevimeline could interfere with desirable antimuscarinic effects of medications used concomitantly.

Similar to pilocarpine, there is evidence to support the use of cevimeline for treatment of dry mouth symptoms. Again, the largest studies have been in patients with head and neck cancer treated with radiation therapy and patients with Sjogren's syndrome. A dose of 30 mg three times per day has been shown

to provide relief of dry mouth symptoms in both of these populations [25]. While it is encouraging that this medication and pilocarpine are effective at decreasing patient-reported symptoms of dry mouth (xerostomia), it is unknown whether they actually result in increased salivary flow or impact other outcomes, like oral health. Additionally, like pilocarpine, use of cevimeline has not been systematically tested in patients with chronic neurologic conditions.

7.4 Treatment Options for Hypersalivation/Sialorrhea

7.4.1 Non-Pharmacological Treatments for Hypersalivation/Sialorrhea

7.4.1.1 Behavioural Modifications

A variety of behavioural modifications for management of sialorrhea have been suggested in order to improve salivary clearance, but only in paediatric populations and with little evidence to support their use. Silvestre-Rangil and colleagues describe the use of myofunctional therapy for sialorrhea management, which includes improving lip seal and oral closure [33]. A systematic review by Arvedson and colleagues in 2011 identified five studies examining the efficacy of oral motor exercises for treatment of feeding and swallowing in children and concluded that these studies were of poor methodologic quality, limiting their value [34]. A variety of approaches to increase the frequency of swallowing have been proposed, including auditory cues provided at regular intervals, biofeedback via electromyography paired with an auditory prompt, and vestibular as well as lingual stimulators. Similar to oral motor therapy approaches, studies of these approaches are sparse and limited to the paediatric population [35]. In the adult population, Dand and Sakel describe the use of positioning in patients with motor neuron disease, especially supporting or stabilizing the head to ensure an upright position, for saliva management, but there is no evidence to support these approaches [36].

7.4.1.2 Radiotherapy

Given the known radiosensitivity of the salivary structures, external beam radiation therapy (RT) has been used as a treatment for patients with chronic neurologic conditions suffering from sialorrhea. Adverse effects of RT include more viscous saliva, facial and skin erythema, aching cheek, temporary or chronic xerostomia, sore throat, and nausea. Additionally, RT increases the risk of cancer in the irradiated field. However, given that conditions like ALS and PD have a poor prognosis and the time to malignancy development post RT is long, this may not be a valid concern for these patient populations suffering with sialorrhea [36].

A thorough systematic review completed in 2015 identified 10 studies (four prospective and six retrospective) examining use of electron or photon RT for treatment of sialorrhea in patients with ALS or PD. The median dose was 12 Gy with a wide range of fractionation schemes. Patients were treated with both photons (72%) and electrons (28%). The most common field arrangement included bilateral submandibular and parotid glands. Most studies reported subjective outcomes that included patient interviews, while a smaller number included objective measures for assessing drooling. Among patients, 40% experienced short-term toxicities of RT, while 12% experienced long-term toxicities. Outcomes showed that 81% of patients reported subjective improvement of symptoms with improvement occurring within two months of RT. It did not appear that either electron or photon therapy was superior. There was no apparent dose response and an increase in field size did not affect outcomes. However, improvement lasted from three months to five years, indicating that the long-term effects were variable. Objective measures demonstrated improvement (decreased salivation) in 72% of patients. Given the wide variability in treatment parameters, the authors were unable to outline an ideal treatment scheme. However, they concluded with caution that bilateral parallel opposed radiation is the recommended beam arrangement with a median dose of 12 Gy in two fractions [37].

7.4.2 Pharmacological Treatments for Hypersalivation/Sialorrhea

A variety of pharmacological interventions are available for treatment of hypersalivation/sialorrhea. As mentioned earlier, salivation is mainly mediated through parasympathetic stimulation and acetylcholine is the active neurotransmitter that binds at muscarinic receptors in the salivary glands. Therefore, cholinergic muscarinic receptor antagonists can be used to treat sialorrhea. The medications of this class that are most commonly prescribed for this purpose are atropine, scopolamine, and glycopyrrolate.

Intraoral tropicamide films (1 mg) were found to provide short-term relief of sialorrhea in a small study of non-demented PD patients, but further research is needed to determine the efficacy of these films [43].

Unfortunately, efficacy data for treating sialorrhea in adults with long-term neurologic conditions are sparse [36]. The majority of studies examining the effects of medications on drooling have been carried out in children with neurological conditions such as cerebral palsy. Additionally, any benefit of these medications may be short lived as the body becomes accustomed to the medication or as side effects become intolerable [38].

7.4.2.1 Botox Injections

Botulinum toxin (BoNT) injections have also been used for treatment of sialorrhea in patients with ALS and PD. BoNT is a neurotoxin produced by the bacterium *Clostridium botulinum*. It has several clinical uses, including the off-label use to treat drooling. BoNT injections are often recommended for patients who do not improve and/or have serious side effects with anticholinergic medications. BoNT results in reduced salivary production by decreasing the release of acetylcholine at the neurosecretory junction. The blockade is irreversible and recovery only occurs when the axons regrow and new acetylcholine receptors are formed. This procedure can be repeated to manage symptoms [38]. Injections are performed under ultrasound guidance into the parotid and submandibular glands.

Currently, three type A and one type B toxins are approved for use in the United States. These include Onabotulinumtoxin A (A/Ona), Abobotulinumtoxin A (A/Abo), Incobotulinumtoxin A (A/Inco), and Rimabotulinumtoxin B (B/Rima) [39]. See Figure 7.2 for a typical regimen for BoNT administration [40]. Generally, the duration of action varies from six weeks to six months with relapse time being variable [38, 39]. Reduction in sialorrhea is known to occur three to seven days after the injection and maximum reduction occurs after two to four weeks [39].

The dose of botulinum toxin must be titrated with care, as too much can result in side effects like severe dry mouth and thick secretions [38]. The facial nerve is very close to the parotid gland, so caution must be taken when injecting to avoid this nerve [39]. Other reported side effects include weakness of adjacent muscles, producing difficulty of chewing and swallowing due to BoNT diffusion into masseter or

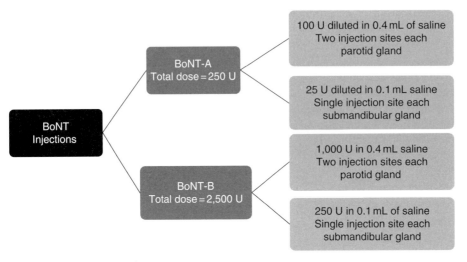

Figure 7.2 Administration of Botox injections

pharyngeal muscles, local infection, hematoma, salivary duct calculi, local injuries of the carotid arteries or branches of the facial nerve, and recurrent jaw [35, 38]. The possibility of increased dysphagia means that BoNT is often considered only when there is an alternative route for feeding. In addition, there is some question as to whether BoNT can enter the bloodstream in sufficient concentration to affect distal muscles [36].

There is strong evidence that both BoNT-A and BoNT-B are effective in treatment of sialorrhea with a low profile of side effects [39]. A 2012 meta-analysis study that reviewed all randomized placebo-controlled trials concluded that BoNT resulted in statistically significant decreases in the severity of drooling for adult and paediatric patients with sialorrhea [39, 41]. A recent Cochrane review of all management approaches for sialorrhea in patients with motor neuron disease identified a study of a single session of BoNT-B as the only randomized controlled trial and study to describe data in adequate detail [42]. Despite these positive outcomes, there are limitations to the studies of BoNT for sialorrhea management in that they use varying serotypes, routes of administration (direct or transductal), and treatment regimens with varying outcome measures (subjective and objective) [39]. In general, efficacy studies have shown BoNT-A and BoNT-B to be equally efficacious and safe [39]. The costs of these two treatments do differ, however, with the BoNT-B treatment costing approximately half of BoNT-A [39].

7.4.2.2 Atropine

While atropine is indicated for temporary blockade of life-threatening muscarinic effects, it has been used off label for treatment of hypersalivation as well as secretions of the airway. Atropine is an anticholinergic agent, thus it inhibits smooth muscle and glands innervated by postganglionic cholinergic nerves [44]. An oral dose of 0.4–0.6 mg is suggested, which is then repeated every four to six hours as needed. As an injection, 0.4–0.6 mg may be administered over 30 minutes and repeated every four to six hours as needed. A 1% ophthalmic solution of atropine administered sublingually is also used [44].

The antimuscarinic action of atropine is responsible for most of its side effects. For a list of these effects, see Table 7.3. Heart rate, blood pressure, and mental status should be monitored closely if on an extended and high daily dose of this medication, particularly in older adults [45]. See Table 7.4 for a list of contraindications for atropine or conditions for which caution should be taken when prescribing it.

Sublingual atropine does have several advantages over the injection administration route, including improved bioavailability, rapid onset, and ready availability in the form of ophthalmic drops. Sublingual atropine has been shown to be effective in reducing the amount of saliva produced in patients with Parkinson's disease who suffer from sialorrhea, patients with clozapine-induced sialorrhea, and cancer patients [45–47]. However, these studies consisted

Table 7.3 Adverse effects of anticholinergic medications for treatment of sialorrhea*

Atropine	Scopolamine	Glycopyrolate
• Dry mouth	• Dry mouth (most common)	• Dry mouth
• Blurred vision	• Drowsiness	• Decreased sweating
• Photophobia	• Dizziness	• Urinary retention
• Tachycardia	• Blurred vision	• Blurred vision
• Anhidrosis	• Dilation of pupils	• Tachycardia
• Constipation	• Urinary retention	• Palpitations
• Urinary retention	• Agitation/restlessness	• Dilatation of the pupil
• Palpitation	• Confusion	• Cycloplegia
• Dilated pupils	• Mydriasis	• Increased ocular tension
• Difficulty swallowing	• Pharyngitis	• Loss of taste
• Hot dry skin		• Headaches
• Thirst		• Vomiting
• Dizziness		• Constipation
• Restlessness		• Bloated feeling
• Tremor		• Suppression of lactation
• Fatigue		
• Ataxia		

* Adverse effects may be exacerbated in older adults, with chronic medication administration, and/or in excessive doses.

of small sample sizes. There is a need for larger, well-designed clinical trials to examine its use in treatment of sialorrhea in patients with PD and ALS.

7.4.2.3 Scopolamine

Scopolamine hydrobromide also is an anticholinergic medication that has been shown to reduce the secretions of various organs in the body, including the stomach and intestines. It also decreases nerve signals that trigger vomiting. Therefore, an FDA indication is for the treatment of motion sickness and postoperative nausea/vomiting. Scopolamine also has been found to decrease saliva production through a similar mechanism as atropine.

This medication is available in several formulations for its various indications. When used as an antiemetic medication, it is administered at a dose of 0.6–1 mg as a subcutaneous injection (SubQ). Preoperatively, the dose administered is 0.3–0.65 mg as a SubQ, intramuscular (IM), or intravenous (IV) injection. When used as sedation, the dose administered is 0.6 mg three to four times per day as a SubQ, IV, or IM injection. It can also be administered transdermally (one or two patches every three days). The transdermal system is formulated to deliver in vivo approximately 1 mg of scopolamine at an approximately constant rate to the systemic circulation over three days. It is applied to the post-auricular skin and is well absorbed percutaneously.

Scopolamine has similar side effects as atropine that are attributable to its anticholinergic action (see Table 7.3). See Table 7.4 for a list of contraindications for scopolamine and conditions for which caution should be taken when prescribing it.

A reduction in salivary secretion may be noted as soon as 15 minutes after application of the scopolamine patch, and benefits are maintained for about 72 hours [48]. One randomized controlled trial of 30 patients with disabilities and a variety of diagnoses, including cerebral palsy, demonstrated a significant reduction in saliva after one week, but four patients dropped out due to side effects [38]. A nebulized route of medication administration can be more effective as swallowing oral medication becomes more challenging for patients with progressive bulbar weakness. The use of nebulized scopolamine may successfully reduce sialorrheam, but further investigation is necessary [38].

7.4.2.4 Glycopyrrolate

Glycopyrrolate, also an anticholinergic medication, has been used off label for treatment of sialorrhea in patients with Parkinson's disease, those taking clozapine for schizophrenia, and in children with developmental disabilities. It is indicated for adjunctive therapy in the treatment of peptic ulcer, to reduce salivation under anaesthesia, and for maintenance treatment of airflow in patients with chronic

Table 7.4 Recommendations regarding prescribing of anticholinergic medications for treatment of sialorrhea*

Anticholinergic medications for treatment of sialorrhea are contraindicated for patients with these conditions*		
Atropine	Scopolamine	Glycopyrrolate
• Cognitive impairment • Dementia • Narrow-angle glaucoma • Tachycardia • Obstructive gastrointestinal disease • Paralytic ileus • Intestinal atrony of elderly or debilitated patient • Severe ulcerative colitis • Toxic megacolon complicating ulcerative colitis • Obstructive uropathy	• Narrow angle glaucoma • Tachycardia	• Glaucoma • Obstructive uropathy • Obstructive disease of the gastrointestinal tract • Paralytic ileus • Intestinal atony of the elderly or debilitated patient • Unstable cardiovascular status in acute haemorrhage • Severe ulcerative colitis • Toxic megacolon complicating ulcerative colitis • Myasthenia gravis
Use caution when prescribing anticholinergic medications to patients with these conditions or characteristics*		
Atropine	Scopolamine	Glycopyrrolate
• Older adults • Arrhythmia • Autonomic neuropathy • Cardiovascular disease • Gastrointestinal disease • Hepatic impairment • Hiatal hernia • Hyperthyroidism • Myasthenia gravis • Renal disease	• Older adults • Open angle glaucoma • Pyloric or urinary bladder neck obstruction • Seizures or psychosis • Impaired renal or hepatic functions • Coronary artery disease • Tachyarrythmias • Heart failure • Hypertension • Gastrointestinal obstruction • Hiatal hernia with reflux esophagitis • Hyperthyroidism • Ulcerative colitis	• Autonomic neuropathy • Hepatic or renal disease • Ulcerative colitis • Hyperthyroidism • Coronary artery disease • Congestive heart failure • Tachyarrhythmias • Tachycardia • Hypertension • Prostatic hypertrophy • Hiatal hernia associated with reflux esophagitis

* See medication insert for more information

obstructive pulmonary disease (COPD). In 2010, the FDA approved a glycopyrrolate oral solution (Cuvposa®) for the treatment of patients aged 3–16 years with chronic severe drooling associated with neurologic conditions, such as cerebral palsy.

Glycopyrrolate has similar adverse effects as the other anticholinergic medications described previously (see Table 7.3). However, since glycopyrrolate is chemically a quaternary ammonium compound, its passage across lipid membranes, such as the blood–brain barrier, is limited in contrast to atropine and scopolamine (scopolamine). As a result, the occurrence of CNS-related side effects is lower, in comparison to their incidence following administration of anticholinergics which are chemically tertiary amines that can cross this barrier readily. See Table 7.4 for a list of contraindications for glycopyrrolate and conditions for which caution should be taken when prescribing it.

As with the other medications in this category, efficacy data to support the use of glycopyrrolate to treat sialorrhea in patients with chronic neurologic conditions are minimal. Arbouw and colleagues reported that oral glycopyrrolate (1 mg, three times a day) was effective and safe in reducing drooling in 23 patients with Parkinson's disease [38, 49]. Strutt and colleagues described the use of nebulized glyco-pyrrolate for one individual with motor neuron disease, which may be preferred as swallowing becomes affected and medications cannot be taken orally [50].

7.4.3 Surgical Interventions for Treatment of Hypersalivation /Sialorrhea

Another therapeutic option for the management of sialorrhea is surgical intervention. However, all studies are in the paediatric population with no clinical studies focused on adults with neurologic conditions in the literature [40]. A variety of different procedures have been described, with the Wilkie procedure being the most commonly used. This procedure involves retropositioning of the parotid ducts into the tonsillar fossa region along with bilateral submandibular gland resection. By relocating the papillae of the submandibular ducts from the anterior oral cavity to the base of the tongue, saliva from the submandibular glands can flow directly into the oropharynx.

Several variants of this procedure have been proposed, including transposition of the submandibular gland duct into the tonsillar fossa, instead of resection; ligation of the parotid ducts, instead of repositioning; deviation of both submandibular and parotid ducts behind the anterior pillar of the soft palate (four-duct diversion); bilateral submandibular duct relocation with or without sublingual gland excision; and ligation of both parotid and submandibular ducts (four-duct ligation) [40]. Other procedures may include transtympanic neurectomy (severing the parasympathetic supply to the salivary glands at the tympanic plexus in the middle ear) and submandibular gland excision [36]. A meta-analysis of surgical management for drooling found bilateral submandibular gland excision and parotid duct rerouting to have the highest success rate in the paediatric population, but these studies are limited by their sample sizes and mostly subjective outcomes.

Potential complications of salivary gland surgeries include post-operative cysts, salivary fistulae and wound dehiscence, swelling of the glands wherein ducts are tied off, subsequent infections, and xerostomia. Stenosis may occur where the ducts are rerouted, leading to the equivalent of a ductal tie off [38]. The Wilkie procedure is not indicated for patients with recurrent aspiration pneumonia as it can increase the risk of aspiration by directing the saliva posteriorly [40].

Given that all studies have been in the paediatric population, there is no known safe and effective surgical treatment for adult patients [40]. While other approaches proving ineffective may lead to consideration of more aggressive approaches, patients with long-term neurologic conditions may not be ideal surgical candidates [38]. However, if the patient has a short life expectancy, a surgical approach may be worth considering depending upon the patient's severity and clinical status [35].

7.5 Summary

In patients with long-term neurologic conditions, several salivary disorders are likely to occur. A variety of non-pharmacological and pharmacological approaches can be taken to the treatment of both hyposalivation/xerostomia and hypersalivation/sialorrhea. Prior to engaging in management techniques, identification of factors associated with the salivary disorder should be conducted through careful assessment. The clinical utility of the available approaches to management will depend on the severity of the salivary disorder(s). A multidisciplinary approach to evaluation and treatment is recommended. While current evidence-based approaches have not been shown to enact lasting change in salivary gland physiology, they will likely alleviate the patient's symptoms to some extent, thereby improving quality of life. Regardless of the chosen treatment, regular follow-up with the patient is necessary to ensure continued success of the approach and to avoid any adverse effects.

References

1. Humphrey SP, Williamson RT. A review of saliva: Normal composition, flow, and function. *Journal of Prosthetic Dentistry* 2001 Feb; **85**(2): 162–9.

2. Affoo RH, Foley N, Garrick R, Siqueira WL, Martin RE. Meta-analysis of salivary flow rates in young and older adults. *Journal of the American Geriatrics Society* 2015; **63**(10): 2142–51.

3. Affoo, RH, Foley C, Garrick R, Siquiera WL, Martin RE. Meta-analysis of salivary flow rates in young and older adults. *Journal of the American Geriatrics Society* 2015; **63**(10): 2142–51.

4. Mese H, Matsuo R. Salivary secretion, taste and hyposalivation. *Journal of Oral Rehabilitation* 2007; **34** (10): 711–23.

5. Nederfors T. Xerostomia and hyposalivation. *Advances in Dental Research* 2000; **14**: 48–56.

6. Castro I, Sepúlveda D, Cortés J, Quest AFG, Barrera MJ, Bahamondes V, et al. Oral dryness in Sjögren's syndrome patients. Not just a question of water. *Autoimmune Reviews*. 2013; **12**(5): 567–74.

7. Boros I, Keszler P. Sialorrhea: Hypersalivation and drooling. An underestimated problem in medical practice. *Fogorvosi szemle* 2006; **99**(3): 99–108.

8. Zlotnik Y, Balash Y, Korczyn AD, Giladi N, Gurevich T. Disorders of the oral cavity in Parkinson's disease and parkinsonian syndromes. *Parkinsons Disease* 2015; **2015**: 379482.

9. Dubow JS. Autonomic dysfunction in Parkinson's disease. *Disease a Month* 2007; **53**(5): 265–74.

10. Trocello JM, Osmani K, Pernon M, Chevaillier G, de Brugière C, Remy P, et al. Hypersialorrhea in Wilson's disease. *Dysphagia* 2015; **30**(5): 489–95.

11. ALS Association [Internet]. [cited 27 November 2016]. Available from: www.alsa.org/als-care/resources/publications-videos/factsheets/epidemiology.html.

12. Freudenreich O. Drug-induced sialorrhea. *Drugs of Today (Barcelona, Spain)* (1998)2005; **41**(6): 411–18.

13. Lakraj AA, Moghimi N, Jabbari B. Sialorrhea: Anatomy, pathophysiology and treatment with emphasis on the role of botulinum toxins. *Toxins* 2013; **5**(5): 1010–1031.

14. Kalf JG, Bloem BR, Munneke M. Diurnal and nocturnal drooling in Parkinson's disease. *Journal of Neurology* 2012; **259**(1): 119–23.

15. Bagheri H, Damase-Michel C, Lapeyre-Mestre M, Cismondo S, O'Connell D, Senard JM, et al. A study of salivary secretion in Parkinson's disease. *Clinical Neuropharmacology* 1999; **22**(4): 213–15.

16. Johnston BT, Li Q, Castell JA, Castell DO. Swallowing and esophageal function in Parkinson's disease. *American Journal of Gastroenterology* 1995; **90**(10): 1741–6.

17. Reeve A, Simcox E, Turnbull D. Ageing and Parkinson's disease: Why is advancing age the biggest risk factor? *Ageing Research Reviews* 2014;**14**: 19–30.

18. Scully C. Drug effects on salivary glands: Dry mouth. *Oral Diseases* 2003;**9**(4): 165–76.

19. Cersosimo MG, Raina GB, Calandra CR, Pellene A, Gutiérrez C, Micheli FE, et al. Dry mouth: An overlooked autonomic symptom of Parkinson's disease. *Journal of Parkinson's Disease* 2011; **1**(2): 169–73.

20. Cersósimo MG, Tumilasci OR, Raina GB, Benarroch EE, Cardoso EM, Micheli F, et al. Hyposialorrhea as an early manifestation of Parkinson disease. *Autonomic Neuroscience* 2009; **150**(1–2): 150–1.

21. Del Tredici K, Hawkes CH, Ghebremedhin E, Braak H. Lewy pathology in the submandibular gland of individuals with incidental Lewy body disease and sporadic Parkinson's disease. *Acta Neuropathologica*. 2010; **119**(6): 703–13.

22. Squires N, Wills A, Rowson J. The management of drooling in adults with neurological conditions. *Current Opinions in Otolaryngology Head and Neck Surgery* 2012; **20**(3): 171–6.

23. Dand P, Sakel M. The management of drooling in motor neurone disease. *International Journal of Palliative Nursing*. 2010; **16**(11): 560–4.

24. Meningaud J-P, Pitak-Arnnop P, Chikhani L, Bertrand J-C. Drooling of saliva: A review of the etiology and management options. *Oral Surgery Oral Medicine Oral Pathology Oral Radiology and Endodontics* 2006; **101**(1): 48–57.

25. Wolff A, Fox PC, Porter S, Konttinen YT. Established and novel approaches for the management of hyposalivation and xerostomia. *Current Pharmaceutical Design* 2012; **18**(34): 5515–21.

26. Furness S, Worthington HV, Bryan G, Birchenough S, McMillan R. Interventions for the management of dry mouth: Topical therapies. *Cochrane Database of Systematic Reviews* 2011; **12**: CD008934.

27. O'Sullivan EM, Higginson IJ. Clinical effectiveness and safety of acupuncture in the treatment of irradiation-induced xerostomia in patients with head and neck cancer: A systematic review. *Acupuncture Medicine* 2010; **28**(4): 191–9.

28. Furness S, Bryan G, McMillan R, Birchenough S, Worthington HV. Interventions for the management of dry mouth: Non-pharmacological interventions. *Cochrane Database of Systematic Reviews* 2013; **5**: CD009603.

29. Hargitai IA, Sherman RG, Strother JM. The effects of electrostimulation on parotid saliva flow: A pilot study. *Oral Surgery Oral Medicine Oral Pathology Oral Radiology and Endodontics* 2005; **99**(3): 316–20.

30. Strietzel FP, Lafaurie GI, Mendoza GRB, Alajbeg I, Pejda S, Vuletić L, et al. Efficacy and safety of an intraoral electrostimulation device for xerostomia relief: A multicenter, randomized trial. *Arthritis and Rheumatology* 2011; **63**(1): 180–90.

31. Wiseman LR, Faulds D. Oral pilocarpine: A review of its pharmacological properties and clinical potential in xerostomia. *Drugs* 1995; **49**(1): 143–55.

32. Hunt T. A double-blind, placebo-controlled, multiple-dose, tolerance and pharmacokinetic study of oral pilocarpine hydrochloride (HCL) in healthy male

subjects. *MGI Pharma. (Minneapolis)* Data on File. 1993; 91–3.

33. Silvestre-Rangil J, Silvestre F-J, Puente-Sandoval A, Requeni-Bernal J, Simó-Ruiz J-M. Clinical-therapeutic management of drooling: Review and update. *Oral Medicine and Pathology* 2011; **16**(6): e763–6.

34. Arvedson J, Clark H, Lazarus C, Schooling T, Frymark T. The effects of oral-motor exercises on swallowing in children: An evidence-based systematic review. *Developmental Medicine and Child Neurology* 2010; **52**(11): 1000–13.

35. Meningaud J-P, Pitak-Arnnop P, Chikhani L, Bertrand J-C. Drooling of saliva: A review of the etiology and management options. *Oral Surgery Oral Medicine Oral Pathology Oral Radiology and Endodontics* 2006; **101**(1): 48–57.

36. Dand P, Sakel M. The management of drooling in motor neurone disease. *International Journal of Palliative Nursing* 2010; **16**(11): 560–4.

37. Hawkey NM, Zaorsky NG, Galloway TJ. The role of radiation therapy in the management of sialorrhea: A systematic review. *Laryngoscope* 2016; **126**(1): 80–5.

38. Squires N, Wills A, Rowson J. The management of drooling in adults with neurological conditions. *Current Opinion on Otolaryngology and Head Neck Surgery* 2012; **20**(3): 171–6.

39. Lakraj AA, Moghimi N, Jabbari B. Sialorrhea: Anatomy, pathophysiology and treatment with emphasis on the role of botulinum toxins. *Toxins (Basel)* 2013; **5**(5): 1010–31.

40. Banfi P, Ticozzi N, Lax A, Guidugli GA, Nicolini A, Silani V. A review of options for treating sialorrhea in amyotrophic lateral sclerosis. *Respiratory Care* 2015; **60**(3): 446–54.

41. Vashishta R, Nguyen SA, White DR, Gillespie MB. Botulinum toxin for the treatment of sialorrhea: A meta-analysis. *Otolaryngology and Head Neck Surgery* 2013; **148**(2): 191–6.

42. Young CA, Ellis C, Johnson J, Sathasivam S, Pih N. Treatment for sialorrhea (excessive saliva) in people with motor neuron disease/amyotrophic lateral sclerosis. *Cochrane Database of Systematic Reviews* 2011; **5**: CD006981.

43. Lloret SP, Nano G, Carrosella A, Gamzu E, Merello M. A double-blind, placebo-controlled, randomized, crossover pilot study of the safety and efficacy of multiple doses of intra-oral tropicamide films for the short-term relief of sialorrhea symptoms in Parkinson's disease patients. *Journal of Neurological Sciences* 2011; **310**(1–2): 248–50.

44. Hyson HC, Johnson AM, Jog MS. Sublingual atropine for sialorrhea secondary to parkinsonism: A pilot study. *Movement Disorders* 2002; **17**(6): 1318–20.

45. Meningaud JP, Pitak-Arnnop P, Chikhani L, Bertrand JC. Drooling of saliva: A review of the etiology and management options. *Oral Surgery Oral Medicine Oral Pathology Oral Radiology and Endodontics* 2006; **101**(1): 48–57.

46. Squires N, Wills A, Rowson J. The management of drooling in adults with neurological conditions. *Current Opinions in Otolaryngology Head Neck Surgery* 2012; **20**(3): 171–6.

47. De Simone GG, Eisenchlas JH, Junin M, Pereyra F, Brizuela R. Atropine drops for drooling: A randomized controlled trial. *Palliative Medicine* 2006; **20**(7): 665–71.

48. Reddihough D, Erasmus CE, Johnson H, McKellar GMW, Jongerius PH, Cerebral Palsy Institute. Botulinum toxin assessment, intervention and aftercare for paediatric and adult drooling: International consensus statement. *European Journal of Neurology* 2010; **17** Suppl. 2: 109–21.

49. Arbouw MEL, Movig KLL, Koopmann M, Poels PJE, Guchelaar H-J, Egberts TCG, et al. Glycopyrrolate for sialorrhea in Parkinson disease: A randomized, double-blind, crossover trial. *Neurology* 2010; **74**(15): 1203–7.

50. Strutt R, Fardell B, Chye R. Nebulized glycopyrrolate for drooling in a motor neuron patient. *Journal of Pain and Symptom Management* 2002; **23**(1): 2–3.

Chapter 8

Management of Upper Limb Impairment in Neurorehabilitation

Preeti Raghavan and Manuel Wilfred

8.1 Introduction

More than 85% of individuals with post-stroke upper limb paresis show persistent deficits in dexterity six months later [1], which often leads to long-term dependence on caregivers for activities of daily living [2, 3]. Damage to the corticospinal tract as a result of stroke produces muscle weakness. Weakness leads to reduced force generation in muscles, abnormal synergy patterns of movement [4], and reduced fractionation of movements in the upper limb segments [5] and fingers [6, 7]. Restoration of active isolated range of motion of the upper limb segments, particularly at the shoulder and fingers early on, predicts functional recovery [8, 9]. However, recovery of function typically lags behind the recovery of neurological impairments, as practice is required to capitalize on the neurological recovery and incorporate the improvements into functional activities [10]. A complicating factor in translating neurological gains into strength and function is the onset of spasticity and muscle stiffness [11]. The incidence of spasticity and muscle stiffness increases over time, particularly in the most severely impaired patients, and is a major barrier to restoration of isolated active range of motion and function despite gains in strength or the ability to produce muscle force [12, 13].

Upper limb motor impairment and function are associated not only with the degree of upper limb weakness and spasticity but also with deficits in visual fields, visual attention, tactile sensitivity, proprioception, cognitive and emotional function, and motor learning [1, 14–22]. Thus restoration of upper limb function also requires strategies to overcome or substitute for these deficits and promote motor relearning. Without a comprehensive and targeted set of strategies that addresses the collective impairments in a personalized manner for each individual, upper limb function may remain compromised long term.

Recently, several studies have shown that patients with mild-moderate stroke show approximately 70% improvement in upper limb impairment at six months, relative to their initial deficit at 72 hours [23–25]. The proportional recovery rule appears to apply in a similar fashion to visuospatial deficits as well [26]. These studies suggest that spontaneous recovery mechanisms drive initial recovery across neural systems. The major questions pertaining to upper limb recovery are: how can spontaneous recovery be enhanced, and what rehabilitation regimens promote recovery beyond what occurs spontaneously in patients with both mild-moderate and severe deficits?

In a recent Cochrane review of physical rehabilitation approaches to recovery of function after stroke, physical rehabilitation was found to have a beneficial effect compared to no treatment on functional recovery after stroke, and this effect was noted to persist beyond the length of the intervention period [27]. Subgroup analyses suggested that a dose of at least 30 to 60 minutes per day delivered five to seven days per week is effective, and there is a significant benefit to those receiving the rehabilitation interventions earlier after stroke. However, several studies have shown that no one physical rehabilitation approach is more (or less) effective than any other approach in improving independence in activities of daily living or motor function [27, 28]. These studies suggest that there is clearly a role for physical rehabilitation in promoting recovery, but the mechanisms by which such approaches promote recovery are multifactorial and not yet clearly understood.

8.2 Treatment: Timing, Intensity, and Setting of Rehabilitation

Stroke care begins with admission to the stroke unit. The median length of stay in a stroke unit is four days for patients with ischemic stroke [29]. During the acute hospital stay, the primary focus is on stabilizing the patient. Data strongly suggest that a multidisciplinary rehabilitation evaluation, which includes occupational therapy, physical therapy, and speech and language therapy, should be initiated as soon as the patient can tolerate it [30]. Following the acute hospital stay patients are transitioned to post-acute care services for further rehabilitation. These services can be provided at inpatient rehab facilities (IRFs), skilled nursing facilities (SNF), outpatient physical therapy centres, or at home. Stroke patients in the United States stay an average of 16–17 days in the acute inpatient rehabilitation unit [31, 32]. The length of stay allowed by insurance companies for post-stroke rehab in IRFs is inadequate given the complex needs of these patients [33]. As a result, rehabilitation of the upper limbs in IRFs is necessarily focused on compensatory techniques using the unaffected hand to allow self-care and basic activities of daily living in order to let the patient return home [31], and less time is spent rehabilitating the affected upper limb [34]. Methods to initiate rehabilitation early in the affected upper limb are therefore warranted and may interact with spontaneous recovery mechanisms to facilitate improved upper limb recovery and reduce disability. However, recent multicentre rehabilitation trials conducted during the first few weeks after stroke, for the upper and lower limbs, suggested that initiating rehabilitation very early may be detrimental [28, 35–37]. Timing of rehabilitation must also take into account readiness of the nervous system for recovery.

Motivation is an important determinant of rehabilitation outcome, and the rehabilitation environment or setting can affect patients' motivation both positively and negatively [38, 39]. While personal goals and attitudes, such as the desire to be independent, contribute to a patient's motivation, social factors have been found to be especially important [40]. The Northern Manhattan Stroke study, which investigated a cohort of more than 1,000 participants, revealed that lack of social support [41], depression [42], and poor subjective well-being [43] are common post stroke, and are associated with increased arm motor impairment, mental distress [44], and risk of future stroke [45, 46]. At least one in three individuals suffers from mood disorders after a stroke [47], including depression, feelings of detachment, fatigue, and anxiety, all of which detract from one's sense of well-being and recovery [48]. A greater sense of satisfaction with social support networks can improve subjective well-being and motivation [49]. Positive mood is associated with higher motor and cognitive status post stroke, and recovery is more likely when there is a positive perception of well-being [48, 50–52]. Indeed, it has been demonstrated that fluoxetine, a serotonin-selective reuptake inhibitor, given from nine days to three months after stroke, was more effective in improving motor scores on the Fugl-Meyer Scale than placebo [20]. Hence environments, both external and internal, that restore mood and well-being are important in providing motivation for individuals to participate actively in their rehabilitation.

Animal studies suggest that post-stroke recovery is enhanced in environments that facilitate meaningful physical and mental activity in socially interactive contexts [53–55]. Environments that simultaneously provide physical, mental, and social stimulation constitute 'enriched environments'. In animal studies, the environment is enriched by animals living in groups, with physical and mental challenges (e.g., large multilevel cages, tubes, and ramps), appropriate animal-specific sensory stimuli (e.g., darkness in nocturnal animals), and engagement in activities through social interaction and play. Physical and mental training and social enrichment have distinct but complementary effects on neurogenesis, integration of new cells into existing circuits, and learning in adult animals, mediated by neuromodulators such as Brain-Derived Neurotrophic Factor (BDNF) [55–59]. Physical activity, especially aerobic exercise, greatly increases the number of new neurons, although very high-intensity exercise may also increase stress hormone levels [60]. Mental training via skill learning increases the survival of new neurons and their integration into existing circuits, particularly when the training goals are challenging [61]. Social enrichment does not refer merely to increasing the numbers of animals housed together, but rather to a positive and stimulating social environment. Social neuropeptides such as oxytocin are thought to play an important role in the development of social bonding [62], and mediate neuroprotective effects such as reduced infarct size, neuroinflammation, and oxidative stress [63], which may contribute to recovery processes post stroke. An additional important consideration is intensity of training; there appears to be a threshold of intensity for recovery even in enriched environments – rats that practised reaching but did not attain the intensity threshold did not recover significantly [64]. Thus the synergistic effects of physical, mental, and social stimulation at sufficient intensity are crucial for recovery in animal models [65–68].

Training environments that integrate physical, cognitive, and social development are known to facilitate human learning [69, 70]. The synergistic effects of physical, mental, and social stimulation also appear to be important for relearning and recovery in humans post stroke [65–68]. Although social isolation is a significant problem after stroke [41], addressing social isolation alone has not been shown to increase functional recovery [71]. However, addressing social isolation and physical activity by engaging individuals physically and socially post stroke, for example with adaptive physical therapy, reduced physical impairment and depression over six months compared to a control group [72]. Aerobic physical exercise, separate from task-specific practice, has been shown to have clear effects on mood and learning [73], but few programmes are available to facilitate aerobic exercise on a long-term basis for individuals with disability [60]. Furthermore, the intensity of task-specific training is much higher in enriched animal protocols than that provided in traditional rehabilitation units [74]. Providing a high intensity of therapy in one-hour sessions that is comparable to those in animal studies has been found to be feasible in inpatient stroke rehabilitation units post stroke [75]; however, much post-stroke rehabilitation now occurs once individuals are back in their own communities due to shortened lengths of stay in rehabilitation facilities. Intense rehabilitation is even more difficult to provide in the community as outpatient therapy sessions are restricted by insurance and community-based rehabilitation programmes are not well developed [76]. In an attempt to create an enriched environment comparable to those used in animal models, a collaborative group music-making intervention was developed for upper limb rehabilitation [77]. The Music Upper Limb Therapy–Integrated (MULT-I) intervention involved music making in a group setting supervised by an occupational therapist and music therapists and was designed to engage subjects with chronic post-stroke hemiparesis physically, mentally, and socially at sufficient intensity twice a week for six weeks. The results showed reduced upper extremity impairment on the Fugl-Meyer Scale, reduced disability on the Modified Rankin Scale, and an increased sense of well-being on the World Health Organization (WHO) well-being

scale at six weeks which persisted one year later. Qualitative analyses of subjects' conversations during the intervention suggested that the MULT-I intervention helped to energize, direct, and sustain movement during and after the intervention, and inspired positive behavioural change that spilled over into activities of daily living. These results suggest that outpatient enriched environments are feasible for post-stroke rehabilitation, and may be created by collaboration between patients and therapists from more than one discipline to engage the patients holistically. The effectiveness of enriched rehabilitation environments on post-stroke recovery needs to be tested in larger controlled trials.

8.3 Treatment: Non-Pharmacological Treatments

A number of interventions/techniques to address post-stroke deficits exist in the literature. These techniques have been used alone or in combination with other modalities to improve function and are summarized in Table 8.1. Note that no one approach to physical rehabilitation appears to be more (or less) effective in promoting recovery of function and mobility after stroke. Some meta-analyses and systematic reviews even propose contradictory recommendations. At present, the major challenge in the field is to figure out how to tailor evidence-based treatment strategies to the needs of the individual stroke patient. Motor skill learning appears to be the key ingredient to recovery and can be fostered in several ways. But which technique is particularly useful in a given patient and why is still not clearly understood.

Most activities of daily living (ADLs), including donning clothes, tying shoelaces, bathing, etc., require the skilful and cooperative use of both upper extremities. The performance of instrumental activities of daily living (IADLs) is better when both hands are used together, which emphasizes the need for training bimanual movements [94]. Studies have shown that the ability to coordinate both upper limbs is partially retained post stroke [95–97], suggesting that therapeutic methods can capitalize on such preserved mechanisms. In an observational study which examined the degree of use of the paretic arm in unimanual and bimanual activities during daily tasks, patients used their paretic side almost exclusively only in bimanual activities, although at a much lower capacity, suggesting that they tend not to use the paretic

Table 8.1 Non-Pharmacological Treatments for post stroke deficits

Technique or Modality	Description	Evidence	Conclusion
Biofeedback	Electromyography (EMG) biofeedback electrodes are placed on the surface of the skin or through needle electrodes, which pick up electric activity and provide feedback to the patient through a display unit or auditory signals. This feedback can be used to enhance movement and function.	Woodford et al., 2007, meta-analysis (78)	Inconclusive due to small studies.
Augmented feedback	Auditory, sensory and/or visual feedback can be provided alone or in combination to enhance motor performance and motor relearning in the hemiparetic arm.	Molier et al., 2010, systematic review (79)	Has an added value, but exact combinations are not known.
Bobath approach	The Bobath approach focuses on hands-on techniques to decrease abnormal muscle tone and facilitate normal movement.	Kollen et al., 2009 (80); Hatem et al., 2016, systematic review (81)	Not superior to other treatment approaches.
Brain stimulation	The two common techniques used to stimulate the brain are transcranial direct current stimulation (tDCS) and transcranial magnetic stimulation (TMS). tDCS uses surface electrodes while TMS uses rapidly changing magnetic fields to stimulate the brain. A form of TMS known as repetitive pulse TMS (rTMS) has been proposed as a treatment option for inducing excitability of the motor cortex in stroke patients.	Hesse et al., 2011(82); Khedr et al., 2013 (83) Hatem et al., 2016, systematic review (81)	tDCS may be a useful adjunct to therapy. rTMS may be useful as an adjuvant therapy; however, theta-burst stimulation has insufficient evidence.
Complimentary interventions	Of the complimentary interventions used to treat stroke, acupuncture, a technique in which needles are inserted into meridian points, has been researched extensively. Other complimentary therapies include traditional Chinese medicine and homeopathy.	Yang et al., 2016 (84)	Inconclusive due to small studies, but may have benefits on global neurological deficiency.
Constraint-induced movement therapy (CIMT)	CIMT prevents movement in the unaffected arm to encourage the use of the paretic arm. Some authors call constraint-induced therapy without motor skill learning 'forced use'. Motor skill learning, not constraint, appears to be the key ingredient in motor improvement.	Janssen et al., 2013, meta-analysis (85); Hatem et al., 2016, systematic review (81)	No benefit of constraint in animal models; raises uncertainty about effectiveness in humans. Insufficient arguments for integrating forced use into stroke rehabilitation.

Table 8.1 (cont.)

Technique or Modality	Description	Evidence	Conclusion
Electrical stimulation	Functional electrical stimulation (FES) is provided through surface electrodes. The stimulation assists involuntary muscle contraction and can be used while a patient is performing a functional task.	Gu et al., 2016, systematic review and meta-analysis (86); Eraifej et al., 2017, systematic review and meta-analysis (87);	Useful to prevent or reduce shoulder subluxation early after stroke. Improved ADLs when applied within two months post stroke.
Mental practice	Mental practice is a training method used to promote skill acquisition through mental rehearsal followed by the practice of the movement. Mental practice with motor imagery can be used in combination with other rehabilitation techniques.	Machado et al., 2015, systematic review and meta-analysis (88); Hatem et al., 2016, systematic review (81);	Not effective as adjunct therapeutic strategy for upper limb motor restoration after stroke. Mental practice with motor imagery appears to be valuable.
Mirror therapy	Mirror therapy is a visual-stimulation-based therapy using mirrors to promote functional movement.	Deconinck et al., 2015, systematic review (89); Hatem et al., 2016, systematic review (81)	Mirror visual feedback increases neural activity in areas involved with allocation of attention and cognitive control. Appears to be valuable.
Music therapy	Music therapy uses acoustic stimulation to promote functional movement.	Magee et al., 2017, Cochrane review (90); Hatem et al., 2016, systematic review (81)	May be beneficial for gait, timing of upper limb function, communication, and quality of life. High-quality randomized controlled trials are needed.
Repetitive task training	Repetitive task training involves practising a task repeatedly to enhance learning and reduce muscle weakness.	French et al., 2016, Cochrane review (91)	Low- to moderate-quality evidence. Number of repetitions need to be measured.
Robotics	Robotic devices are electromechanical devices that can provide assistance or resistance to movement.	Veerbeek et al., 2017, meta-analysis (92)	Effects on motor control are small and specific to targeted joints without generalization.
Sensory interventions	Somatosensory awareness can improve upper limb function and movement. Techniques such as sensory re-education, tactile-kinaesthetic guiding, repetitive sensory practice, or desensitization may be used to improve somatosensory awareness.	Doyle et al., 2010, Cochrane review (93)	Inconclusive due to high degree of clinical heterogeneity in both interventions and outcomes.

Table 8.1 (cont.)

Technique or Modality	Description	Evidence	Conclusion
Strength training	Strength training muscles may be performed with assistance from a therapist or by using weights and gym equipment.	Hatem et al., 2016, systematic review (81)	Muscle strengthening is valuable to improve motor impairments.
Stretching and positioning	Stretching and positioning techniques can involve the use of splints and orthoses. Orthoses are devices used in patients to provide stability and prevent or limit movement.	Pollock et al., 2014, Cochrane review (27) Hatem et al., 2016, systematic review (81)	Low-quality evidence of no benefit or harm. Non-superiority of stretching therapy.
Bilateral arm training	Bilateral arm training uses activities that facilitate the use of both arms to perform identical movements simultaneously. This training may be achieved either by therapeutic activities, mechanical devices or by the use of robotic devices.	Hatem et al., 2016, systematic review (81)	Non-superiority of bilateral training.

arm at all in unimanual tasks [98]. Unimanual training on its own may not improve bilateral coordination; therefore, upper limb rehabilitation must incorporate the use of both hands to accomplish task-related goals [99, 100]. Healthy adults also tend to use both hands in functional tasks more frequently than they would either hand alone [101, 102]. Targeting activities with both arms may thus help increase the amount of use of the paretic limb and address learned non-use. However, when patients do not regain adequate paretic upper limb function post stroke, functional movements are usually achieved by using compensatory movements (learned bad-use) and/or with the use of adaptive equipment (which can reinforce non-use). These compensations may allow for completion of functional tasks, but at the expense of efficiency and fluidity of these movements and tasks [17]. Hence, it is important to not only promote use of the paretic upper limb in bimanual tasks, but also to retrain it so it is used optimally.

How can training facilitate optimal use of the paretic upper limb? Optimal use can be defined as using the right muscles at the right time for a given task. Optimal use requires skill, where movements are planned and executed precisely. Both planning and execution can be impaired to varying degrees depending on the location of the lesion and its size [18, 19, 103, 104]. Assessment of performance with motion analysis can reveal aspects of movement that

are specifically impaired so that an appropriate training approach can be selected, enabling personalization of rehabilitation. For example, in a single session study, patients were stratified based on simple movement kinematics (wrist extension and speed) into three groups: (1) those with predominant paresis, who showed impaired planning and execution; (2) those with spastic co-contraction, who still had impaired planning but showed better execution (higher Fugl-Meyer scores); and (3) those with minimal paresis, who showed better planning and execution [105]. Transfer of learning from the unaffected to the affected wrist with bimanual-to-unimanual training was measured in the three groups under various auditory conditions. The three groups showed diametrically opposite effects: the predominantly paretic group improved motor execution and planning on the affected wrist with rhythmic auditory stimulation, but the other groups did not. The group with spastic co-contraction showed reduced co-contraction without auditory stimulation of any kind. Thus a data-driven evaluation of deficits and training strategies may greatly assist with selection of therapeutic strategies for individual patients for skill relearning. These effects may be further modulated or enhanced with functional electrical stimulation [86, 106] or non-invasive brain stimulation techniques [107], although the evidence is still not conclusive.

8.4 Pharmacological Treatment

The most common indication for pharmacologic intervention post stroke is to re-perfuse the brain and limit stroke-related damage (reperfusion therapies) and management of co-morbidities such as diabetes, hypercholesterolemia, and depression. Post-stroke depression affects one-third of individuals. Post-stroke depression impedes the rehabilitation and recovery process, and adversely impacts quality of life [108, 109]. However, even in the absence of post-stroke depression, early treatment with selective serotonin reuptake inhibitor (SSRI) antidepressants can promote motor recovery, which is strongly supported by several clinical trials [20, 110–112]. In a double-blinded placebo-controlled trial which used Fluoxetine for Motor Recovery after Acute Ischemic Stroke (FLAME) [20], 118 non-depressed stroke patients with hemiplegia or hemiparesis were randomized to receive fluoxetine (20 mg/day) or placebo for three months starting 5–10 days after stroke onset. In the fluoxetine group, the change score on the Fugl-Meyer Scale was significantly higher in the treatment group than in the placebo group. While the motor recovery effects of SSRIs may be due to the antidepressant effect [113], other mechanisms of action may include reduced neural inflammation [114, 115], enhancing neurotrophin activity [116], and increasing neurogenesis [117]. Fluoxetine increases intracortical facilitation [118] and reduces intracortical inhibition [119], and these changes are similar to those that occur in critical periods during development [119, 120]. In addition, serotonin modulates spinal motor control through multiple effects on spinal motor circuits, including regulation of rhythmic activity and control of excitability, by acting on intrasynaptic and extrasynaptic receptors; this may help locomotor function but can also worsen spasticity [121].

For neuromodulation and motor recovery, the role of the dopaminergic neurotransmitter is well established. Dopaminergic terminals in the motor cortex contribute to cortical plasticity and are necessary for motor skill learning [122–124]. A randomized, double-blind, placebo-controlled study of 53 patients within six months of stroke onset found that 100 mg L-dopa/day, given as Sinemet and combined with physical therapy, was significantly better than placebo plus physical therapy on motor recovery after three weeks, measured using the Rivermead Motor Assessment [125]. Prolonged treatment with L-dopa in the chronic stage after stroke may also lead to improvement in dexterity, walking speed, and lengthening of the cortical silent period over the affected hemisphere [126]. However, not all studies have shown a benefit [127–129]. For example, a placebo-controlled, double-blind study of 33 patients 1–12 months after stroke did not find a difference between a nine-week course of ropinirole plus physical therapy compared with placebo plus physical therapy on gait velocity [127]. These differences might reflect small sample sizes, or represent other effects of dopaminergic neurotransmitters [130]. Genetic factors may also be important in modulating dopamine neurotransmission [131–133]. Thus one must be cautious in interpreting the results of initial pharmacological studies as later better-designed studies may contradict conclusions from earlier ones, for example in the study of amphetamines for stroke recovery. Initial clinical trials showed promising results in hemiparetic stroke patients when amphetamine was combined with physical therapy [134, 135]. However, other randomized controlled clinical trials revealed concerns regarding safety and long-term efficacy [136–138]. Other antidepressant or neuro-modulating agents have been examined as well with positive benefits. For instance, clinical trials utilizing cholinesterase inhibitors and glutaminergic medications suggest improvements in aphasic patients, especially when combined with therapy of adequate intensity and duration [139–142]. These have not been tested for upper limb recovery.

Spasticity is another indication for pharmacologic management. In a survey from the National Stroke Association, 57% of 504 stroke survivors reported tight or stiff muscles, suggesting the presence of spasticity [143, 144]. Furthermore, the prevalence of spasticity increases over time post stroke [145–148]. Commonly used systemic oral antispasmodic medications are baclofen and tizanidine, although their use is often limited by side effects such as sedation and weakness [149]. They are typically prescribed in divided doses throughout the day, due to their short duration of effect (usually four to six hours), but single dosing at bedtime is an option if the primary treatment goal is to control night-time spasticity. Antiepileptic drugs, such as gabapentin and pregabalin, are not considered first-line options for spasticity, but can be used especially when central neuropathic pain is present [150]. Cannabis derivatives have been tested to treat spasticity in multiple sclerosis; however, there is a concern of potential cognitive impairment [151].

The advantages of local treatments for spasticity are the absence of sedation, and the ability to selectively treat specific muscles. Local anaesthetics may be injected to produce transient neuromuscular blockade to differentiate between contractures and severe spasticity, but their effect is short term. Injections of phenol or alcohol (chemical neurolysis) may be given selectively in motor nerves, such as the musculocutaneous, obturator, and tibial nerves, to paralyse the muscle and thereby reduce muscle tone [152]. It is important to select the nerves appropriately as injection to sensory nerves can cause dysesthesia. Botulinum toxin, when injected intramuscularly, causes chemo-denervation by blocking the release of acetylcholine at the neuromuscular junction. The effect is reversible muscle paralysis, and it is the most widely used local treatment for spasticity, with a large body of evidence supporting its efficacy in reducing muscle tone but with limited data on its functional impact [153, 154]. Several preparations of botulinum toxin type A and one preparation of type B are available, although there is no fully reliable dosing conversion factor between these preparations. A relatively recent local treatment for spastic muscle stiffness is the use of the enzyme hyaluronidase intramuscularly, which showed safety and potential efficacy in improving active movement in an open-label study [155].

Intrathecal baclofen (ITB) therapy allows the delivery of baclofen intrathecally via a catheter whose distal end is inserted into the spinal canal, and whose proximal end is inserted into a programmable pump implanted subcutaneously in the abdomen. ITB therapy is indicated in patients with severe spasticity refractory to other treatments, and higher thoracic and cervical catheter tip locations may be considered for individuals with severe upper limb spasticity. Compared with oral baclofen, ITB therapy has a more potent effect on spasticity and is less sedative; however, its efficacy has to be balanced with potentially lethal adverse effects such as baclofen withdrawal, intrathecal infection, and paralytic ileus [156–158].

8.5 Surgical Treatment, Stem Cell Therapy, and Brain–Machine Interfaces

Surgical intervention to the upper limbs can include tendon transfers, which are more common in individuals with tetraplegia [159], and in children with cerebral palsy [160]. A variety of procedures such as transfer of the brachioradialis-to-extensor digitorum communis, tendon lengthening of the flexor pollicis longus, and release of the flexor–pronator tendons is used, and have shown favourable outcomes on hand function [161].

Stem cells have the capacity to differentiate into various types of cells, including neurons and glial cells, and possibly to replace the brain tissue damaged by stroke [162]. Alternatively, trophic factors that are by-products of stem cells, such as vascular endothelial growth factor (VEGF), fibroblast growth factor (FGF), glial cell-derived neurotrophic factor (GDNF), and BDNF, may play a role in supporting existing neurons by enhancing synaptogenesis and angiogenesis [163]. Studies in animal models suggest that stem cells may be promising in improving motor function, decreasing stroke volume, promoting neurogenesis and angiogenesis, and exerting immunomodulatory, anti-inflammatory effects in the brain of stroke-affected rodents [164]. However, a meta-analysis of seven clinical studies performed until 2015 revealed that stem cell treatment did not significantly reduce the mortality of ischemic stroke patients or improve scores on the National Institutes of Health Stroke Scale. However, the European Stroke Scale score was significantly improved using the stem cell treatment. The authors concluded that further research is needed to discover more effective stem cell-based therapies for ischemic stroke treatment [165]. An open-label phase 1/2a study, published in 2016, of modified bone marrow-derived mesenchymal stem cells in 18 patients showed that all patients experienced at least one treatment-emergent adverse event. Six patients experienced six serious treatment-emergent adverse events; two were probably or definitely related to surgical procedure; none was related to cell treatment. All serious treatment-emergent adverse events resolved without sequelae. There were no dose-limiting toxicities or deaths. Sixteen patients completed the 12 months of follow-up, and significant improvements from baseline were reported on the European Stroke Scale, the National Institutes of Health Stroke Scale, and the Fugl-Meyer total score, but no changes were observed on the modified Rankin Scale [166].

Another emerging technology is brain–computer interface (BCI) or brain–machine interface (BMI). In stroke survivors with motor impairments, the cortical neural circuitry can be disconnected from the spinal neural circuitry needed to perform a motor task. The goal of BCI technology is to bridge this disconnect by recording neural signals from the brain, decoding the signals, and using them to control an external device [167]. The components required include a sensor to record cortical signals (usually an electroencephalogram [EEG] or invasive microelectrodes), a processor to extract the appropriate signals (such as for hand movement) and decode them, and an effector to carry out the intended signal (usually a computer-screen cursor, robotic limb, or wheelchair). In some BMI paradigms, motor cortical output and input may be simultaneously activated, for instance by translating motor cortical activity associated with the attempt to move the paralysed fingers into actual exoskeleton-driven finger movements, resulting in contingent visual and somatosensory feedback [168]. Real-time feedback can allow patients to learn to control the amplitude of a particular frequency of the neural signal between 8 Hz and 13 Hz called the sensorimotor rhythm (SMR) (or mu-rhythm) [169]. The SMR modulations can be quantified and used to control hand orthoses or FES systems. Rehabilitation using these BMI-controlled devices, called BMI motor rehabilitation training, has demonstrated feasibility in randomized controlled trials [170–173]. More recently it has been shown that the EEG activity of the healthy contralesional motor cortex during attempts to move the paretic arm in chronic stroke patients can be used as a natural, easy, and intuitive way to achieve control of BMIs or robot-assisted rehabilitation devices [174].

8.6 Conclusions

The management of upper limb weakness in neurorehabilitation remains challenging despite decades of work. The main takeaways of the positive and negative trials are: (1) Upper limb weakness is not a static condition. The status of the limb changes over time, requiring rehabilitation strategies to be tailored to the individual. (2) The brain–machine interface trials reveal that even small improvements in the neural signal are important, and if detected, may be harnessed for motor training and recovery. (3) Many promising ideas are currently being tested that bring hope for upper limb recovery.

References

1. Kwakkel G, Kollen BJ, Van der Grond J, Prevo AJ. Probability of regaining dexterity in the flaccid upper limb: Impact of severity of paresis and time since onset in acute stroke. *Stroke* 2003; **34**(9): 2181–6.

2. Anderson CS, Linto J, Stewart-Wynne EG. A population-based assessment of the impact and burden of caregiving for long-term stroke survivors. *Stroke* 1995; **26**(5): 843–9.

3. Miller EL, Murray L, Richards L, Zorowitz RD, Bakas T, Clark P, et al. Comprehensive overview of nursing and interdisciplinary rehabilitation care of the stroke patient: A scientific statement from the American Heart Association. *Stroke* 2010; **41**(10): 2402–48.

4. Dewald JP, Pope PS, Given JD, Buchanan TS, Rymer WZ. Abnormal muscle coactivation patterns during isometric torque generation at the elbow and shoulder in hemiparetic subjects. *Brain* 1995; **118**(Pt. 2): 495–510.

5. Beebe JA, Lang CE. Absence of a proximal to distal gradient of motor deficits in the upper extremity early after stroke. *Clin. Neurophysiol.* 2008; **119**(9): 2074–85.

6. Schieber MH, Lang CE, Reilly KT, McNulty P, Sirigu A. Selective activation of human finger muscles after stroke or amputation. *Adv. Exp. Med. Biol.* 2009; **629**: 559–75.

7. Raghavan P, Petra E, Krakauer JW, Gordon AM. Patterns of impairment in digit independence after subcortical stroke. *J. Neurophysiol.* 2006; **95**(1): 369–78.

8. Beebe JA, Lang CE. Active range of motion predicts upper extremity function 3 months after stroke. *Stroke* 2009; **40**(5): 1772–9.

9. Nijland RH, Van Wegen EE, Harmeling-Van der Wel BC, Kwakkel G. Presence of finger extension and shoulder abduction within 72 hours after stroke predicts functional recovery: Early prediction of functional outcome after stroke: The EPOS cohort study. *Stroke* 2010; **41**(4): 745–50.

10. Lang CE, Bland MD, Bailey RR, Schaefer SY, Birkenmeier RL. Assessment of upper extremity impairment, function, and activity after stroke: Foundations for clinical decision making. *J. Hand Ther.* 2013; **26**(2): 104–14, quiz 15.

11. Kong KH, Chua KS, Lee J. Symptomatic upper limb spasticity in patients with chronic stroke attending a rehabilitation clinic: Frequency, clinical correlates and predictors. *J. Rehabil. Med.* 2010; **42**(5): 453–7.

12. Ward AB. A literature review of the pathophysiology and onset of post-stroke spasticity. *Eur. J. Neurol.* 2012; **19**(1): 21–7.

13. Burke D, Wissel J, Donnan GA. Pathophysiology of spasticity in stroke. *Neurology* 2013; **80**(3 Suppl. 2): S20–6.

14. Kenzie JM, Semrau JA, Findlater SE, Yu AY, Desai JA, Herter TM, et al. Localization of impaired kinesthetic processing post-stroke. *Front. Hum. Neurosci.* 2016; **10**: 505.

15. Dos Santos GL, Salazar LF, Lazarin AC, de Russo TL. Joint position sense is bilaterally reduced for shoulder abduction and flexion in chronic hemiparetic individuals. *Top Stroke Rehabil.* 2015; **22**(4): 271–80.

16. Meyer S, Karttunen AH, Thijs V, Feys H, Verheyden G. How do somatosensory deficits in the arm and hand relate to upper limb impairment, activity, and participation problems after stroke? A systematic review. *Phys. Ther.* 2014; **94**(9): 1220–31.

17. Raghavan P. Upper limb motor impairment after stroke. *Phys. Med. Rehabil. Clin. N. Am.* 2015; **26**(4): 599–610.

18. Raghavan P. The nature of hand motor impairment after stroke and its treatment. *Curr. Treat. Options Cardiovasc. Med.* 2007; **9**(3): 221–8.

19. Raghavan P, Krakauer JW, Gordon AM. Impaired anticipatory control of fingertip forces in patients with a pure motor or sensorimotor lacunar syndrome. *Brain.* 2006; **129**(Pt. 6): 1415–25.

20. Chollet F, Tardy J, Albucher JF, Thalamas C, Berard E, Lamy C, et al. Fluoxetine for motor recovery after acute ischaemic stroke (FLAME): A randomised placebo-controlled trial. *Lancet Neurol.* 2011; **10**(2): 123–30.

21. Mullick AA, Subramanian SK, Levin MF. Emerging evidence of the association between cognitive deficits and arm motor recovery after stroke: A meta-analysis. *Restor. Neurol. Neurosci.* 2015; **33**(3): 389–403.

22. Bolognini N, Russo C, Edwards DJ. The sensory side of post-stroke motor rehabilitation. *Restor. Neurol. Neurosci.* 2016; **34**(4): 571–86.

23. Prabhakaran S, Zarahn E, Riley C, Speizer A, Chong JY, Lazar RM, et al. Inter-individual variability in the capacity for motor recovery after ischemic stroke. *Neurorehabil. Neural. Repair.* 2008; **22**(1): 64–71.

24. Byblow WD, Stinear CM, Barber PA, Petoe MA, Ackerley SJ. Proportional recovery after stroke depends on corticomotor integrity. *Ann. Neurol.* 2015; **78**(6): 848–59.

25. Winters C, Van Wegen EE, Daffertshofer A, Kwakkel G. Generalizability of the proportional recovery model for the upper extremity after an ischemic stroke. *Neurorehabil. Neural Repair* 2015; **29**(7): 614–22.

26. Winters C, Van Wegen EE, Daffertshofer A, Kwakkel G. Generalizability of the maximum proportional recovery rule to visuospatial neglect early poststroke. *Neurorehabil. Neural Repair* 2017; **31**(4): 334–42.

27. Pollock A, Baer G, Campbell P, Choo PL, Forster A, Morris J, et al. Physical rehabilitation approaches for the recovery of function and mobility following stroke. *Cochrane Database Syst. Rev.* 2014; **22**(4): CD001920.

28. Winstein CJ, Wolf SL, Dromerick AW, Lane CJ, Nelsen MA, Lewthwaite R, et al. Effect of a task-oriented rehabilitation program on upper extremity recovery following motor stroke: The ICARE randomized clinical trial. *JAMA.* 2016; **315**(6): 571–81.

29. Prvu Bettger JA, Kaltenbach L, Reeves MJ, Smith EE, Fonarow GC, Schwamm LH, et al. Assessing stroke patients for rehabilitation during the acute hospitalization: Findings from the get with the guidelines stroke program. *Arch. Phys. Med. Rehabil.* 2013; **94**(1): 38–45.

30. Winstein CJ, Stein J, Arena R, Bates B, Cherney LR, Cramer SC, et al. Guidelines for adult stroke rehabilitation and recovery: A guideline for healthcare professionals from the American Heart Association/American Stroke Association. *Stroke* 2016; **47**(6): e98–e169.

31. Dobkin BH. Clinical practice: Rehabilitation after stroke. *N. Engl. J. Med.* 2005; **352**(16): 1677–84.

32. Gassaway J, Horn SD, DeJong G, Smout RJ, Clark C, James R. Applying the clinical practice improvement approach to stroke rehabilitation: Methods used and baseline results. *Arch. Phys. Med. Rehabil.* 2005; **86**(12 Suppl. 2): S16–S33.

33. O'Brien SR, Xue Y, Ingersoll G, Kelly A. Shorter length of stay is associated with worse functional outcomes for Medicare beneficiaries with stroke. *Phys. Ther.* 2013; **93**(12): 1592–1602.

34. West T, Bernhardt J. Physical activity in hospitalised stroke patients. *Stroke Res. Treat.* 2012. http://dx.doi.org/10.1155/2012/81376535

35. Bernhardt J, English C, Johnson L, Cumming TB. Early mobilization after stroke: Early adoption but limited evidence. *Stroke* 2015; **46**(4): 1141–6.

36. English C, Bernhardt J, Crotty M, Esterman A, Segal L, Hillier S. Circuit class therapy or seven-day week therapy for increasing rehabilitation intensity of therapy after stroke (CIRCIT): A randomized controlled trial. *Int. J. Stroke.* 2015; **10**(4): 594–602.

37. Bernhardt J, Langhorne P, Lindley RI, Thrift AG, Ellery F, Collier J, et al. Efficacy and safety of very early mobilisation within 24 h of stroke onset (AVERT): A randomised controlled trial. *Lancet* 2015; **386**(9988): 46–55.

38. Maclean N, Pound P, Wolfe C, Rudd A. Qualitative analysis of stroke patients' motivation for rehabilitation. *BMJ* 2000; **321**(7268): 1051–4.

39. Chang LH, Hasselkus BR. Occupational therapists' expectations in rehabilitation following stroke: Sources of satisfaction and dissatisfaction. *Am. J. Occup. Ther.* 1998; **52**(8): 629–37.

40. Maclean N, Pound P, Wolfe C, Rudd A. The concept of patient motivation: A qualitative

analysis of stroke professionals' attitudes. *Stroke* 2002; **33**(2): 444–8.

41. Boden-Albala B, Litwak E, Elkind MS, Rundek T, Sacco RL. Social isolation and outcomes post stroke. *Neurology* 2005; **64**(11): 1888–92.

42. Willey JZ, Disla N, Moon YP, Paik MC, Sacco RL, Boden-Albala B, et al. Early depressed mood after stroke predicts long-term disability: The Northern Manhattan Stroke Study (NOMASS). *Stroke* 2010; **41**(9): 1896–900.

43. Wyller TB, Sveen U, Sodring KM, Pettersen AM, Bautz-Holter E. Subjective well-being one year after stroke. *Clinical Rehabilitation.* [Research Support, Non-US Gov't]. 1997; **11**(2): 139–45.

44. Wiltink J, Beutel ME, Till Y, Ojeda FM, Wild PS, Munzel T, et al. Prevalence of distress, comorbid conditions and well being in the general population. *J. Affect Disord.* 2011; **130**(3): 429–37.

45. Ostir GV, Markides KS, Peek MK, Goodwin JS. The association between emotional well-being and the incidence of stroke in older adults. *Psychosom. Med.* [Research Support, US Gov't, PHS]. 2001; **63**(2): 210–15.

46. Araki A, Murotani Y, Kamimiya F, Ito H. Low well-being is an independent predictor for stroke in elderly patients with diabetes mellitus. *J. American Geriatr. Soc.* 2004; **52**(2): 205–10.

47. Hackett M, Yapa C, Parag V, Anderson C. Frequency of depression after stroke: A systematic review of observational studies. *Stroke* 2005; **36**: 1330–40.

48. Ostir GV, Berges IM, Ottenbacher ME, Clow A, Ottenbacher KJ. Associations between positive emotion and recovery of functional status following stroke. *Psychosomatic Medicine.* [Research Support, NIH, Extramural]. 2008; **70**(4): 404–9.

49. Clarke P, Marshall V, Black SE, Colantonio A. Well-being after stroke in Canadian seniors: Findings from the Canadian Study of Health and Aging. *Stroke* 2002; **33**(4): 1016–21.

50. Whitson HE, Thielke S, Diehr P, O'Hare AM, Chaves PH, Zakai NA, et al. Patterns and predictors of recovery from exhaustion in older adults: The Cardiovascular Health Study. *J. Am. Geriatr. Soc.* 2011; **59**(2): 207–13.

51. Hall NC, Chipperfield JG, Heckhausen J, Perry RP. Control striving in older adults with serious health problems: A 9-year longitudinal study of survival, health, and well-being. *Psychol. Aging* 2010; **25**(2): 432–45.

52. Carod-Artal FJ, Egido JA. Quality of life after stroke: The importance of a good recovery. *Cerebrovasc. Dis.* 2009; **27** Suppl. 1: 204–14.

53. Maclellan CL, Keough MB, Granter-Button S, Chernenko GA, Butt S, Corbett D. A critical threshold of rehabilitation involving brain-derived neurotrophic factor is required for poststroke recovery. *Neurorehabil Neural Repair.* 2011; **25**(8): 740–8.

54. Shono Y, Yokota C, Kuge Y, Kido S, Harada A, Kokame K, et al. Gene expression associated with an enriched environment after transient focal ischemia. *Brain Res.* 2011; **28**(1376): 60–5.

55. Johansson BB. Functional and cellular effects of environmental enrichment after experimental brain infarcts. *Restor. Neurol. Neurosci.* 2004; **22**(3–5): 163–74.

56. Madronal N, Lopez-Aracil C, Rangel A, del Rio JA, Delgado-Garcia JM, Gruart A. Effects of enriched physical and social environments on motor performance, associative learning, and hippocampal neurogenesis in mice. *PloS One.* 2010; **5**(6): e11130.

57. Curlik DM, 2nd, Shors TJ. Training your brain: Do mental and physical (MAP) training enhance cognition through the process of neurogenesis in the hippocampus? *Neuropharmacology* 2013; **64**: 506–14.

58. Olson AK, Eadie BD, Ernst C, Christie BR. Environmental enrichment and voluntary exercise massively increase neurogenesis in the adult hippocampus via dissociable pathways. *Hippocampus* 2006; **16**(3): 250–60.

59. Clark PJ, Bhattacharya TK, Miller DS, Kohman RA, DeYoung EK, Rhodes JS. New neurons generated from running are broadly recruited into neuronal activation associated with three different hippocampus-involved tasks. *Hippocampus* 2012; **22**(9): 1860–7.

60. Ploughman M. Exercise is brain food: The effects of physical activity on cognitive function. *Dev. Neurorehabil.* 2008; **11**(3): 236–40.

61. Churchill JD, Galvez R, Colcombe S, Swain RA, Kramer AF, Greenough WT. Exercise, experience and the aging brain. *Neurobiol. Aging.* 2002; **23**(5): 941–55.

62. Israel S, Lerer E, Shalev I, Uzefovsky F, Reibold M, Bachner-Melman R, et al. Molecular genetic studies of the arginine vasopressin 1a receptor (AVPR1a) and the oxytocin receptor (OXTR) in human behaviour: From autism to altruism with some notes in between. *Prog. Brain Res.* 2008; **170**: 435–49.

63. Karelina K, Stuller KA, Jarrett B, Zhang N, Wells J, Norman GJ, et al. Oxytocin mediates social neuroprotection after cerebral ischemia. *Stroke* [Research Support, NIH, Extramural Research Support, Non-US Gov't]. 2011; **42**(12): 3606–11.

64. MacLellan CL, Keough MB, Granter-Button S, Chernenko GA, Butt S, Corbett D. A critical threshold of rehabilitation involving brain-derived neurotrophic

factor is required for poststroke recovery. *Neurorehabil. Neural Repair.* 2011; **25**(8): 740–8.

65. Belanger L, Bolduc M, Noel M. Relative importance of after-effects, environment and socio-economic factors on the social integration of stroke victims. *Int. J. Rehabil. Res.* 1988; **11**(3): 251–60.

66. Bronstein KS. Psychosocial components in stroke: Implications for adaptation. *Nurs. Clin. North Am.* 1991; **26**(4): 1007–17.

67. Fuhrer MJ. Subjective well-being: Implications for medical rehabilitation outcomes and models of disablement. *Am. J. Phys. Med. Rehabil.* 1994; **73**(5): 358–64.

68. White MA, Johnstone AS. Recovery from stroke: Does rehabilitation counselling have a role to play? *Disabil. Rehabil.* 2000; **22**(3): 140–3.

69. Blair C, Diamond A. Biological processes in prevention and intervention: The promotion of self-regulation as a means of preventing school failure. *Dev. Psychopathol.* 2008; **20**(3): 899–911.

70. Diamond A, Lee K. Interventions shown to aid executive function development in children 4 to 12 years old. *Science* 2011; **333**(6045): 959–64.

71. Glass TA, Berkman LF, Hiltunen EF, Furie K, Glymour MM, Fay ME, et al. The Families In Recovery from Stroke Trial (FIRST): Primary study results. *Psychosom. Med.* 2004; **66**(6): 889–97.

72. Stuart M, Benvenuti F, Macko R, Taviani A, Segenni L, Mayer F, et al. Community-based adaptive physical activity program for chronic stroke: Feasibility, safety, and efficacy of the Empoli model. *Neurorehabil. Neural Repair.* 2009; **23**(7): 726–34.

73. Ploughman M, Attwood Z, White N, Dore JJ, Corbett D. Endurance exercise facilitates relearning of forelimb motor skill after focal ischemia. *Eur. J. Neurosci.* 2007; **25**(11): 3453–60.

74. Krakauer JW, Carmichael ST, Corbett D, Wittenberg GF. Getting neurorehabilitation right: What can be learned from animal models? *Neurorehabil. Neural Repair.* 2012; **26**(8): 923–31.

75. Birkenmeier RL, Prager EM, Lang CE. Translating animal doses of task-specific training to people with chronic stroke in 1-hour therapy sessions: A proof-of-concept study. *Neurorehabil. Neural Repair.* 2010; **24**(7): 620–35.

76. Graven C, Brock K, Hill K, Joubert L. Are rehabilitation and/or care co-ordination interventions delivered in the community effective in reducing depression, facilitating participation and improving quality of life after stroke? *Disabil. Rehabil.* 2011; **33**(17–18): 1501–20.

77. Raghavan P, Geller D, Guerrero N, Aluru V, Eimicke JP, Teresi JA, et al. Music Upper Limb

78. Woodford H, Price C. EMG biofeedback for the recovery of motor function after stroke. *Cochrane Database Syst. Rev.* 2007; **18**(2): CD004585.

79. Molier BI, Van Asseldonk EH, Hermens HJ, Jannink MJ. Nature, timing, frequency and type of augmented feedback: Does it influence motor relearning of the hemiparetic arm after stroke? A systematic review. *Disabil. Rehabil.* 2010; **32**(22): 1799–1809.

80. Kollen BJ, Lennon S, Lyons B, Wheatley-Smith L, Scheper M, Buurke JH, et al. The effectiveness of the Bobath concept in stroke rehabilitation: What is the evidence? *Stroke* 2009; **40**(4): e89–97.

81. Hatem SM, Saussez G, Della Faille M, Prist V, Zhang X, Dispa D, et al. Rehabilitation of motor function after stroke: A multiple systematic review focused on techniques to stimulate upper extremity recovery. *Front. Hum. Neurosci.* 2016; **10**: 442.

82. Hesse S, Waldner A, Mehrholz J, Tomelleri C, Pohl M, Werner C. Combined transcranial direct current stimulation and robot-assisted arm training in subacute stroke patients: An exploratory, randomized multicenter trial. *Neurorehabil. Neural Repair.* 2011; **25**(9): 838–46.

83. Khedr EM, Shawky OA, El-Hammady DH, Rothwell JC, Darwish ES, Mostafa OM, et al. Effect of anodal versus cathodal transcranial direct current stimulation on stroke rehabilitation: A pilot randomized controlled trial. *Neurorehabil. Neural Repair.* 2013; **27**(7): 592–601.

84. Yang A, Wu HM, Tang JL, Xu L, Yang M, Liu GJ. Acupuncture for stroke rehabilitation. *Cochrane Database Syst. Rev.* 2016; **26**(8): CD004131.

85. Janssen H, Speare S, Spratt NJ, Sena ES, Ada L, Hannan AJ, et al. Exploring the efficacy of constraint in animal models of stroke: Meta-analysis and systematic review of the current evidence. *Neurorehabil. Neural Repair.* 2013; **27**(1): 3–12.

86. Gu P, Ran JJ. Electrical stimulation for hemiplegic shoulder function: A systematic review and meta-analysis of 15 randomized controlled trials. *Arch. Phys. Med. Rehabil.* 2016; **97**(9): 1588–94.

87. Eraifej J, Clark W, France B, Desando S, Moore D. Effectiveness of upper limb functional electrical stimulation after stroke for the improvement of activities of daily living and motor function: A systematic review and meta-analysis. *Syst. Rev.* 2017; **6**(1): 40.

88. Machado S, Lattari E, de Sa AS, Rocha NB, Yuan TF, Paes F, et al. Is mental practice an effective adjunct therapeutic strategy for upper limb motor restoration after stroke? A systematic review and meta-analysis. *CNS Neurol. Disord. Drug Targets.* 2015; **14**(5): 567–75.

89. Deconinck FJ, Smorenburg AR, Benham A, Ledebt A, Feltham MG, Savelsbergh GJ. Reflections on mirror therapy: A systematic review of the effect of mirror visual feedback on the brain. *Neurorehabil. Neural Repair*. 2015; **29**(4): 349–61.

90. Magee WL, Clark I, Tamplin J, Bradt J. Music interventions for acquired brain injury. *Cochrane Database Syst. Rev.* 2017; **1**: CD006787.

91. French B, Thomas LH, Coupe J, McMahon NE, Connell L, Harrison J, et al. Repetitive task training for improving functional ability after stroke. *Cochrane Database Syst. Rev.* 2016; **11**: CD006073.

92. Veerbeek JM, Langbroek-Amersfoort AC, Van Wegen EE, Meskers CG, Kwakkel G. Effects of robot-assisted therapy for the upper limb after stroke. *Neurorehabil. Neural Repair* 2017; **31**(2): 107–21.

93. Doyle S, Bennett S, Fasoli SE, McKenna KT. Interventions for sensory impairment in the upper limb after stroke. *Cochrane Database Syst. Rev.* 2010; **16**(6): CD006331.

94. Haaland KY, Mutha PK, Rinehart JK, Daniels M, Cushnyr B, Adair JC. Relationship between arm usage and instrumental activities of daily living after unilateral stroke. *Arch. Phys. Med. Rehabil.* 2012; **93**(11): 1957–62.

95. Harris-Love ML, McCombe Waller S, Whitall J. Exploiting interlimb coupling to improve paretic arm reaching performance in people with chronic stroke. *Arch. Phys. Med. Rehabil.* 2005; **86**(11): 2131–7.

96. Rose DK, Winstein CJ. The co-ordination of bimanual rapid aiming movements following stroke. *Clin. Rehabil.* 2005; **19**(4): 452–62.

97. McCombe Waller S, Whitall J. Bilateral arm training: Why and who benefits? *NeuroRehabilitation* 2008; **23**(1): 29–41.

98. Michielsen ME, Selles RW, Stam HJ, Ribbers GM, Bussmann JB. Quantifying nonuse in chronic stroke patients: A study into paretic, nonparetic, and bimanual upper-limb use in daily life. *Arch. Phys. Med. Rehabil.* 2012; **93**(11): 1975–81.

99. Kantak S, McGrath R, Zahedi N. Goal conceptualization and symmetry of arm movements affect bimanual coordination in individuals after stroke. *Neurosci. Lett.* 2016; **626**: 86–93.

100. Sainburg R, Good D, Przybyla A. Bilateral synergy: A framework for post-stroke rehabilitation. *J. Neurol. Transl. Neurosci.* 2013; **1**(3): 1025.

101. Kilbreath SL, Heard RC. Frequency of hand use in healthy older persons. *Aust. J. Physiother.* 2005; **51**(2): 119–22.

102. Stone KD, Bryant DC, Gonzalez CL. Hand use for grasping in a bimanual task: Evidence for different roles? *Exp. Brain Res.* 2013; **224**(3): 455–67.

103. Raghavan P, Santello M, Gordon AM, Krakauer JW. Compensatory motor control after stroke: An alternative joint strategy for object-dependent shaping of hand posture. *J. Neurophysiol.* 2010; **103**(6): 3034–43.

104. Schaefer SY, Mutha PK, Haaland KY, Sainburg RL. Hemispheric specialization for movement control produces dissociable differences in online corrections after stroke. *Cereb. Cortex* 2012; **22**(6): 1407–19.

105. Aluru V, Lu Y, Leung A, Verghese J, Raghavan P. Effect of auditory constraints on motor performance depends on stage of recovery post-stroke. *Front Neurol.* 2014; **5**: 106.

106. Howlett OA, Lannin NA, Ada L, McKinstry C. Functional electrical stimulation improves activity after stroke: A systematic review with meta-analysis. *Arch. Phys. Med. Rehabil.* 2015; **96**(5): 934–43.

107. Rothwell JC. Can motor recovery in stroke be improved by non-invasive brain stimulation? *Adv. Exp. Med. Biol.* 2016; **957**: 313–23.

108. Gaete JM, Bogousslavsky J. Post-stroke depression. *Expert Rev. Neurother.* 2008; **8**(1): 75–92.

109. Carson AJ. Impact commentaries: Mood disorder as a specific complication of stroke. *J. Neurol. Neurosurg. Psychiatry.* 2012; **83**(9): 859.

110. Pariente J, Loubinoux I, Carel C, Albucher JF, Leger A, Manelfe C, et al. Fluoxetine modulates motor performance and cerebral activation of patients recovering from stroke. *Ann. Neurol.* 2001; **50**(6): 718–29.

111. Zittel S, Weiller C, Liepert J. Citalopram improves dexterity in chronic stroke patients. *Neurorehabil. Neural Repair* 2008; **22**(3): 311–14.

112. Acler M, Robol E, Fiaschi A, Manganotti P. A double blind placebo RCT to investigate the effects of serotonergic modulation on brain excitability and motor recovery in stroke patients. *J. Neurol.* 2009; **256**(7): 1152–8.

113. Saxena SK, Ng TP, Koh G, Yong D, Fong NP. Is improvement in impaired cognition and depressive symptoms in post-stroke patients associated with recovery in activities of daily living? *Acta. Neurol. Scand.* 2007; **115**(5): 339–46.

114. Walker FR. A critical review of the mechanism of action for the selective serotonin reuptake inhibitors: Do these drugs possess anti-inflammatory properties and how relevant is this in the treatment of depression? *Neuropharmacology* 2013; **67**: 304–17.

115. Maes M, Leonard B, Fernandez A, Kubera M, Nowak G, Veerhuis R, et al. (Neuro)inflammation and neuroprogression as new pathways and drug targets in depression: From antioxidants to kinase

inhibitors. *Prog. Neuropsychopharmacol. Biol. Psychiatry* 2011; **35**(3): 659–63.

116. Duman RS, Monteggia LM. A neurotrophic model for stress-related mood disorders. *Biol. Psychiatry.* 2006; **59**(12): 1116–27.

117. Santarelli L, Saxe M, Gross C, Surget A, Battaglia F, Dulawa S, et al. Requirement of hippocampal neurogenesis for the behavioral effects of antidepressants. *Science* 2003; **301**(5634): 805–9.

118. Gerdelat-Mas A, Loubinoux I, Tombari D, Rascol O, Chollet F, Simonetta-Moreau M. Chronic administration of selective serotonin reuptake inhibitor (SSRI) paroxetine modulates human motor cortex excitability in healthy subjects. *Neuroimage* 2005; **27**(2): 314–22.

119. Maya Vetencourt JF, Sale A, Viegi A, Baroncelli L, De Pasquale R, O'Leary OF, et al. The antidepressant fluoxetine restores plasticity in the adult visual cortex. *Science* 2008; **320**(5874): 385–8.

120. Guirado R, Perez-Rando M, Sanchez-Matarredona D, Castren E, Nacher J. Chronic fluoxetine treatment alters the structure, connectivity and plasticity of cortical interneurons. *Int. J. Neuropsychopharmacol.* 2014; **17**(10): 1635–46.

121. Perrier JF, Cotel F. Serotonergic modulation of spinal motor control. *Curr. Opin. Neurobiol.* 2015; **33**: 1–7.

122. Molina-Luna K, Pekanovic A, Rohrich S, Hertler B, Schubring-Giese M, Rioult-Pedotti MS, et al. Dopamine in motor cortex is necessary for skill learning and synaptic plasticity. *PLoS One* 2009; **4**(9): e7082.

123. Rioult-Pedotti MS, Pekanovic A, Atiemo CO, Marshall J, Luft AR. Dopamine promotes motor cortex plasticity and motor skill learning via PLC activation. *PLoS One* 2015; **10**(5): e0124986.

124. Hosp JA, Pekanovic A, Rioult-Pedotti MS, Luft AR. Dopaminergic projections from midbrain to primary motor cortex mediate motor skill learning. *J. Neurosci.* 2011; **31**(7): 2481–7.

125. Scheidtmann K, Fries W, Muller F, Koenig E. Effect of levodopa in combination with physiotherapy on functional motor recovery after stroke: A prospective, randomised, double-blind study. *Lancet* 2001; **358** (9284): 787–90.

126. Acler M, Fiaschi A, Manganotti P. Long-term levodopa administration in chronic stroke patients: A clinical and neurophysiologic single-blind placebo-controlled cross-over pilot study. *Restor. Neurol. Neurosci.* 2009; **27**(4): 277–83.

127. Cramer SC, Dobkin BH, Noser EA, Rodriguez RW, Enney LA. Randomized, placebo-controlled, double-blind study of ropinirole in chronic stroke. *Stroke* 2009; **40**(9): 3034–8.

128. Restemeyer C, Weiller C, Liepert J. No effect of a levodopa single dose on motor performance and motor excitability in chronic stroke: A double-blind placebo-controlled cross-over pilot study. *Restor. Neurol. Neurosci.* 2007; **25**(2): 143–50.

129. Sonde L, Lokk J. Effects of amphetamine and/or L-dopa and physiotherapy after stroke – a blinded randomized study. *Acta. Neurol. Scand.* 2007; **115**(1): 55–9.

130. Cramer SC. Drugs to enhance motor recovery after stroke. *Stroke* 2015; **46**(10): 2998–3005.

131. Pearson-Fuhrhop KM, Cramer SC. Pharmacogenetics of neural injury recovery. *Pharmacogenomics* 2013; **14**(13): 1635–43.

132. Pearson-Fuhrhop KM, Dunn EC, Mortero S, Devan WJ, Falcone GJ, Lee P, et al. Dopamine genetic risk score predicts depressive symptoms in healthy adults and adults with depression. *PLoS One* 2014; **9** (5): e93772.

133. Pearson-Fuhrhop KM, Minton B, Acevedo D, Shahbaba B, Cramer SC. Genetic variation in the human brain dopamine system influences motor learning and its modulation by L-dopa. *PLoS One* 2013; **8**(4): e61197.

134. Crisostomo EA, Duncan PW, Propst M, Dawson DV, Davis JN. Evidence that amphetamine with physical therapy promotes recovery of motor function in stroke patients. *Ann. Neurol.* 1988; **23**(1): 94–7.

135. Gladstone DJ, Danells CJ, Armesto A, McIlroy WE, Staines WR, Graham SJ, et al. Physiotherapy coupled with dextroamphetamine for rehabilitation after hemiparetic stroke: A randomized, double-blind, placebo-controlled trial. *Stroke* 2006; **37**(1): 179–85.

136. Martinsson L, Wahlgren NG. Safety of dexamphetamine in acute ischemic stroke: A randomized, double-blind, controlled dose-escalation trial. *Stroke* 2003; **34**(2): 475–81.

137. Martinsson L, Wahlgren NG, Hardemark HG. Amphetamines for improving recovery after stroke. *Cochrane Database Syst. Rev.* 2003; **3**: CD002090.

138. Martinsson L, Hardemark H, Eksborg S. Amphetamines for improving recovery after stroke. *Cochrane Database Syst. Rev.* 2007; **1**: CD002090.

139. Hong JM, Shin DH, Lim TS, Lee JS, Huh K. Galantamine administration in chronic post-stroke aphasia. *J. Neurol. Neurosurg. Psychiatry.* 2012; **83**(7): 675–80.

140. Berthier ML, Green C, Lara JP, Higueras C, Barbancho MA, Davila G, et al. Memantine and constraint-induced aphasia therapy in chronic poststroke aphasia. *Ann. Neurol.* 2009; **65**(5): 577–85.

141. Barbancho MA, Berthier ML, Navas-Sanchez P, Davila G, Green-Heredia C, Garcia-Alberca JM, et al.

Bilateral brain reorganization with memantine and constraint-induced aphasia therapy in chronic post-stroke aphasia: An ERP study. *Brain Lang.* 2015; 145–6: 1–10.

142. Berthier ML, Pulvermuller F, Davila G, Casares NG, Gutierrez A. Drug therapy of post-stroke aphasia: A review of current evidence. *Neuropsychol. Rev.* 2011; **21**(3): 302–17.

143. Bethoux F. Spasticity management after stroke. *Phys. Med. Rehabil. Clin. N Am.* 2015; **26**(4): 625–39.

144. National Stroke Association. Stroke Perceptions Study. 2006. http://support.stroke.org/site/DocServer/StrokePerceptions_FinalSurveyResults_2006.pdf?docID=1941.

145. Wissel J, Manack A, Brainin M. Toward an epidemiology of poststroke spasticity. *Neurology* 2013; **80**(3 Suppl. 2): S13–19.

146. Opheim A, Danielsson A, Alt Murphy M, Persson HC, Sunnerhagen KS. Upper-limb spasticity during the first year after stroke: Stroke arm longitudinal study at the University of Gothenburg. *Am. J. Phys. Med. Rehabil.* 2014; **93**(10): 884–96.

147. Wissel J, Schelosky LD, Scott J, Christe W, Faiss JH, Mueller J. Early development of spasticity following stroke: A prospective, observational trial. *J. Neurol.* 2010; **257**(7): 1067–72.

148. Welmer AK, Widen Holmqvist L, Sommerfeld DK. Location and severity of spasticity in the first 1–2 weeks and at 3 and 18 months after stroke. *Eur. J. Neurol.* 2010; **17**(5): 720–5.

149. Montane E, Vallano A, Laporte JR. Oral antispastic drugs in nonprogressive neurologic diseases: A systematic review. *Neurology* 2004; **63**(8): 1357–63.

150. Finnerup NB. A review of central neuropathic pain states. *Curr. Opin. Anaesthesiol.* 2008; **21**(5): 586–9.

151. Chohan H, Greenfield AL, Yadav V, Graves J. Use of cannabinoids for spasticity and pain management in MS. *Curr. Treat. Options Neurol.* 2016; **18**(1): 1.

152. Kocabas H, Salli A, Demir AH, Ozerbil OM. Comparison of phenol and alcohol neurolysis of tibial nerve motor branches to the gastrocnemius muscle for treatment of spastic foot after stroke: A randomized controlled pilot study. *Eur. J. Phys. Rehabil. Med.* 2010; **46**(1): 5–10.

153. Simpson DM, Gracies JM, Graham HK, Miyasaki JM, Naumann M, Russman B, et al. Assessment: Botulinum neurotoxin for the treatment of spasticity (an evidence-based review): Report of the Therapeutics and Technology Assessment Subcommittee of the American Academy of Neurology. *Neurology* 2008; **70**(19): 1691–8.

154. Foley N, Pereira S, Salter K, Fernandez MM, Speechley M, Sequeira K, et al. Treatment with botulinum toxin improves upper-extremity function post stroke: A systematic review and meta-analysis. *Arch. Phys. Med. Rehabil.* 2013; **94**(5): 977–89.

155. Raghavan P, Lu Y, Mirchandani M, Stecco A. Human recombinant hyaluronidase injections for upper limb muscle stiffness in individuals with cerebral injury: A case series. *EBioMedicine* 2016; **9**: 306–13.

156. Ivanhoe CB, Francisco GE, McGuire JR, Subramanian T, Grissom SP. Intrathecal baclofen management of poststroke spastic hypertonia: implications for function and quality of life. *Arch. Phys. Med. Rehabil.* 2006; **87**(11): 1509–15.

157. Francisco GE, Yablon SA, Schiess MC, Wiggs L, Cavalier S, Grissom S. Consensus panel guidelines for the use of intrathecal baclofen therapy in poststroke spastic hypertonia. *Top Stroke Rehabil.* 2006; **13**(4): 74–85.

158. Francisco GE, McGuire JR. Poststroke spasticity management. *Stroke* 2012; **43**(11): 3132–6.

159. Dunn JA, Hay-Smith EJ, Keeling S, Sinnott KA. Decision-making about upper limb tendon transfer surgery by people with tetraplegia for more than 10 years. *Arch. Phys. Med. Rehabil.* 2016; **97**(6 Suppl.): S88–96.

160. Seruya M, Dickey RM, Fakhro A. Surgical treatment of pediatric upper limb spasticity: The wrist and hand. *Semin. Plast. Surg.* 2016; **30**(1): 29–38.

161. Eliasson AC, Ekholm C, Carlstedt T. Hand function in children with cerebral palsy after upper-limb tendon transfer and muscle release. *Dev. Med. Child. Neurol.* 1998; **40**(9): 612–21.

162. Bliss T, Guzman R, Daadi M, Steinberg GK. Cell transplantation therapy for stroke. *Stroke* 2007; **38**(2 Suppl.): 817–26.

163. Luo Y. Cell-based therapy for stroke. *J. Neural Transm (Vienna).* 2011; **118**(1): 61–74.

164. Zents K, Copray S. The therapeutic potential of induced pluripotent stem cells after stroke: Evidence from rodent models. *Curr. Stem Cell Res. Ther.* 2016; **11**(2): 166–74.

165. Wang Q, Duan F, Wang MX, Wang XD, Liu P, Ma LZ. Effect of stem cell-based therapy for ischemic stroke treatment: A meta-analysis. *Clin. Neurol. Neurosurg.* 2016; **146**: 1–11.

166. Steinberg GK, Kondziolka D, Wechsler LR, Lunsford LD, Coburn ML, Billigen JB, et al. Clinical outcomes of transplanted modified bone marrow-derived mesenchymal stem cells in stroke: A phase 1/2a study. *Stroke* 2016; **47**(7): 1817–24.

167. Lee B, Liu CY, Apuzzo ML. A primer on brain–machine interfaces, concepts, and technology: A key element in the future of functional

neurorestoration. *World Neurosurg.* 2013; **79**(3–4): 457–71.

168. Ushiba J, Soekadar SR. Brain–machine interfaces for rehabilitation of poststroke hemiplegia. *Prog Brain Res.* 2016; **228**: 163–83.

169. Ono T, Kimura A, Ushiba J. Daily training with realistic visual feedback improves reproducibility of event-related desynchronisation following hand motor imagery. *Clin. Neurophysiol.* 2013; **124**(9): 1779–86.

170. Ang KK, Chua KS, Phua KS, Wang C, Chin ZY, Kuah CW, et al. A randomized controlled trial of EEG-based motor imagery brain–computer interface robotic rehabilitation for stroke. *Clin. EEG Neurosci.* 2015; **46**(4): 310–20.

171. Ang KK, Guan C, Phua KS, Wang C, Zhou L, Tang KY, et al. Brain–computer interface-based robotic end effector system for wrist and hand

rehabilitation: Results of a three-armed randomized controlled trial for chronic stroke. *Front. Neuroeng.* 2014; 7: 30.

172. Pichiorri F, Morone G, Petti M, Toppi J, Pisotta I, Molinari M, et al. Brain–computer interface boosts motor imagery practice during stroke recovery. *Ann. Neurol.* 2015; **77**(5): 851–65.

173. Ramos-Murguialday A, Broetz D, Rea M, Laer L, Yilmaz O, Brasil FL, et al. Brain–machine interface in chronic stroke rehabilitation: A controlled study. *Ann. Neurol.* 2013; **74**(1): 100–8.

174. Antelis JM, Montesano L, Ramos-Murguialday A, Birbaumer N, Minguez J. Decoding upper limb movement attempt from EEG measurements of the contralesional motor cortex in chronic stroke patients. *IEEE Trans. Biomed. Eng.* 2017; **64**(1): 99–111.

Management of Vestibular Disorders in Neurorehabilitation

Adolfo M. Bronstein and Marousa Pavlou

9.1 Introduction

Postural control is mediated by central processes dependent on the integration of peripheral sensory inputs, mostly arising from the visual, proprioceptive, and vestibular systems. When balance is disrupted by illness, patients usually report unpleasant *subjective feelings* of dizziness, vertigo, and unsteadiness, which create considerable disability and disruption to working and social life. Patients may also suffer *objective loss* of balance and gait disorder, which, in extreme cases, may completely curtail a patient's autonomy. Subjective symptoms of dizziness or vertigo are more prominent in patients with peripheral vestibular disorders whereas objective gait unsteadiness is more prominent in central lesions.

Vertigo, dizziness, and postural as well as gait instability due to a vestibular impairment are highly prevalent [1]. Vestibular-related vertigo is a common symptom, with a one-year prevalence of 8.4% [2] and a lifetime prevalence of 7.8%, a female preponderance, and a three times increased likelihood in older versus younger adults [3]. The most common cause of recurrent vertigo is benign paroxysmal positional vertigo (BPPV). Posterior semicircular canal BPPV (PC-BPPV) is the most common type, accounting for 85–95% of patients [4]. However, the importance of BPPV remains underestimated due to low recognition rates at the primary care level and a lack of epidemiological studies [1]. In community samples, the commonest causes of vertigo also include migrainous vertigo and vestibular neuritis [3, 5]. Between 2001 and 2004, a national US audit identified that 35.4% of the population (69 million people) aged 40 years and older experienced a vestibular disorder [6]. However, this finding was based on a single test of standing on a foam surface with eyes closed, which has no validity or reliability information available [1], and therefore the accuracy of these findings is ambiguous.

In traumatic brain injury (TBI), dizziness due to trauma of the labyrinth and/or other vestibular structures is the most common symptom, followed closely by headache and cognitive-type symptoms [7]. Dizziness and imbalance due to trauma of the labyrinth and/or other vestibular structures after TBI are considered adverse prognostic factors that may lead to functional limitations and psychological distress, poor quality of life, and inability to return to work [8].

Vestibular dysfunction is also a major contributor to falls in older adults, with a prevalence of 80% in older adults over the age of 65 who have experienced two or more falls in the past 12 months and for which other falls causes have been excluded [9]. Recent literature reports a significantly higher risk of fractures, especially of the vertebra, ribs, and pelvis, in people with vertigo, particularly men and those over the age of 65 [10].

Vestibular dysfunction results in functional limitations with significant difficulties in performing activity of daily living tasks, particularly those involving a cognitive component (i.e., calculating finances) [11], and significantly increases falls risk [6]. Furthermore, older adults with vestibular disease predominately report difficulty walking, a constant anxiety, and fear of falling, resulting in limitation of and decreased participation in activities and increased social isolation, to the point of social withdrawal [11]. However, it is not just older adults who are negatively affected by vestibular dysfunction. In Germany, 80% of adults with a vestibular disorder require sick leave from work [12], while in a UK- and Italy-based study, 48% of people with dizziness report that they either have to change their occupation or give up work, in addition to significant disruption in their ability to travel and to participate in social and family life [13]. There is also a continuously growing body of evidence to support the association between vestibular disease and cognitive impairment [14].

Despite the high prevalence of vestibular impairment across a wide range of patient populations, healthcare service provision to address vestibular disease, and its impacts on the individual as well as its socio-economic costs, remains inadequate [15]. It is important that people reporting dizziness, vertigo, and/or instability are assessed for the presence of a vestibular impairment so that appropriate management can be instigated early, thus avoiding chronic illness.

9.2 Treatment Types

Treatment for dizziness and vestibular disorders varies according to the specific disease and stage. For instance, whereas a patient with vestibular neuritis may need intravenous (IV) hydration and anti-vertiginous drugs in the first couple of days of the acute phase of the illness, rehabilitation is the only useful treatment in the sub-acute and chronic stages.

9.2.1 Vestibular Rehabilitation

Vestibular rehabilitation (VR) should be the standard of care for persons with vestibular disease. An evidence-based clinical practice guideline from the American Physical Therapy Association (APTA) neurology sections states that VR should be offered to persons with unilateral and bilateral hypofunction [16]. A recent Cochrane review states that there is moderate-to-strong evidence to support VR as a safe, effective management for persons with vestibular disease [17], while Quantam-Yates et al. [18] reported that VR is a physical rehabilitation option with minimal risk for negative outcomes for individuals with continuing symptoms post mild TBI [18]. Vestibular rehabilitation strategies, though, are wide-ranging and vary from generic booklet-based care with no or minimal supervision [19] to customized VR incorporating virtual reality [20, 21].

The provision of VR varies widely depending on a clinician's professional background [22], resources, and healthcare service funding available while individualized assessment of deficits and specific VR programmes for different disorders are rare [22]. In addition, despite a strong body of evidence supporting the use of VR for the management of peripheral vestibular disorders, referrals to VR remain low. A qualitative study evaluating clinicians' (neurologists, primary care, otolaryngologists) perspectives regarding the factors which influenced their management of people with vestibular disorders found that they were often unaware of the concept of VR and wanted to learn more to improve healthcare delivery to their patients [23].

9.2.2 Repositioning Manoeuvres for the Management of BPPV

Repositioning manoeuvres to treat BPPV are highly effective, inexpensive, and easy to perform. As therapeutic efficacy is comparable amongst the manoeuvres available for each canal, the treatment chosen should be based on clinician preference, the patient's age, any musculoskeletal conditions, including arthritis or reduced range of motion of the cervical spine, and poor response to a specific manoeuvre/s [24]. Repeated manoeuvres in one session are superior to a single manoeuvre [24]. Clinicians also need to be aware that in approximately 6% of patients, PC-BPPV may convert to horizontal canal BPPV (HC-BPPV) [25]. Patients who suffer frequent recurrence of symptoms and who do not immediately respond to the manoeuvres or live a long distance away or in a remote area may be provided with a modified self-Epley to do at home [26].

It is important to note that BPPV often resolves without treatment with spontaneous resolution in untreated patients, although the time taken for this varies between weeks to years after onset. However, repositioning manoeuvres can be used to treat BPPV promptly and effectively.

9.2.3 Pharmacotherapy

Pharmacotherapy has been investigated for the management of symptoms in people with vestibular disorders. Low-quality evidence suggests that betahistine administered for three months or less may have a slight positive effect in reducing vertigo symptoms when compared to a placebo [27]. Few studies, though, compare VR with medication management for people with vestibular disorders. Horak et al. [28] reported that customized VR was superior to medication (valium or meclizine) for improving subjective symptoms of dizziness as well as objective postural sway in people with a unilateral peripheral vestibular disorder, with no improvements noted for the medication group. Shepard and Telian [29] found that using medication, such as vestibular suppressants, antidepressants, tranquilizers, and anticonvulsants, prolonged VR duration, and a longer period of time was required in order to achieve the same level of improvement as patients who were not using medication. For this reason, most specialists recommend that use of antiemetics for the acute phase of vertigo is only restricted to three or four days maximum. Recent reviews state that there is currently insufficient evidence to support the use of corticosteroids for management of symptoms in people with idiopathic acute vestibular dysfunction, such as vestibular neuritis; although there is some evidence showing that corticosteroids improve the recovery of vestibular function, this does not hold for clinical outcome in these patients [30]. No studies have systematically investigated the treatment of vestibular migraine and therefore no recommendations can be made [31]. However, acute attacks of vestibular migraine may respond to antimigraine medications such as triptans, and VR should be considered for patients with inter-ictal symptoms [32], including imbalance, dizziness, and/or visually induced dizziness. There is no evidence to support the use of symptomatic drug treatment as a substitute form of management for BPPV [33]. Medications may be used, though, for people with BPPV to relieve severe symptoms of nausea or vomiting, sometimes selectively used before proceeding to repositioning treatment manoeuvres in susceptible patients.

Non-operative therapy continues to be the mainstay of treatment of persons with Ménière's disease. Since the exact pathogenesis of Ménière's disease – characterized by acute attacks of rotational vertigo, transient fluctuations in hearing, tinnitus, and, many times, aural fullness – remains unknown and poorly understood, most treatments are aimed at controlling symptoms. A number of therapies have been utilized, ranging from dietary measures (e.g., a low-salt diet) and medication (e.g., betahistine, diuretics) to surgery (e.g., endolymphatic sac surgery). Betahistine is a licensed drug for Ménière's disease–like symptom complexes. A recent meta-analysis of published and unpublished placebo-controlled clinical studies using betahistine in people with vestibular vertigo or Ménière's disease supports the therapeutic benefit in both [34]. However, a Cochrane review reported that although it was acceptable to those who used it, there was insufficient evidence to show whether it had any effect on Ménière's disease [35] and a long-term, multicentre, double-blind, randomized controlled trial showed that betahistine treatment is ineffective in people with Ménière's disease [36]. Findings have shown a beneficial effect of intra-tympanic gentamicin in aggressive phases with frequent and severe vertigo episodes. This treatment is a minimally invasive outpatient procedure; however, as the therapeutic effects rely on gentamicin's ototoxic properties,

patients sustain a permanent vestibular deficit and hearing loss occurs in up to 20% of individuals. No definitive results were available for intra-tympanic corticosteroids until recently when a randomized controlled trial showed that the corticosteroid methylprednisolone administered via intra-tympanic injections is a non-ablative, effective treatment for refractory unilateral Ménière's disease [37]. Methylprednisolone and gentamicin were found to be equally effective (approximately 90% reduction in the number of vertigo attacks) and the decision regarding choice should be made based on individual clinical circumstances [37].

9.2.4 Surgery

Surgical procedures have been developed to reduce the symptoms of Ménière's disease and to treat intractable BPPV. A Cochrane review which considered interventions that either aim to conserve or abolish vestibular function in persons with Ménière's disease noted only two randomized controlled trials, both of which studied endolymphatic sac surgery. They concluded that there was insufficient evidence of the beneficial effect of endolymphatic sac surgery in Ménière's disease [38].

Repositioning manoeuvres, when performed correctly, are almost always effective. However, surgical procedures, including transection of the posterior ampullary nerve or fenestration and occlusion of the posterior semicircular canal, may occasionally be used as a last resort for people with severe and protracted symptoms of BPPV. Evidence regarding the efficacy of these surgical interventions is limited to case reports and series.

Due to the undoubted effectiveness of repositioning manoeuvres for BPPV and intra-tympanic injection for refractory Ménière's disease, the numbers of patients with these conditions requiring surgery are exceptionally small. As a consequence, there is insufficient evidence to support the use of surgery in the management of either Ménière's disease or BPPV, and therefore no further discussion on surgical interventions will be included.

9.3 Non-Pharmacological Treatments: Rationale, Technique, and Evidence

The APTA practice guidelines state that there is moderate evidence to support the use of specific exercise techniques to target identified impairments or functional limitations and for the provision of supervised VR [16]. This section focuses on a range of VR techniques, their rationale, and their evidence base.

9.3.1 Generic Booklet or Internet-Based VR

Generic booklet-based VR provides a generic set of eye, head, and body movement exercises in sitting, standing, and walking. A freely available generic VR booklet may be found at www.menieres.org.uk/information-and-support/treatment-and-management/vestibular-rehabilitation. The first part of the booklet aims to optimize adherence by explaining symptoms, addressing common concerns, and reporting positive outcomes in people with similar issues. Instructions are provided on how to carry out the exercises, for how long, and how to monitor progress and modify the exercises as appropriate. Yardley et al. [39] showed that generic booklet-based VR can be effectively implemented at the primary care level. Recently, this booklet has been developed into an Internet-based VR programme available at https://balance.lifeguidehealth.org/player/play/balance?thiz=meet-the-team, which may have additional advantages compared to a paper-based method, including provision of video instructions, automated tailoring, and symptom-related feedback. Initial findings show high user acceptance.

Generic booklet-based VR with additional telephone support (30 minutes at the start of the programme and two subsequent 15-minute sessions at weeks 1 and 3) provides some level of improvement to subjective symptoms [19]. The drop-out rate, though, is very high at approximately 60% versus 10% for customized VR programmes [40, 41], and improvements are not as significant. A clinically meaningful change is 18 points on a widely used subjective outcome measure, the Dizziness Handicap Inventory [42]. Customized VR studies achieve between a 17- and 24-point change [43, 44] compared with a 7-point change for booklet-based care with and without telephone support.

Minimal research exists into the cost-effectiveness of VR and is limited to analysis of generic booklet-based care to no intervention standard care [19]. However, the APTA VR practice guidelines [16] state that it is already known that vestibular exercises are beneficial when compared to no intervention, and

therefore this cost-analysis does not provide any true insight into value for money of VR interventions and further research is needed.

A multitude of studies in fact supports the use of customized, individualized VR [40, 43, 44]. This includes a comprehensive assessment of sensory systems involved in balance and the provision of exercises to treat each individual's identified impairment or functional limitations, address their individual goals, and focus on the concepts of habituation, adaptation, and sensory reweighting [16]. Therefore, the following section focuses on providing an overview of customized VR, including: (1) the physiologic basis and rationale; (2) customized VR, including novel techniques; (3) factors that may affect outcome; and (4) its efficacy for peripheral and central vestibular disorders.

9.3.2 Customized VR

9.3.2.1 Neurophysiological Basis and Rationale for VR

Habituation, adaptation, substitution, and/or sensory reweighting comprise the neurophysiological basis for vestibular compensation and the rationale for improvements noted following a VR programme, with recent findings showing structural changes in gray matter volume in certain brain areas after people with vestibular neuritis have recovered functionally [45].

Habituation is a decrease in the magnitude of the response to repetitive sensory stimuli [46]. Initial generic VR programmes such as the Cawthorne-Cooksey exercises are a type of habituation and involve repeating the provoking movement at regular intervals until symptoms are no longer experienced. However, although components of this exercises programme may still be used today, customized VR programmes which focus on an individual's deficits and incorporate exercises based on multiple neurophysiological components are more widely advocated.

The vestibulo-ocular reflex (VOR) is responsible for our ability to maintain fixation on a target during head movement. The VOR functions to stabilize images on the retina during head movement by producing compensatory eye movements, simultaneously and at the same rate, in the direction opposite to head movement. In people with a peripheral vestibular disorder, the VOR gain can be impaired, resulting in retinal image slip with visual blurring during head rotations. Retinal image slip provides an error signal which generates VOR response changes that decrease (i.e., improve) the gaze error. Adaptation exercises [47] (please refer to Section 9.3.2.2) incorporating gaze fixation and head movements are prescribed to simulate retinal slip to promote VOR improvement with a reduction in blurring of the visual image during head movement. Saccadic substitution and specifically compensatory saccades (the substitution of a saccade in the direction of the deficient VOR) also contribute to improvements in VOR performance with a decrease in gaze instability [48].

Sensory reweighting is the central nervous system's ability to adapt its relative reliance on a specific sensory modality for orientation depending on environment conditions, task demands, and/or pathology [6]. Therefore, if a sensory input is reduced, absent, or unreliable, other sensory inputs are centrally up-regulated or weighted-up. For instance, in the dark or in the presence of unstable visual surroundings, when visuo-postural responses are unavailable or unreliable, respectively, the efficiency of vestibulo-proprioceptive responses increases whereas, visuo-postural responses are down-regulated. Similarly, a patient with uni- or bilateral vestibular failure will develop increased postural responses to visual motion stimulation. It is thought that by performing exercises in environments with altered sensory information, vestibular rehabilitation is able to affect a person's use of sensory information or sensory reweighting.

Visually induced dizziness, or visual vertigo, is a term which refers to feelings of discomfort, imbalance, or dizzy symptom exacerbation that occurs in challenging visual environments such as supermarkets. It is believed that improvements noted in visually induced dizziness following a customized VR programme incorporating exposure to optokinetic stimulation is due to a decreased over-reliance on visual input for perceptual and postural responses and a more effective use of vestibulo-proprioceptive cues through sensory reweighting [49]. Overall, however, the central mechanisms mediating sensory reweighting in postural control remain poorly understood.

9.3.2.2 Customized VR Techniques

A thorough assessment is required prior to the onset of customized VR. Treatment goals are then devised to address each person's individual subjective (i.e., dizziness, oscillopsia, nausea) and objective

symptoms (postural and gait instability, falls). These goals often include to (1) improve functional balance, gait, and ability to perform daily activities; (2) decrease falls risk; (3) decrease symptom severity; (4) improve VOR function; (5) improve sensory integration and reweighting ability; and (6) patient education.

Adaptation Exercises

VR should be based on the eye, head, and postural exercises that provoke a patient's symptoms. Adaptation exercises [47] (see Figures 9.1a and 9.1b) incorporating gaze fixation and head movements and postural exercises are prescribed to promote recovery of VOR and vestibulo-spinal reflex function. Gaze fixation exercises are practised with varying target distances (i.e., 2 m, 1 m, 1/2 m) since VOR gain varies with target distance (closer targets require slightly higher gains). Fixation exercises are given to patients with oscillopsia and/or decreased VOR gain, most often seen in peripheral vestibular disorders.

Gaze transfer

Gaze stability (VOR)

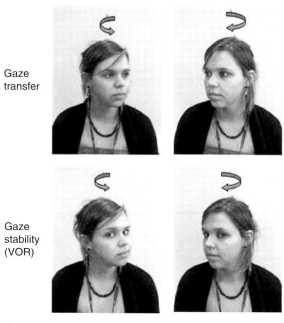

Figures 9.1a and 9.1b Gaze transfer and adaptation exercises [84] included within a vestibular rehabilitation programme. During 'gaze transfer' (a), the normal head and eye movement required for transferring gaze from one object to another is practised.
The exercise can initially be practised without head movements with objects placed approximately 40 cm apart at eye level. During adaptation exercises (b), the vestibulo-ocular reflex (VOR) is being stimulated, which is responsible for maintaining a steady gaze on a fixated object with progressively faster head movements.

Saccades can support higher-speed functional eye movements in people with bilateral vestibular hypofunction in whom the VOR gain is extremely reduced or absent. Patients are asked to practise saccadic or gaze transfer exercises whereby they quickly shift their gaze between two horizontal or vertical targets. As the VR programme progresses, the complexity and difficulty of exercises should increase and therefore exercises will be practised sitting, standing, and walking on level ground or compliant surfaces, e.g., foam. Table 9.1 includes examples of commonly prescribed exercises, which can be viewed on a DVD [50].

Retraining Postural Alignment and Movement Strategies

Many people with a vestibular disorder will experience some level of balance and gait dysfunction. Exercises which focus on retraining postural alignment, and movement strategies, may need to be incorporated whereby patients learn to maintain an upright posture during progressively more difficult tasks, including eyes closed and standing on compliant surfaces, with progressively reduced feedback about position [51]. The goal when retraining movement strategies is to develop those successful in moving the centre of gravity relative to a stationary base of support (ankle or hip strategy) and changing the base of support relative to the centre of gravity (stepping strategy). Retraining a coordinated ankle or hip strategy involves practising voluntary anterio-posterior and lateral sway, without taking a step. Facilitating a hip strategy involves faster and larger displacements than an ankle strategy and may include activities such as tandem or single-leg stance. Retraining externally induced postural responses involves pushes or pulls of various amplitudes, speed, and direction applied at the hips or shoulders, or the use of moving surfaces. Stepping can be practised by shifting the patient's weight to one side and then quickly bringing the centre of gravity back towards the unweighted leg, or in response to large anterio-posterior or lateral

Table 9.1 Examples of commonly prescribed exercises in vestibular rehabilitation

Head exercises (performed with eyes open and eyes closed)
Bend head backwards and forwards
Turn head from side to side
Eye movement exercises
Head stationary, follow movement of finger left and right/up and down
Head movement to look back and forth between two vertical or horizontal targets
Visual fixation exercises
Perform head exercises while fixating on a stationary target
Perform head exercises while fixating on a moving target
Positioning exercises (performed with eyes open and closed)
While seated, bend down to touch the floor
While seated, turn to look over shoulder both to the left and the right
Bend down with head turned first to one side and then the other
Lying down, roll from one side to the other
Sit up from lying supine and on each side
Postural exercises (performed eyes open; eyes closed under supervision)
Practise static stance with feet as close together as possible
Practise standing on one leg, and heel-to-toe
Repeat head and fixation exercises while standing and then walking
Practise walking in circles, pivot turns, up slopes, stairs, around obstacles
Stand and walk in environments with altered surface and/or visual conditions with and without head and fixation exercises
Aerobic exercises, e.g., alternative touching the fingers to the toes, trunk bends, and rotation.

perturbations. Multidirectional stepping and stepping over a visual target or obstacle can also be practised [51]. The simplest way of eliciting corrective stepping postural responses is by pushing or pulling at the hip or shoulder level. Patient safety has to be carefully monitored; initially, an assistant may be needed. Delivering trunk pulls from behind the patient in a corner of the room may be sufficient (Figures 9.2a and 2b). If after a trunk pull the patient falls backwards, the clinician has to be prepared to catch them, but if they fall forwards, the patient can use their arms to steady themselves. Patients with peripheral vestibular disorders are not at risk of falling during this training; only patients with severe central nervous system disorders will show a clear tendency to fall.

Sensory Reweighting

When the ability to select appropriate sensory input for postural stability is disrupted, exercises focus on asking patients to maintain balance in situations where the availability and accuracy of one or more sensory inputs is varied [52].

Sensory strategy retraining aims to help people with a vestibular disorder learn to effectively select appropriate sensory information for balance in various environments. Treatment focuses on maintaining balance during progressively more difficult static and dynamic balance and gait exercises while the availability and accuracy of sensory input is systematically varied. People with vestibular lesions who over-rely on somatosensory cues for orientation – i.e. difficulty when walking on uneven surfaces, changing between different types of floor surface – practise tasks while sitting, standing, or walking on surfaces with disrupted somatosensory cues such as compliant foam, moving platforms, or tilt boards. For people with a visual dependency, this involves exercises where visual input is incorrect, conflicting, or absent, in order to learn to rely more on proprioceptive and available vestibular cues [49]. Guerraz et al. [53] suggested that rehabilitation programmes promoting desensitization and increased tolerance to visual stimuli through exposure to visual motion (i.e., optokinetic

A

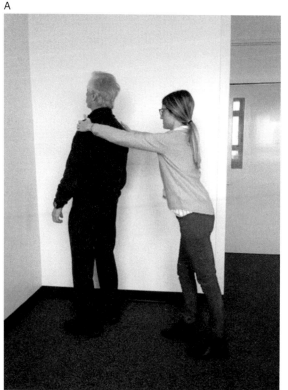

B

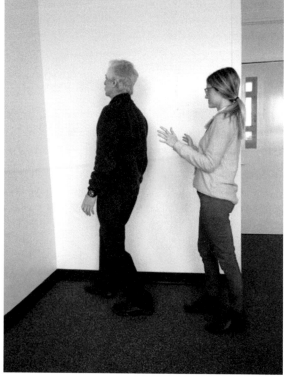

Figures 9.2a and 9.2b The clinician stands behind the patient and pulls him back from the trunk (a). This subject shows a normal, single-step response (b). The clinician remains ready to catch the patient should he show excessive retropulsion or fall risk.

A

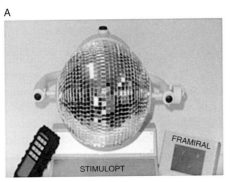

B

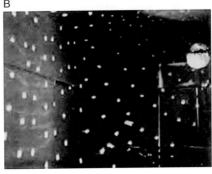

Figures 9.3a and 9.3b Apparatus used for full-field optokinetic stimulation-based intervention [5]. (a). A photo of the visual environment rotator apparatus (Stimulopt, Framiral, France) (b). Participants are asked to stare ahead while the apparatus rotates in different directions and at differing speeds. Participants practise exercises sitting, standing, and walking either towards or away from the stimulus or alongside it with or without vertical or horizontal head movements.

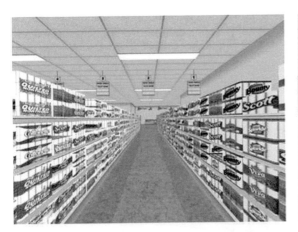

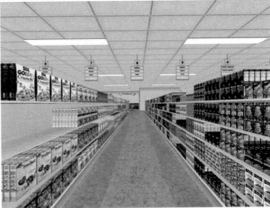

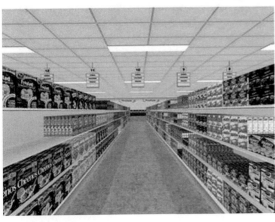

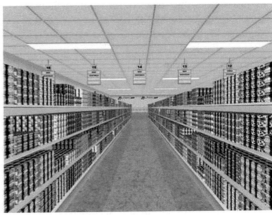

Figure 9.4 Four aisles from a virtual reality supermarket are shown [56]. The four images show a progression in visual complexity.

stimulation) would be specifically beneficial for patients with visual vertigo. Advanced techniques in VR incorporate exposure to optokinetic stimuli (Figures 9.3a and 9.3b) [40] or virtual reality (Figure 9.4) [54] environments. When optokinetic stimulation has been incorporated into both the treatment session and home programme, improvements have been noted in postural and gait stability, visually induced dizziness, and psychological state, including depression and anxiety [40]. Easily accessible and economical computer games, YouTube videos, or a DVD including visual stimulation recorded from the clinical equipment, i.e. optokinetic test in neuro-otology departments [55], can also be used. Regardless of the type of optokinetic or virtual reality stimulus employed, exposure should be gradual and progressive.

Dual-Task Activities

People with a vestibular disorder may complain of poor concentration and memory impairment, and a cognitive–vestibular function interaction has been highlighted in this population [11]. People with a vestibular disorder appear to have decreased attentional resources available when simultaneously performing a cognitive and posture or gait tasks (i.e., dual tasking), with priority given to maintaining the motor task to the detriment of performance on the cognitive task [56]. More recent studies investigating gait performance while performing a simultaneous cognitive task (dual-task) consistently show a significantly decreased gait speed and greater ataxia and deviation from a linear path in this population when dual-tasking [57]. Although no studies have specifically assessed the impact of incorporating dual-task training within a VR programme, findings in older adults with increased falls risk show an increase in dual-task gait speed after training [58], and clinicians often include dual-task training in VR programmes when a functional deficit is noted in this area. Dual-task training involves practising progressive balance exercises, e.g., tandem standing or walking with or without upper limb activities, while simultaneously performing a secondary cognitive task such as counting backwards by three, recounting daily activities, or writing a text message [59]. During training, patients are asked to either constantly maintain attention on both tasks or focus attention on one of them [59].

Motor, sensory, and cognitive strategy retraining should occur in parallel rather than sequentially. General characteristics of VR include specificity, repetition, progression, and patient education, e.g., initially symptoms may worsen and improvement may be uneven. Patients should be aware that even after symptoms have largely resolved, a temporary reoccurrence may occur during periods of stress, fatigue, or illness. Patients should be advised to stop exercising and seek advice if they experience neck pain, loss of consciousness or vision, sensations of numbness, weakness, or tingling in the face or limbs, or increased migraine frequency.

Virtual Reality-Based Techniques

Various authors have discussed the potential benefit of virtual reality as a therapeutic protocol to improve postural and gait stability, VOR gain, and subjective symptoms [16]. Using a limited field-of-view head-mounted device, improvements have been noted in VOR gain and symptoms in patients with a peripheral vestibular disorder. Two randomized controlled trials comparing customized VR and virtual reality-based VR reported no significant pre-post treatment between-group differences in gait speed, functional gait performance, computerized dynamic posturography, or subjective symptoms despite one study using a full-field immersive virtual environment consisting of a grocery store model [54] while in the other, the low-cost Nintendo Wii Fit Plus (Figure 9.5) was

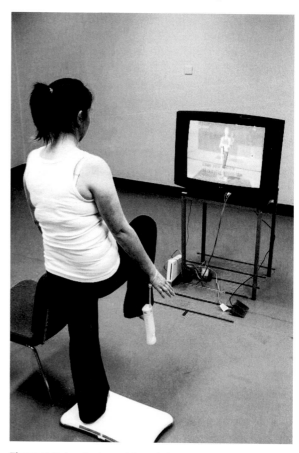

Figure 9.5 A patient practising a balance exercise using the Nintendo Wii Fit Plus® system [21]

employed [21]. The lack of difference in findings between the two types of virtual reality may be due to the fact that both small- and large-field optokinetic stimulation show similar reciprocally inhibitory visual–vestibular interactions, indicating that sensory reweighting occurs independent of visual field size and other factors, including frequency, velocity, texture, stimulus area, and position within the visual field. Pavlou et al. [40] reported that this may explain why significant improvements were noted for both full and limited field-of-view optokinetic stimulation without significant between-group differences in their study.

Sessoms et al. [60], however, reported that 12 sessions of virtual reality exposure without additional VR provided greater benefit in gait speed and weight shift in people with TBI and vestibular dysfunction compared to virtual reality (six sessions) plus VR (six sessions). It is important to note that balance and vestibular exercises were practised during exposure to the virtual reality environment, thus providing multidimensional tasking. Multitasking provides a more demanding form of VR. Therefore, it may possibly be more appropriate than traditional techniques for people who need more challenging tasks or are required to operate at a higher level of performance in their profession (e.g., athletes, military servicemen) [61].

Current literature therefore suggests that virtual reality is beneficial and may offer a more enjoyable exercise method, particularly with regard to the Nintendo Wii system [21]. Further work, however, is needed to identify the specific role of virtual reality within VR with regard to the patients groups it is most suitable for and optimal virtual reality format.

Factors Affecting Outcome

The relationship between psychological and dizziness symptoms is well documented as is the significant correlation between depression and anxiety in people with vestibular dysfunction [62, 63]. People who experience higher levels of somatic anxiety report greater handicap [64] and show a delay in recovery [65]. Every effort should be made to identify and act on these negative factors, referring the patient for counselling and/or adding psychopharmacological medication as appropriate. Studies combining VR with explicit cognitive behavioural therapy demonstrate improvements in patients' ability to cope, function, subjective symptoms, and satisfaction with care

[66, 67]. However, the clear additional effect of combining cognitive behavioural therapy with VR remains unknown.

People with peripheral or central vestibular disorders may experience visuo-motor symptoms, such as oscillopsia or diplopia, which are capable of disrupting recovery and rehabilitation. Rehabilitation specialists should enquire directly about such symptoms. It has recently been reported that binocular vision abnormalities may affect the improvement of visually induced dizziness symptoms, and these findings may have important implications for the management of subjects with refractory vestibular symptoms [68]. Clinicians need to be aware of the possible negative effect of this type of binocular abnormality on visually induced dizziness treatment outcome in order to manage their own and the client's expectations from treatment.

Patients with vestibular migraine can adhere to and benefit from VR [69]. However, Bronstein and Pavlou [51] reported that in their experience of treating patients with migraine-associated dizziness, an initial exercise programme including fewer exercises, i.e. three maximum, is better tolerated and adhered to. The exercises should be practised only once daily initially and gradually increased to twice daily. As symptoms and tolerance improve, the number and total duration of daily exercises progressively increases. It is important for improvement to be noted with exercises such as those in Table 9.1 before progressing to the inclusion of optokinetic stimuli.

Other factors that may impact VR treatment outcome may be found in Table 9.2.

Efficacy of Customized VR

Customized VR programmes provide greater benefit than generic ones (Cawthorne-Cooksey) [16]. A recent Cochrane review validated the safety and effectiveness of VR for the management of unilateral vestibular dysfunction [17].

People with bilateral vestibular hypofunction (BVH) have an increased falls risk. In one study, a significant percentage of participants with BVH reported that they had to alter or change their professional activities and/or required the presence of another person due to the level of disability they experienced [70]. A number of studies report significant improvements in gaze, postural and gait stability, balance confidence, subjective symptoms, and perceived handicap from dizziness in people with BVH

Table 9.2 Factors that may delay vestibular compensation

- Fluctuating vestibular disorder (i.e., Ménière's disease)
- Migraine
- Additional disorder:
  - Central Nervous System
  - Peripheral nerve
  - Cervical spine
  - Visual (reduced visual acuity, modified optics [e.g., cataract operation], strabismus, diplopia)
- Age
- Lack of mobility (orthopaedic problem, forced bedrest, psychological/fear)
- Medication (anti-vertiginous drugs)
- Psychosocial
- Visually induced dizziness

Adapted from Bronstein and Pavlou [55]

with a systematic review stating that there is moderate-strength evidence to support VR for improvements in gaze and postural stability [71]. Further work is needed, though, to identify its benefit for ICF-Participation outcome measures.

In people with Ménière's disease, management has been challenging due to recurring vertigo episodes. Specifically for VR, significant improvements in postural stability, subjective symptoms, and quality of life have been noted with customized VR physical exercises [72] or incorporating balance exercises with exposure to a virtual reality platform [73].

Some studies report similar responses for patients with peripheral, central, and mixed pathology, but others claim poorer outcomes for the latter two groups. Differing results may be due to individual study variations regarding treatment duration (patients with central deficits are expected to require a longer duration for improvement), extent and location of central deficit (cerebellar dysfunction appears to reduce the effect of rehabilitation), and any additional cognitive or neuromuscular deficits. Cerebellar and vascular disease and traumatic brain injuries (including concussion) are examples of central vestibular disorders associated with dizziness.

Current evidence suggests VR can improve dizziness, gait, and postural stability after mild TBI (or concussion) [74]. In people with persistent neck pain, headaches, and/or dizziness following a sports-related concussion, the time to return to sports is reduced following a programme of VR

combined with cervical exercises [75]. McCulloch et al. [76] published clinical guidelines for rehabilitation providers regarding progressive return to activity after mild TBI, and VR was recommended for those experiencing persistent dizziness and/or balance symptoms.

As stated earlier, people with vestibular migraine significantly benefit from a VR programme [69]. Patients with vestibular migraine or migraine history and a peripheral vestibular disorder can also tolerate and benefit from customized VR incorporating optokinetic exposure; surprisingly, migraineurs report significantly greater improvements for visually induced dizziness compared to non-migraineurs [40]. It has been suggested that medication may help control visually induced dizziness symptoms in migraineurs, enabling them to better tolerate the exercises, leading to greater improvement [69]. However, Vitkovic et al. [77] reported that a six-month VR programme without optokinetic exposure showed similar improvements in both participants with vestibular migraine and those with vestibular symptoms without migraine, and for the former, improvements were noted regardless of medication regime, although medication was not controlled for.

9.3.3 Repositioning Manoeuvres for BPPV: Rationale, Techniques, and Evidence Base

Posterior canal (PC) BPPV can be treated effectively with an Epley or Semont manoeuvre, which induces the return of otolithic debris from the posterior canal back into the utricle, where the debris no longer produces positional vertigo. The procedure can be repeated immediately to see if positional vertigo and nystagmus are still present as this increases the success rate to more than 90%. In patients with, for example, vertebrobasilar insufficiency, cervical spondylosis, or lower back problems, certain aspects of the Epley or Semont are contraindicated, including neck hyperextension or the rapid lateral motion of the Semont. The Gans repositioning manoeuvre, a hybrid treatment incorporating elements of both the Semont and Epley manoeuvres, but avoiding the neck hyperextension part of the Epley, was developed for these individuals. Outcomes for all three manoeuvres are comparable [78]. The efficacy of repositioning manoeuvres is not improved by post-treatment postural restrictions. Repositioning manoeuvres in 360° rotating devices can also be implemented successfully [79] and do not produce neck or back strain on the patient.

Manoeuvres that can be used to treat horizontal canal (HC) BPPV with geotropic (i.e., beating towards the ground) nystagmus include: (a) the patient lies on their healthy side for 12 consecutive hours [80] (NB: the healthy side is usually the one that elicits less vertigo and nystagmus); (b) Gufoni's manoeuvre, whereby a patient will quickly lie down on the side of the unaffected ear, remain in this position for one to two minutes, until the nystagmus subsides, followed by the head being quickly rotated 45° towards the floor and maintained in this position for a further two minutes, after which the patient returns to an upright position; and (c) the 'barbecue rotation' whereby the patient lies supine and is rotated 270° in the horizontal canal plane towards the healthy ear in three successive 90° steps at 30-second intervals and is then brought to a sitting position. Horizontal canal BPPV resolves in approximately 70% of patients after one session using any of these approaches with no treatment found to be superior over the others regarding success rate [81]. In geotropic nystagmus, the Gufoni manoeuvre is, however, considered superior for ease of performance.

A modified Gufoni or Semont manoeuvre may be used for BPPV involving the horizontal canal with apogeotropic (away from the ground) nystagmus as well as a barbeque manoeuvre, supine head roll, or head shaking. Supine head roll involves turning the head approximately 90° to each side left and right while the patients is in a supine position. The head-shaking method involves shaking the head side to side for two cycles/s for 15 seconds. The barbecue and Gufoni manoeuvres have comparable success rates for HC-BPPV with ageotrophic nystagmus.

Although repositioning manoeuvres are highly effective, post-traumatic BPPV appears more difficult to treat than idiopathic BPPV and has a higher recurrence rate [82]. Randomized trials have compared the effectiveness of various manoeuvres for specific types of BPPV; it is not clear which manoeuvre is the most effective for each type. It is also unclear what strategy should be pursued if the initial manoeuvre is not effective. It is currently unknown whether (a) the same or a different manoeuvre should be performed if one is unsuccessful; (b) vitamin D supplementation has a preventative effect for the risk of incident as well as recurrence; and (c) the efficacy of repositioning manoeuvres for the more rare anterior canal BPPV [83].

9.4 Conclusion

Vestibular impairment is highly prevalent across a wide range of patient populations and has a significant impact on quality of life, ability to work or attend to educational activities, school, travel, or social interactions. VR is the mainstay of treatment for people with peripheral vestibular disorder, although pharmacological treatment has been shown to be beneficial under certain circumstances, particularly the acute phase of a vertigo attack. BPPV repositioning manoeuvres are highly effective. Evidence is emerging for the benefit of VR in people with central vestibular disorders, particularly mild TBI. Vestibular rehabilitation should be informed by assessment and individually designed based on each person's impairments. Further work is needed regarding optimum interventions, treatment duration, long-term outcome, and the efficacy and the potential benefit of novel techniques, like virtual reality.

References

1. Neuhauser HK. The epidemiology of dizziness and vertigo. *Handb. Clin. Neurol.* 2016; **137**: 67–82.

2. Bigelow RT, Semenov YR, du Lac S, Hoffman HJ, Agrawal Y.Vestibular vertigo and comorbid cognitive and psychiatric impairment: The 2008 National Health Interview Survey. *J. Neurol. Neurosurg. Psychiatry* 2016; **87**(4): 367–72.

3. Neuhauser HK, von Brevern M, Radtke A, et al. Epidemiology of vestibular vertigo: A neurotologic survey of the general population. *Neurology* 2005; **65**(6): 898–904.

4. Parnes LS, Agrawal SK, Atlas J. Diagnosis and management of benign paroxysmal positional vertigo (BPPV). *CMAJ* 2003; **169**(7): 681–93.

5. Sekitani TIY, Noguchi T, Inokuma T. Vestibular neuritis: Epidemiological survey by questionnaire in Japan. *Acta Oto-Laryngologica* (Suppl.) 1993; **503**: 9–12.

6. Agrawal Y, Carey JP, Della Santina CC, Schubert MC, Minor LB. Disorders of balance and vestibular function in US adults: Data from the National Health and Nutrition Examination Survey, 2001–2004. *Arch. Intern. Med.* 2009; **169**(10): 938–44.

7. Hoffer ME. Mild traumatic brain injury: Neurosensory effects. *Curr. Opin. Neurol.* 2015; **28**(1): 74–7.

8. Maskell F, Chiarelli P, Isles R. Dizziness after traumatic brain injury: Results from an interview study. *Brain Inj.* 2007; **21**(7): 741–52.

9. Liston MB, Bamiou DE, Martin F, et al. Peripheral vestibular dysfunction is prevalent in older adults

experiencing multiple non-syncopal falls versus age-matched non-fallers: A pilot study. *Age Ageing* 2014; **43**(1): 38–43.

10. Liao WL, Chang TP, Chen HJ, Kao CH. Benign paroxysmal positional vertigo is associated with an increased risk of fracture: A population-based cohort study. *J. Orthop. Sports Phys. Ther.* 2015; **45**(5): 406–12.

11. Harun A, Semenov YR, Agrawal Y. Vestibular function and activities of daily living: Analysis of the 1999 to 2004 National Health and Nutrition Examination Surveys. *Gerontol. Geriatr. Med.* 2015; 1.

12. von Brevern M, Radtke A, Lezius F, et al. Epidemiology of benign paroxysmal positional vertigo: A population based study. *J. Neurol. Neurosurg. Psychiatry* 2007; **78** (7): 710–15.

13. Bronstein AM, Golding JF, Gresty MA, et al. The social impact of dizziness in London and Siena. *J. Neurol.* 2010; **257**(2): 183–90.

14. Harun A, Oh ES, Bigelow RT, Studenski S, Agrawal Y. Vestibular impairment in dementia. *Otol. Neurotol.* 2016; **37**(8): 1137–42.

15. Royal College of Physicians. Hearing and balance disorders: Achieving excellence in diagnosis and management. Report of a working party. London, UK, 2007.

16. Hall CD, Herdman SJ, Whitney SL, et al. Vestibular rehabilitation for peripheral vestibular hypofunction: An evidence-based clinical practice guideline: From the American Physical Therapy Association Neurology Section. *J. Neurol. Phys. Ther.* 2016; **40**(2): 124–55.

17. Hillier S, McDonnell M. Is vestibular rehabilitation effective in improving dizziness and function after unilateral peripheral vestibular hypofunction? An abridged version of a Cochrane Review. *Eur. J. Phys. Rehabil. Med.* 2016; **52**(4): 541–56.

18. Quatman-Yates C, Cupp A, Gunsch C, Haley T, Vaculik S, Kujawa D. Physical rehabilitation interventions for post-mTBI symptoms lasting sreater than 2 weeks: Systematic review. *Phys. Ther.* 2016; **96** (11): 1753–63.

19. Yardley L, Barker F, Muller I, et al. Clinical and cost effectiveness of booklet based vestibular rehabilitation for chronic dizziness in primary care: Single blind, parallel group, pragmatic, randomised controlled trial. *BMJ* 2012; **344**: e2237.

20. Pavlou M, Kanegaonkar RG, Swapp D, Bamiou DE, Slater M, Luxon LM. The effect of virtual reality on visual vertigo symptoms in patients with peripheral vestibular dysfunction: A pilot study. *J. Vestib. Res.* 2012; **22**(5–6): 273–81.

21. Meldrum D, Herdman S, Vance R, et al. Effectiveness of conventional versus virtual reality-based balance exercises in vestibular rehabilitation for unilateral peripheral vestibular loss: results of a randomized controlled trial. *Arch. Phys. Med. Rehabil.* 2015; **96**(7): 1319–28 e1311.

22. Tjernstrom F, Zur O, Jahn K. Current concepts and future approaches to vestibular rehabilitation. *J. Neurol.* 2016; **263** Suppl. 1: S65–70.

23. Polensek SH, Tusa RJ, Sterk CE. The challenges of managing vestibular disorders: A qualitative study of clinicians' experiences associated with low referral rates for vestibular rehabilitation. *Int. J. Clin. Pract.* 2009; **63**(11): 1604–12.

24. Gold DR, Morris L, Kheradmand A, Schubert MC. Repositioning maneuvers for benign paroxysmal positional vertigo. *Curr. Treat. Options. Neurol.* 2014; **16**(8): 307.

25. Bhattacharyya N, Baugh RF, Orvidas L, et al. Clinical practice guideline: Benign paroxysmal positional vertigo. *Otolaryngol. Head Neck Surg.* 2008; **139**(5 Suppl. 4): S47–81.

26. Radtke A, von Brevern M, Tiel-Wilck K, Mainz-Perchalla A, Neuhauser H, Lempert T. Self-treatment of benign paroxysmal positional vertigo: Semont maneuver vs Epley procedure. *Neurology* 2004; **63**(1): 150–2.

27. Murdin L, Hussain K, Schilder AG. Betahistine for symptoms of vertigo. *Cochrane Database of Systematic Reviews* 2016; **6**: CD010696.

28. Horak FB, Jones-Rycewicz C, Black FO, Shumway-Cook A. Effects of vestibular rehabilitation on dizziness and imbalance. *Otolaryngol. Head Neck Surg.* 1992; **106**(2): 175–80.

29. Shepard NT, Telian SA, Smith-Wheelock M. Habituation and balance retraining therapy: A retrospective review. *Neurol. Clin.* 1990; **8**(2): 459–75.

30. Fishman JM, Burgess C, Waddell A. Corticosteroids for the treatment of idiopathic acute vestibular dysfunction (vestibular neuritis). *Cochrane Database of Systematic Reviews.* 2011; **5**: CD008607.

31. Strupp M, Zwergal A, Feil K, Bremova T, Brandt T. Pharmacotherapy of vestibular and cerebellar disorders and downbeat nystagmus: Translational and back-translational research. *Ann. N. Y. Acad. Sci.* 2015; **1343**: 27–36.

32. Furman JM, Balaban CD. Vestibular migraine. *Ann. N. Y. Acad. Sci.* 2015; **1343**: 90–6.

33. National Institute for Health and Care Excellence (NICE). *Benign paroxysmal positional vertigo: Clinical knowledge summaries.* London, UK: National Institute for Health and Care Excellence, 2013.

34. Nauta JJ. Meta-analysis of clinical studies with betahistine in Ménière's disease and vestibular vertigo. *Eur. Arch. Otorhinolaryngol.* 2014; **271**(5): 887–97.

35. James ALBM. Betahistine for Ménière's disease or syndrome. *Cochrane Database of Systematic Reviews* 2001. Issue 1. Art. No.: CD001873. doi:10.1002/14651858.CD001873

36. Adrion C, Fischer CS, Wagner J, et al. Efficacy and safety of betahistine treatment in patients with Meniere's disease: Primary results of a long term, multicentre, double blind, randomised, placebo controlled, dose defining trial (BEMED trial). *BMJ* 2016; **352**: h6816.

37. Patel M, Agarwal K, Arshad Q, et al. Intratympanic methylprednisolone versus gentamicin in patients with unilateral Ménière's disease: A randomised, double-blind, comparative effectiveness trial. *Lancet* 2016; **388** (10061): 2753–62.

38. Pullens B, Verschuur HP, van Benthem PP. Surgery for Ménière's disease. *Cochrane Database of Systematic Reviews* 2013; **2**: CD005395.

39. Yardley L, Donovan-Hall M, Smith HE, Walsh BM, Mullee M, Bronstein AM. Effectiveness of primary care-based vestibular rehabilitation for chronic dizziness. *Ann. Intern. Med.* 2004; **141**(8): 598–605.

40. Pavlou M, Bronstein AM, Davies RA. Randomized trial of supervised versus unsupervised optokinetic exercise in persons with peripheral vestibular disorders. *Neurorehabil. Neural Repair.* 2013; **27**(3): 208–18.

41. Pavlou M, Lingeswaran A, Davies RA, Gresty MA, Bronstein AM. Simulator based rehabilitation in refractory dizziness. *J. Neurol.* 2004; **251**(8): 983–95.

42. Jacobson GP, Newman CW. The development of the Dizziness Handicap Inventory. *Arch. Otolaryngol. Head Neck Surg.* 1990; **116**(4): 424–7.

43. AlMohiza MA, Sparto PJ, Marchetti GF, et al. A quality improvement project in balance and vestibular rehabilitation and its effect on clinical outcomes. *J. Neurol. Phys. Ther.* 2016; **40**(2): 90–9.

44. Tsukamoto HF, Costa Vde S, Silva RAJ, et al. Effectiveness of a vestibular rehabilitation protocol to improve the health-related quality of life and postural balance in patients with vertigo. *Int. Arch. Otorhinolaryngol.* 2015; **19**(3): 238–47.

45. Hong SK, Kim JH, Kim HJ, Lee HJ. Changes in the gray matter volume during compensation after vestibular neuritis: A longitudinal VBM study. *Restor. Neurol. Neurosci.* 2014; **32**(5): 663–73.

46. Young LR. Models for neurovestibular adaptation. *J. Vestib. Res.* 2003; **13**(4–6): 297–307.

47. Tusa RJHS. Vertigo and disequilibrium. In Johnson RGJ. ed. *Current therapy in neurological disease.* 4th edn. St Louis, MO: Mosby Yearbook, 1983.

48. Schubert MC, Hall CD, Das V, Tusa RJ, Herdman SJ. Oculomotor strategies and their effect on reducing gaze position error. *Otol. Neurotol.* 2010; **31**(2): 228–31.

49. Shumway-Cook A, Horak FB. Rehabilitation strategies for patients with vestibular deficits. *Neurol. Clin.* 1990; **8**(2): 441–57.

50. Bronstein AMLT. *Dizziness with downloadable video: A practical approach to diagnosis and management.* 2nd edn. Cambridge, UK: Cambridge University Press, 2017.

51. Bronstein AM, Pavlou M. Balance. *Handb. Clin. Neurol.* 2013; **110**: 189–208.

52. Pavlou M. The use of optokinetic stimulation in vestibular rehabilitation. *J. Neurol. Phys. Ther.* 2010; **34** (2): 105–10.

53. Guerraz M, Yardley L, Bertholon P, et al. Visual vertigo: Symptom assessment, spatial orientation and postural control. *Brain.* 2001; **124**(Pt. 8): 1646–56.

54. Alahmari KA, Sparto PJ, Marchetti GF, Redfern MS, Furman JM, Whitney SL. Comparison of virtual reality based therapy with customized vestibular physical therapy for the treatment of vestibular disorders. *IEEE Trans. Neural Syst. Rehabil. Eng.* 2014; **22**(2): 389–99.

55. Wrisley DM, Pavlou M. Physical therapy for balance disorders. *Neurol. Clin.* 2005; **23**(3): 855–74, vii–viii.

56. Nascimbeni A, Gaffuri A, Penno A, Tavoni M. Dual task interference during gait in patients with unilateral vestibular disorders. *J. Neuroeng. Rehabil.* 2010; 7: 47.

57. Roberts JC, Cohen HS, Sangi-Haghpeykar H. Vestibular disorders and dual task performance: Impairment when walking a straight path. *J. Vestib. Res.* 2011; **21**(3): 167–74.

58. Silsupadol P, Lugade V, Shumway-Cook A, et al. Training-related changes in dual-task walking performance of elderly persons with balance impairment: S double-blind, randomized controlled trial. *Gait Posture* 2009; **29**(4): 634–9.

59. Silsupadol P, Shumway-Cook A, Lugade V, et al. Effects of single-task versus dual-task training on balance performance in older adults: A double-blind, randomized controlled trial. *Arch. Phys. Med. Rehabil.* 2009; **90**(3): 381–7.

60. Sessoms PH, Gottshall KR, Collins JD, Markham AE, Service KA, Reini SA. Improvements in gait speed and weight shift of persons with traumatic brain injury and vestibular dysfunction using a virtual reality computer-assisted rehabilitation environment. *Mil. Med.* 2015; **180**(3 Suppl.): 143–9.

61. Gottshall KR, Sessoms PH. Improvements in dizziness and imbalance results from using a multi disciplinary and multi sensory approach to vestibular physical therapy: A case study. *Front. Syst. Neurosci.* 2015; **9**: 106.

62. Eagger S, Luxon LM, Davies RA, Coelho A, Ron MA. Psychiatric morbidity in patients with peripheral vestibular disorder: A clinical and neuro-otological study. *J. Neurol. Neurosurg. Psychiatry* 1992; **55**(5): 383–7.

63. Furman JM, Jacob RG. A clinical taxonomy of dizziness and anxiety in the otoneurological setting. *J. Anxiety Disord.* 2001; **15**(1–2): 9–26.

64. Yardley L, Verschuur C, Masson E, Luxon L, Haacke N. Somatic and psychological factors contributing to handicap in people with vertigo. *Br. J. Audiol.* 1992; **26**(5): 283–90.

65. Yardley L. Contribution of symptoms and beliefs to handicap in people with vertigo: a longitudinal study. *Br. J. Clin. Psychol.* 1994; **33** (Pt. 1): 101–13.

66. Naber CM, Water-Schmeder O, Bohrer PS, Matonak K, Bernstein AL, Merchant MA. Interdisciplinary treatment for vestibular dysfunction: The effectiveness of mindfulness, cognitive-behavioral techniques, and vestibular rehabilitation. *Otolaryngol. Head Neck Surg.* 2011; **145**(1): 117–24.

67. Andersson G, Asmundson GJ, Denev J, Nilsson J, Larsen HC. A controlled trial of cognitive-behavior therapy combined with vestibular rehabilitation in the treatment of dizziness. *Behav. Res. Ther.* 2006; **44**(9): 1265–73.

68. Pavlou M, Acheson J, Nicolaou D, Fraser CL, Bronstein AM, Davies RA. Effect of developmental binocular vision abnormalities on visual vertigo symptoms and treatment outcome. *J. Neurol. Phys. Ther.* 2015; **39**(4): 215–24.

69. Whitney SL, Wrisley DM, Brown KE, Furman JM. Physical therapy for migraine-related vestibulopathy and vestibular dysfunction with history of migraine. *Laryngoscope* 2000; **110**(9): 1528–34.

70. Miffon M, Guyot JP. Difficulties faced by patients suffering from total bilateral vestibular loss. *ORL J. Otorhinolaryngol. Relat. Spec.* 2015; **77**(4): 241–7.

71. Porciuncula F, Johnson CC, Glickman LB. The effect of vestibular rehabilitation on adults with bilateral vestibular hypofunction: A systematic review. *J. Vestib. Res.* 2012; **22**(5–6): 283–98.

72. Black FO, Angel CR, Pesznecker SC, Gianna C. Outcome analysis of individualized vestibular rehabilitation protocols. *Am. J. Otol.* 2000; **21**(4): 543–51.

73. Garcia AP, Gananca MM, Cusin FS, Tomaz A, Gananca FF, Caovilla HH. Vestibular rehabilitation with virtual reality in Meniere's disease. *Braz. J. Otorhinolaryngol.* 2013; **79**(3): 366–74.

74. Alsalaheen BA, Whitney SL, Mucha A, Morris LO, Furman JM, Sparto PJ. Exercise prescription patterns in patients treated with vestibular rehabilitation after concussion. *Physiother. Res. Int.* 2013; **18**(2):100–8.

75. Schneider KJ, Meeuwisse WH, Nettel-Aguirre A, et al. Cervicovestibular rehabilitation in sport-related concussion: A randomised controlled trial. *Br. J. Sports Med.* 2014; **48**(17): 1294–8.

76. McCulloch KL, Goldman S, Lowe L, et al. Development of clinical recommendations for progressive return to activity after military mild traumatic brain injury: Guidance for rehabilitation providers. *J. Head Trauma Rehabil.* 2015; **30**(1): 56–67.

77. Vitkovic J, Winoto A, Rance G, Dowell R, Paine M. Vestibular rehabilitation outcomes in patients with and without vestibular migraine. *J. Neurol.* 2013; **260** (12): 3039–48.

78. Hilton MP, Pinder DK. The Epley (canalith repositioning) manoeuvre for benign paroxysmal positional vertigo. *Cochrane Database of Systematic Reviews* 2014; **12**: CD003162.

79. Lempert T, Wolsley C, Davies R, Gresty MA, Bronstein AM. Three hundred sixty-degree rotation of the posterior semicircular canal for treatment of benign positional vertigo: A placebo-controlled trial. *Neurology* 1997; **49**(3): 729–33.

80. Vannucchi P, Giannoni B, Pagnini P. Treatment of horizontal semicircular canal benign paroxysmal positional vertigo. *J. Vestib. Res.* 1997; **7**(1): 1–6.

81. Oron Y, Cohen-Atsmoni S, Len A, Roth Y. Treatment of horizontal canal BPPV: Pathophysiology, available maneuvers, and recommended treatment. *Laryngoscope* 2015; **125**(8): 1959–64.

82. Liu H. Presentation and outcome of post-traumatic benign paroxysmal positional vertigo. *Acta Otolaryngol.* 2012; **132**(8): 803–6.

83. Kim JS, Zee DS. Clinical practice. Benign paroxysmal positional vertigo.*N. Engl. J. Med.* 2014; **370**(12): 1138–47.

84. Bronstein AM, Lempert T, Seemungal BM. Chronic dizziness: A practical approach. *Pract. Neurol.* 2010; **10** (3): 129–39.

Management of Walking Disorders in Neurorehabilitation

Jonathan F. Marsden

10.1 Introduction

Walking is characterized by alternating periods when the leg is on (stance phase) or off (swing phase) the ground. Walking has two periods of double stance for every gait cycle when both feet are on the ground. Stance and swing phases can be further divided into subphases or events; these can help in the clinical analysis and reporting of walking dysfunction (Figure 10.1).

Human bipedal standing is inherently unstable as the base of support is small and the centre of mass is high. While walking, people are not in static equilibrium as the centre of mass is rarely over the base of support (Figure 10.2a) [1]. Instead, walking consists of a controlled fall of the centre of mass away from the stance leg that is stopped by correct placement of the swing leg. Both the movement of the centre of mass leading to the fall and the placement of the leg halting the fall are carefully controlled and coordinated (Figure 10.2b) [2]. Thus primary problems with balance (initiating and controlling the fall) and/or accurate leg motion or the coordination of the two can affect walking. Normally, when walking, people can progress forward efficiently whilst maintaining equilibrium and adapting to changing environmental conditions or different goals (e.g., different support surfaces/inclines or the need to increase speed to cross a road). To do this requires the interaction of multiple systems, including the peripheral and central nervous systems and the musculoskeletal system. Thus walking deficits can have multiple causes. The main systems controlling walking and causes of walking dysfunction are summarized in what follows:

(1) Spinal cord and central pattern generators (CPGs) – by virtue of their interconnectivity and/or neuronal properties, circuits within the spinal cord are able to generate rhythmic activity associated with the alternating swing and stance phases of walking. The properties of these circuits have been mainly assessed in animal models, but there is indirect evidence for their existence in humans [3]. Spinal reflexes such as the short latency mono-synaptic muscle stretch reflex are modulated with the gait cycle. In the ankle plantarflexors, for example, stretch reflexes are higher in stance than swing phase. This modulation is caused by changes in the amount of inhibition in spinal cord circuits caused by phase-dependent changes in sensory and descending inputs [4]. Stretch reflex modulation may allow for rapid adjustment to changing terrain in stance phase and correct foot placement during swing phase. However, the size of the stretch reflex (its gain) is small and its role in balance control is supported by longer latency stretch reflexes, some of which run through the motor cortex. In people with spasticity, the modulation of stretch reflexes with gait cycle is reduced, and this can lead to deficits such as impaired clearance of the foot in swing phase as the ankle plantarflexors are stretched and activated during ankle dorsiflexion in swing phase and in mid-stance [4]. However, the increased tone associated with spasticity may also be beneficial in some cases, aiding antigravity activity.

(2) Multiple sensory systems – normal walking and balance require the integration of somatosensory (cutaneous and proprioceptive), vestibular, and visual information. These sensations are integrated in multiple areas of the central nervous system such as the spinal cord, brainstem, and cerebellum. Some sensations interact with the CPGs to trigger/prolong the stance (e.g., lower limb loading) and swing phases (e.g., stretch of the hip flexors) [5]. Sensory deficits can arise from damage to the end organ, peripheral pathways, or central projections. Poor visual acuity and contrast sensitivity are associated with an increased risk

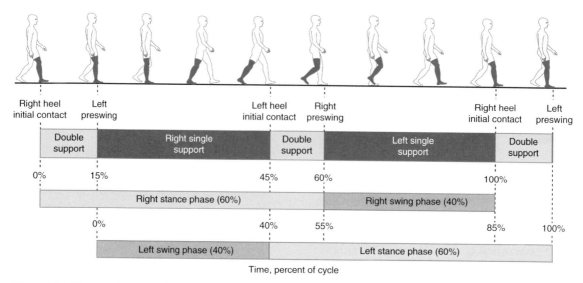

Figure 10.1 Phases and events in the gait cycle

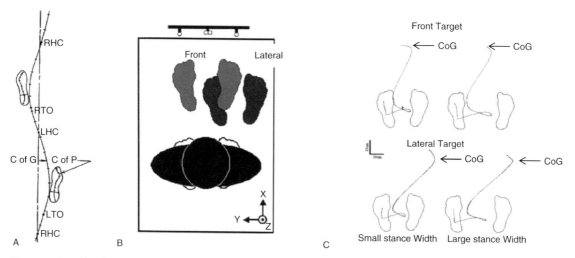

Figure 10.2 A. Plot of the centre of gravity (C of G) and centre of pressure (C of P) while walking, highlighting the fact that the C of G does not move over the base of support as indicated by the foot outline while walking. R/L HC = right/left heel contact R/L TO = right/left toe off B. Experimental setup where a participant had to step onto targets in front or to the side with the right leg leading. C. Plot of the centre of force and C of G (arrow). Note the different trajectory of the C of G when stepping to the front and to the side with a large and small initial stance width. The C of G and foot placement are coordinated; large sideways movements of the C of G accompanying from foot placement would result in imbalance laterally whilst a small C of G motion with a lateral foot movement would result in imbalance medially.

of falls. Vision is particularly important for detecting forthcoming obstacles and guiding proactive avoidance strategies [6]. Deficits in somatosensory information lead to delayed and poorly scaled postural responses to a perturbation [7]. Vestibular deficits can result in balance dysfunction (e.g., poor modulation of postural responses and reduced head control) that can be associated with an over-reliance on

vision for balance. This can further exacerbate balance and walking dysfunction because vision in isolation does not distinguish between self-motion and movement of the external environment [8]. People who are visually dominant (termed 'visual vertigo') will often experience an exacerbation of symptoms in complex visual environments (e.g., supermarket aisles). The symptoms of vertigo and oscillopsia (arising from vestibulo-ocular dysfunction) often result in compensatory reductions in head motion as people try to avoid head movement that precipitates symptoms. This can impair the ability to compensate for the vestibular dysfunction [9].

(3) Subcortical systems – the pedunculopontine nucleus (PPN) in the midbrain, also termed the 'mesencephalic locomotor region', triggers walking when stimulated in animals. A similar function has been proposed in humans [10]. It has inputs directly from the basal ganglia and projects to the reticular nuclei that give rise to the reticulospinal tracts [11]. Nuclei such as the raphe nucleus, vestibular nucleus, and reticular formation have descending projections to the spinal cord that are important for the regulation of postural tone and balance and can be affected in conditions such as a brainstem stroke [11].

(4) The basal ganglia is important in the control of goal-directed and habitual movements. Walking and balance dysfunctions in Parkinson's disease in part arise due to alterations in basal ganglia inputs to the PPN as well as direct degeneration affecting the PPN and dysfunction in cortico-basal ganglia-cortical circuits. Parkinson's disease is associated with a flexed posture (termed 'camptocormia' when extreme) and axial rigidity, poorly scaled postural responses to altered task conditions, festinating gait, and freezing. Freezing is often seen when turning, going through doorways, and initiating gait, and when anxious and performing simultaneous cognitive tasks. The asymmetry in motion between the legs required when turning may exacerbate the left–right asymmetry in symptoms commonly seen in Parkinson's disease. People often turn to their non-affected side and freezing often starts on the inner turning leg that has a longer stance duration [12]. Freezing is a risk factor for falls that most frequently occur in Hoehn and Yahr stage 3. Reductions in walking speed and increased step variability are seen when walking and undertaking another cognitive/motor task (dual tasking). This may be due to increased attentional requirements as movements become less automatic, compounded by associated degeneration of cholinergic projections that are part of attentional circuits [13].

(5) The cerebellum is important for the adaptation of walking when task conditions change (e.g., altered vision or terrain). People with cerebellar dysfunction can show impairments in balance and in limb control and in the coordination of the two components while stepping. The coordination between joints when walking is more variable, and postural responses to a perturbation are hypermetric and do not adapt with repeated presentations [14]. Balance responses to moving visual stimuli are particularly marked. Associated oculo-motor deficits such as dysmetric saccades and impaired smooth pursuit can further impair walking when accurate visual control is required [14].

(6) Cortical areas – neural activity in motor cortical areas modulates with the gait cycle, and long latency transcortical stretch reflexes descending via the corticospinal tract are important for balance. These reflexes are more adaptable to changing conditions (e.g., a slippery surface) than mono-synaptic stretch reflexes [15]. Impairment of these long latency responses as well as dysfunction of cortico-fugal projections to brainstem areas contribute to the balance impairment seen after a hemispheric stroke. Activity in the corticospinal tract seems to be particularly important when accurate, visually driven stepping is required (e.g., using stepping stones). However, the relative importance of the corticospinal tract in the recovery of walking may not be as important as its role in the recovery of hand function [16]. This may reflect the contribution of subcortical areas and/or the fact that it is easier to compensate for associated limb weakness to achieve functional walking compared to functional upper limb movements.

(7) Higher-level gait disorders are walking disorders that are not explained by deficits in strength, tone, sensation, or coordination. Posterior cortical areas such as the parieto-insular areas and secondary somatosensory areas integrate multisensory information and are important in the perception of body motion and verticality. Deficits such as the pusher syndrome, consisting of an active push to the paretic side associated with a stroke, are associated with marked multisensory deficits in verticality perception associated with lesions to thalamic nuclei processing somatosensory and/or vestibular

information. Balance and verticality perceptual deficits are more common with right-sided lesions. Anterior (frontal) cortical dysfunction, commonly associated with microvascular lesions, results in freezing of gait, small steps, and disequilibrium. These arise in part due to lesions affecting the projections to the basal ganglia and/or brainstem. They can be associated with an overcautious gait characterized by a wide base of support, holding onto walls, and fear of falling [17]. Important interactions with other cortical systems and the motor system exist. Navigation of walking around the environment requires interactions with the hippocampus. Damage to this system, as seen in Alzheimer's dementia, can cause problems with navigation, leading to people often getting lost. Attentional systems are particularly important when accurate and precise walking is required, either imposed by a change in the environment or due to an intrinsic change (e.g., associated pathology). The importance of attention can be seen by the degradation of walking when an additional cognitive or motor task is required while walking (termed 'dual tasking') in the elderly or in people with neurological deficits [13].

(8) Multi-linked musculoskeletal system – muscle weakness arising from neuropathies and myopathies results in walking dysfunction. With a peripheral neuropathy, associated sensory deficits will further impact balance and walking. In diabetic peripheral neuropathy, this can be compounded by foot ulceration. Secondary changes following central neurological damage also occur such as increased muscle stiffness and contracture or secondary muscle atrophy [4]. Changes in muscle fibre properties such as a decrease in slow fibres and atrophy of fast fibres have also been described in conditions such as stroke and are associated with changes in walking speed [18]. When neurological deficits are present during development, the abnormal pull of contracted or overactive muscles and/or a lack of physiological loading can result in bony deformity. This is common in conditions such as cerebral palsy where abnormalities such as hip dysplasia and torsional bony deformity of the femur and tibia can occur. This can in turn alter the line of pull of muscles and their lever arm, leading to an alteration in the moment generated at a joint (termed 'lever arm dysfunction').

(9) Fear, anxiety – excessive anxiety often accompanies deficits in balance and walking. A fear of falling is a risk factor for future falls. Anxiety is often associated with dysfunction to peripheral and central vestibular pathways; it is associated with slower and less complete recovery of symptoms. This may result from the interconnections between the vestibular nuclei with autonomic areas (e.g., nucleus tractus solitarius) and parabrachial nuclei that in turn interconnect with limbic circuits (e.g., orbitofrontal cortex and amygdala) and the hypothalamus, which are important for emotional regulation [19].

(10) Functional gait disorders – phobic postural vertigo is a syndrome associated with transient subjective sensations of unsteadiness and fear of falling that are associated with normal balance on clinical examination. It is linked to obsessive-compulsive disorder and high anxiety. People walk slowly, overreact to a perturbation, and often have an excessive increase in unsteadiness when vision is obscured. It is a type of functional movement disorder. Functional movement disorders can account for 1.5% of referrals to a neurology outpatient clinic and gait abnormalities are seen in ~40% of cases. Gait abnormalities can occur with/without other movement disorders. Excessive slowing of walking is seen, with common symptoms being buckling of the knee and an inability to stand independently due to a lack of coordination while walking (astasia-abasia) that is not evident when leg movements are tested when sitting/lying. Women are more affected than men, with a mean age of onset of 37–50 years. Diagnosis relies on clinical signs such as observed variability of movement, alterations in movement when the person is distracted, spread of symptoms to other sites, and the ruling out of organic causes. People with functional disorders have an altered decision-making style as well as an enhanced self-focus. In the presence of a minor injury, these may interact and result in the exaggerated responses seen [20].

10.2 Assessment: Goal Setting and General Principles

10.2.1 Subjective Assessment

It is important to understand a patient's perceived difficulties with walking and balance and their perceived cause as well as the goals of the patient and, in the paediatric population, the goals of the patient's guardians. Aims may vary, such as improving walking speed, endurance, or efficiency, reducing pain associated with walking, or improving the cosmetic aspects of walking to reduce the stigma associated with altered patterns of walking. Often goals and aims of intervention will be expressed in terms of tasks that people would like to achieve. In these cases, it is important to ascertain the perceived factors that prevent that task as this can guide assessment and management. Many difficulties with walking at home and in the community are frequently determined by extrinsic social issues such as poor access. Further, it may be that mobility is the key aim, i.e. getting from A to B, and the mechanisms underlying that are not as important. In such cases, the use of manual or electric wheelchairs as a mobility aid may be appropriate.

10.2.2 Objective Assessment

Assessment should include an observational analysis of walking. Protocols for analysing walking have been described, and several validated scales are available that can aid in recording the movement of joints while walking (kinematics) [21]. These tend to divide the gait cycle into specific phases and to estimate the maximal motion of a joint (e.g., hip, knee, or ankle). In addition, a note should be made about any walking aids and the overall pattern of walking. Clinically, several patterns of walking have been described (Table 10.1). Observational assessment can be complemented by video analysis. Here care must be taken to avoid parallax error. Following a set protocol to capture frontal and sagittal plane views of the whole body and close-up images of the legs/feet is recommended [22].

Observational analysis needs to be supplemented by a static examination assessing impairments such as spasticity; muscle paresis or weakness; sensory loss, extrapyramidal features, or cerebellar signs; balance (sitting and standing); and posture. As walking is a whole-body activity, an assessment should include the control not only of the lower limbs but also of the

Table 10.1 A Gait labels and descriptors

Label	Descriptor
Crouch	Increased hip and knee flexion during stance phase
Recurvatum	Increased knee hyperextension in mid-stance
Stiff knee	Reduced knee flexion in swing phase
Jump	Increased knee flexion at loading response and almost normal knee function later in the gait cycle
Equinus	Increased ankle plantarflexion in mid-stance

head, arms, and trunk [22]. Further, abnormalities in oculomotor control can impact walking accuracy, and abnormal visuospatial attention and verticality perception are associated with walking and balance dysfunction. These should be assessed in people with balance difficulties after vestibular dysfunction or a brainstem or supratentorial lesion (e.g., stroke, head injury).

Although with neurological lesions the primary site of pathology is the central or peripheral nervous system, it is also important to examine the musculoskeletal system [4]. Neurological damage is frequently associated with changes in the visco-elastic properties of muscle and tendon and contractures affecting two joint leg muscles. Therefore, range of motion and limb stiffness at different speeds of passive movement (to distinguish between spasticity and non-neural stiffness) should be assessed [22]. Further, when neurological damage affects people prior to reaching skeletal maturity, bony abnormalities can develop such as leg length discrepancies, scoliosis, and torsional changes in the femur and tibia. These can directly affect walking and are often a target for surgical interventions. In these cases, radiographs may be indicated.

Instrumented gait analysis consists of 3-D motion analysis of joint movement (kinematics) combined with recording of the forces through the stance leg using force plates. These allow the calculation of joint moments and power (kinetics). Such analysis can useful in aiding clinical decision making when combined with subjective history, observational assessment, and static assessment. Standardization of techniques is important and data must be referenced to an age-matched database of healthy children and adults. Data are more reliable in the sagittal and coronal as opposed to the horizontal planes [22]. This technique only reveals net joint moments, and factors such as co-contraction can only be ascertained from additional surface electromyography recordings.

10.2.3 Walking-Related Outcome Measures

A review of measures used for research into walking for people with stroke highlighted that the most commonly used test is self-paced gait speed [23]. Ultimately, the clinical outcome measure chosen should reflect the goals of the patient and the aims of the management strategy. The ecological validity of many of the commonly used tests can be questioned. Clinic-based walking speeds, for example, overestimate community ambulation speed if it is below 0.8 m/s [24]. Few measures explore longer distances (>1 Km), obstacle negotiation, and walking outside and on uneven surfaces, or the frequent need to dual task when walking. Some tests such as the Emory Ambulation Profile and the community balance and mobility scale have tried to address some of these issues. It is important to define where possible what is a minimum detectable change (MDC) and whether this is indeed clinically significant. The MDC for a 10-minute time walk at a usual (not maximal) pace is a speed of 0.15 m/s. The speed required to cross a road varies geographically from 0.8–1.3 m/s [24]. Therefore, a change of 0.15 m/s from 0.40 to 0.55 m/s with an intervention, although indicating an improvement, may not help the person become independent in the community; thus clinical significance also needs to be considered. Patient-reported outcome measures such as the 10-item walking scale provide a subjective rating of walking. Additional subjective scales can ask about the fear of falling or confidence with balance. Direct measures of community walking using accelerometers are increasingly used as outcome measures as well as aids to goal setting.

10.2.4 General Principles of Assessment and Management

Walking dysfunction will frequently be associated with altered movement patterns or kinematics; these can arise from the primary impairment, but also from compensatory mechanisms to maintain

mobility. For example, a high-stepping gait can be a compensatory mechanism associated with a foot drop in peripheral neuropathy. Through clinical assessment, it is important to try to determine the cause of any walking dysfunction as this will help to guide management strategies. When trying to understand the causes of walking dysfunction, it is important to understand the cyclical nature of walking and that patterns of walking in one part of the gait cycle may be caused by events occurring earlier in the gait cycle. A lack of knee flexion during swing phase, for example, can be caused by hypertonia (spasticity or increased passive stiffness) of the knee extensors or by weakness in the hip flexors or ankle plantarflexors that are active at the end of stance phase and help to initiate swing phase.

The management approaches adopted depend on understanding the person's goals, the cause of walking dysfunction, and the current evidence base for interventions. The approach chosen will also be determined by prognostic indicators such as the size of a lesion; the presence of multiple sensorimotor impairments or cognitive and perceptual deficits; and whether a condition is acute or chronic, progressive or a single incident. This will determine whether techniques aimed at maintaining/improving walking should have more emphasis on compensatory techniques (e.g., walking aids) or restorative techniques (e.g., progressive resisted exercise). Some interventions such as task-related training by emphasizing task attainment can be achieved through a combination of compensatory or restorative mechanisms. Although normal walking patterns form the basis for the observational assessment of walking and normative values form the basis of static clinical testing, this does not mean that aiming for a more normal pattern of walking is always the most appropriate approach. It may be that maintenance of walking with a progressive condition requires the adoption of walking aids or compensatory walking patterns.

10.2.5 Goal Setting

Self-management is the cornerstone of rehabilitation, especially in people with long-term chronic conditions. Sustainable improvements in real-world walking are seen in interventions that incorporate health behaviour change techniques rather than just exercise alone [25]. There are several models of behaviour change. Many emphasize the need to understand the need to change (e.g., theory information-motivation-strategy model, health belief model) [26]. Therefore, education about the condition and the underlying causes of gait dysfunction is a first step in collaboratively developing a management strategy. Social cognitive models highlight how a person's beliefs, experiences, and personal attributes influence their responses to new information and will determine the goals they set and the actions they are willing to take to achieve them. Further, environmental factors associated with where people live, work, and socialize will influence the adoption and delivery of goals [26]. Therefore, when collaboratively arriving at realistic and achievable goals, it is important to take these factors into account to maximize success and long-term adherence. Several tools are available that can aid goal setting. Scales such as the goal attainment scale have been used in setting walking-related goals. Further, accelerometers that measure walking distance and activity times have been used (e.g., post stroke) to set and monitor goals [27].

10.3 Non-Pharmacological Treatments

Non-pharmacological interventions may target underlying impairments (e.g., weakness/spasticity) or focus on task-related training or the use of aids and orthoses. Additional interventions such as environmental modifications (e.g., environmental modifications to reduce falls risk and improve accessibility) are not covered in this chapter and are reviewed elsewhere [28].

10.3.1 Progressive Resisted Exercise

Muscle paresis is a primary cause of walking dysfunction in an upper motor neuron lesion. A multitude of studies highlights the association between walking parameters and weakness; for example, weakness in the ankle plantarflexors is associated with slower walking speeds [29]. Paresis can be caused by damage to descending pathways (e.g., the corticospinal tract) and secondary disuse atrophy. Progressive resisted exercises involve repetitive exercises against resistance with the aim of inducing muscle hypertrophy. Changes in the excitability of central descending pathways may also occur. The parameters of training tend to follow the American College of Sports Medicine (ACSM) guidelines advocating 60–80% of the one-repetition maximum: 6–12 repetitions per set and three sets. Progression should occur and training should last at least 8–12 weeks as this is the minimum time before physiological changes occur.

Systematic reviews highlight that progressive resisted exercises in people with an upper motor neuron syndrome and in Parkinson's disease can lead to improvements not only in strength but also in walking parameters (speed, endurance) [30]. Factors to consider with training include: (a) the position of exercise; so-called closed chain exercises where the distal segment is fixed can reproduce more functional tasks; (b) the range of training: is this equivalent to that observed during walking?

10.3.2 Functional Electrical Stimulation (FES)

FES can be a useful adjunct where there is central nervous system damage with preserved peripheral nerve function. Here the peripheral nerve is stimulated to activate a muscle. The stimulation is timed so that the muscle is activated at the appropriate point of the gait cycle. This can be achieved through sensors that detect events of the gait cycle. Most commonly switches are placed in the shoe that detect the onset/offset of loading. i.e. foot contact and toe off, but more recently sensors such as gyroscopes within the stimulator unit are being used to indicate stance/swing onset/offset. The most common form of FES is common peroneal stimulation to achieve ankle dorsiflexion during swing phase and controlled dorsiflexion at the start of stance phase (termed the 'first ankle rocker'). Other muscles active in the stance or swing phase however can be targeted.

FES for the ankle dorsiflexors leads to a small improvement in walking speed and an improvement in energy efficiency as measured by the physiological cost index [31]. These effects occur straightaway. With long-term use in stroke, FES is associated with a carryover effect that there is an improvement in walking even without FES in situ. This carryover effect may not be as marked in progressive conditions such as multiple sclerosis. These carryover effects may be the result of increased walking practice and/or central changes induced by the stimulation.

10.3.3 Stretching and Splinting

Increases in connective tissue, shortening of muscle fascicles, and reductions in sarcomere number have been described in adult and paediatric populations with an upper motor neuron syndrome and is often accompanied by spasticity. Although commonly prescribed, there is no evidence that manual stretches can decrease spasticity or change passive muscle properties, and evidence suggests that increases in range of motion, assessed at the ankle, are of the order of ~5° [32]. There is limited evidence that this leads to an improvement in walking. In contrast, casting or taping the ankle when combined with botulinum toxin injections in adult stroke is associated with improvements in walking speed and six-minute walk tests after a 20-day period, with improvements in the six-minute walk test being maintained at 90 days [33].

10.3.4 Cardiovascular Training

With decreased activity caused by neurological damage, a reduction in aerobic capacity can occur. Further, cardiovascular impairments are risk factors for conditions such as stroke and so frequently co-occur. Reduced aerobic capacity can therefore be an important factor in limiting walking endurance. Addressing cardiovascular fitness is recommended in clinical guidelines of neurological conditions (e.g., stroke, multiple sclerosis, Parkinson's disease), and systematic reviews of aerobic training highlight that training can lead to improvements in walking speed and endurance. Training can be task specific (e.g., walking), but also involve other techniques (e.g., static cycling). Training guidelines suggest that training at 60–80% of the maximal heart rate for periods of 15–40 minutes at least thrice a week over 12 weeks is required to achieve an improvement in aerobic function[34].

10.3.5 Cueing and Dual Task Training

In Parkinson's disease, walking speed can be improved and freezing episodes reduced by using auditory and visual cueing techniques. This may reflect the fact that circuits underlying sensory-driven movements are less affected than circuits underlying self-initiated movements. Rhythmic cues improve stride length and walking speed. Simple verbal instructions (e.g., 'take big steps') can also have short-term effects on walking parameters [35]. Due to a reduction in the automaticity of walking and potential additional cognitive impairments, dual tasking is commonly affected in neurological conditions. Dual task training involves progressive addition of more complex additional tasks whilst undertaking walking

and has been combined with cueing techniques in people with Parkinson's disease with initial small-scale studies showing benefit [36].

10.3.6 Orthotics and Shoes

Orthotics provides mechanical support to a body part. Ankle foot orthoses (AFOs) can be used to increase ankle dorsiflexion during swing phase in people with weakness of the anterior tibial muscles and improve balance by stabilizing the ankle joint [37]. Different types of AFOs are available (e.g., dorsal and elastic), and they vary in their perceived comfort and their impact on walking efficiency [38]. More rigid orthoses may be required for people with significant additional plantarflexor tone.

For bilateral leg paralysis (e.g., following a thoracic, lumbar spinal cord injury [SCI], myelomeningocele), reciprocating orthoses (hip guidance orthosis, reciprocating gait orthosis, and advanced reciprocating gait orthosis) work on the principle of coupling two hip-knee-ankle orthoses together to improve reciprocal leg movement when walking. Although they improve walking speeds, their long-term use can be an issue and adults who cannot climb stairs and have limited walking ability indoors are more likely to abandon them [39]. Powered orthoses incorporate electric motors or pneumatic or hydraulic actuators to aid movement of paretic/paralysed leg joints They reduce energy consumption more than conventional orthoses [40]. Hybrid systems occur where FES is used to control motion at some joints (e.g., knees). However, to date, evidence is limited that they are more efficient or result in greater walking speed compared to mechanical orthoses [41].

In-shoe orthoses may be used to accommodate/correct foot deformity such as pes planus or pes cavus, although there is little evidence that this improves walking parameters. Improvements in balance with in-shoe orthoses have been reported [42]. Some designs aim to improve balance through selective stimulation of cutaneous receptors on the plantar aspects of the feet, although in neurological populations (multiple sclerosis and Parkinson's disease), there is no evidence of an effect [43]. Although often overlooked, shoe design (e.g., improving lateral stability) can aid balance and walking. Wearing slippers indoors is commonly associated with falls in the elderly, and habitual shoe use should be sought during the clinical assessment [44].

10.3.7 Walking Aids

Walking aids such as sticks, crutches, and frames are commonly prescribed to assist balance and off-load limbs to help with pain relief. The effects on balance are not solely due to the application of additional stabilizing forces applied through the arm. Even a light touch on a walking aid can improve balance, possibly by providing additional sensory cues about body motion [45]. Excessive weight bearing through walking aids can be associated with changes in posture and a reduction in postural activity in the legs. Therefore, advocating a reduction in excessive weight bearing (often termed 'fixing') may aid in balance and walking rehabilitation.

10.3.8 Task-Related Training

As highlighted in Section 10.1, walking is a complex interaction between multiple systems and requires coordination between balance and motion. Further, due to the cyclical nature of walking, one phase of walking affects future events. Therefore, practising the whole coordinated task is an essential part of walking rehabilitation. Task-related training has also been associated with plastic, adaptive changes within the brain, although much of the evidence for this derives for upper limb paradigms due to difficulties in using functional imaging in humans during walking tasks and the lack of bipedal animal models.

Task-related training may occur either in an open and unpredictable, natural environment (e.g., overground walking) or within a closed and predictable environment (e.g., treadmill walking). In an open environment, training would also include how the person attends to and responds to the environment and plans their path and navigation. In a closed environment, factors such as the slope, speed, direction, obstacles, and visual scene are controlled; this may be beneficial if the aim is to achieve large amounts of repetitive practice. Treadmill training can be combined with body weight support. Reducing body weight will reduce the strength required to walk. This allows people with mild-to-moderate paresis to practise coordinated walking. This can be aided by a therapist guiding/facilitating correct motion at joints, e.g., correct heel strike or knee position. Fundamental to task-related training is the need for repetitive practice. Systematic reviews highlight that over-ground or treadmill training with/without body weight support after stroke compared to a control condition leads to similar small improvements in walking speed or endurance. However, it does not affect how many people are able to walk independently [46, 47].

Balance is a key component of walking. Systematic reviews highlight that tasks such as Tai Chi that emphasize good standing balance can also lead to improvements in balance but also walking in conditions such as Parkinson's disease [48]. Other exercises emphasizing standing balance in different conditions (e.g., different support surfaces such as carpets/foam) are also associated with improvements in measures of balance and walking ability in a number of neurological conditions. In people with cerebellar dysfunction, for example, intensive training of balance and walking is associated with improvements in walking [49].

10.3.9 Robotics and Electromechanical Training

The use of robotics has the potential advantage of providing repetitive high-intensity task-related training with minimal manual handling. It allows the monitoring of the training and support provided. One disadvantage is the potential cost, and it is important to consider the transferability of training into real-world environments. Randomized controlled trials of electromechanical training after stroke show improvements in walking speed and endurance compared to usual care. People in the first few months following stroke and who are not able to walk seem to benefit the most. With training, there is an increase in the number of independent walkers. This highlights a potential advantage and need for this approach over and above traditional therapies such as treadmill walking with/without body weight support [50].

10.3.10 Virtual Reality

Walking not only involves the progression from A to B but also requires the ability to interact with the environment. When walking is impaired, however, tasks such as crossing roads and walking in crowds can be unsafe and cause anxiety, especially in the early stages of rehabilitation. Virtual reality (VR) allows for the practice of walking in a safe environment. The use of VR is still in its infancy, although there are trials supporting its use in training walking. To date, systematic reviews suggest minimal improvements in walking speed, but other measures such as confidence in real-world situations should be explored in future work [51].

10.3.11 Sensory Rehabilitation

Vestibular compensation describes the central adaptive changes that underlie recovery following a peripheral vestibular nerve lesion. These processes are driven by actively moving the head and whole body to stimulate the vestibular system. With repeated movements, the brain adapts to the deficits in balance, head control and, vestibulo-ocular reflex (VOR). Recovery is in part caused by sensory substitution where remaining sensations compensate for the lost vestibular function. Recovery of dynamic symptoms also involves learning behavioural strategies such as saccadic substitution to compensate for an impaired dynamic VOR. Animal studies highlight that early movement is important for maximizing recovery. The principles of early rehabilitation, actively undertaking movements that precipitate symptoms (e.g., of vertigo, imbalance, or blurred vision), avoiding over-reliance on one sensory input for balance (e.g., vision), combined with education about the causes of symptoms and recovery process, are key components of vestibular rehabilitation [9]. Systematic reviews highlight that the evidence base for VR following a unilateral peripheral lesion is strong and that VR leads to improvements in walking and balance, as well as in specific symptoms such as vertigo [52]. Customized exercises directed to the participants' main difficulties are more effective than generic exercises (e.g., Cawthorne-Cooksey exercises). In people who are very visually dominant, progressive exposure to moving visual stimuli that precipitate symptoms leads to a reduction in symptoms and an improvement in balance and walking. Preliminary work suggests similar techniques could be useful in the rehabilitation of balance in people with cerebellar dysfunction [53].

With peripheral somatosensory loss there is also an increase in the relative effectiveness of remaining sensations such as the vestibular system in controlling balance. This raises the possibility that balance retraining flowing similar principles to VR may be effective, and this is supported by small-scale studies to date in conditions such as diabetic peripheral neuropathy [54], although current evidence is insufficient for this to be currently recommended.

10.4 Pharmacological Treatment

Many symptomatic treatments of movement disorders or motor symptoms (e.g., spasticity) have the potential of improving balance and walking, whilst some medications are associated with an increased incidence of falls.

10.4.1 Management of Spasticity

The evidence that spasticity treatment causes improvements in walking ability is mixed and studies are often of low methodological quality. This may reflect the fact that the measures used (e.g., walking speed) are not responsive to the changes. Assessment of walking kinematics has shown effects such as an improvement in stiff knee gait after stroke with focal treatment using botulinum toxin [55]. Effect sizes are similar to that seen with physiotherapy alone and combined interventions, reflecting real-world practice, produce larger effect sizes [56]. Systematic reviews highlight that side effects such as weakness and lethargy can occur with oral medications. Reductions in functional ability may also reflect the fact that spasticity may not be the primary cause of walking dysfunction after an upper motor neurone syndrome and/or that in some cases the increased tone may aid antigravity function by contributing to stance phase activity.

A systematic review of intrathecal baclofen (ITB) in ambulant children with spasticity or dystonia with a cerebral lesion found that about 30% showed an improvement in ambulatory status. In 12%, there was a deterioration of ambulation transfer ability; this may be due to an effect on antigravity activity. There is no evidence that ITB will lead to a change in someone who is not ambulatory [57]. ITB has been reported to aid walking in people with hereditary spastic paraparesis who present with bilateral spasticity and paresis. In contrast, ITB post stroke led to a deterioration in walking in six out of eight patients due to an impact on paretic antigravity activity [58], and there is limited evidence supporting the use of baclofen to improve walking after SCI [59].

10.4.2 Management of Extrapyramidal Signs

Pharmacological management of extrapyramidal signs with levodopa, dopamine agonists, and dopamine MAO-B inhibitors can lead to improved motor symptoms, balance, and mobility in the early and mid-stages of Parkinson's disease [60, 61]. Donepezil, an acetylcholinesterase inhibitor, has been associated with a reduced risk of falls [62]. This may reflect the importance of cholinergic transmission in movement initiation and also that attentional networks are affected by Parkinson's disease and are important for dual tasking. Methylphenidate is a CNS stimulant that blocks the presynaptic dopamine transporter and the noradrenaline transporter in the striatum and the prefrontal cortex. Methylphenidate reduces gait hypokinesia and freezing of gait in people with advanced Parkinson's disease receiving subthalamic nucleus deep brain stimulation in the off-dopaminergic drug condition [63]. However, these initial findings are yet to be replicated in large randomized studies [60].

The relationship between pharmacological interventions and falls in Parkinson's disease is complex. Increased mobility associated with pharmacological interventions can increase in falls. Further, they can also induce dyskinesias that are also associated with an increased falls risk.

10.4.3 Medications Associated with Falls

Several medications are associated with falls, including antihypertensive agents, diuretics, β-blockers, sedatives and hypnotics, neuroleptics and antipsychotics, antidepressants, benzodiazepines, narcotics, and nonsteroidal anti-inflammatory drugs [64]. Antidepressants, neuroleptics, and antipsychotics (odds ratio 1.50; 95% confidence interval [CI] 1.37–1.83) and benzodiazepines (odds ratio 1.57 95% CI 1.43–1.72) have the strongest association with falls [65]. Mechanisms of action include sedative effects, orthostatic hypotension, confusion, and cardiac arrhythmias.

10.4.4 Ion Channel Modulation

Frampidine (dalfampridine-ER, 4-aminopyridine) acts to restore axonal conduction through the blockade of the potassium channels that become exposed during axonal demyelination. Clinical trials have highlighted that it is associated with an increase in walking speed in 25% and walking ability in 33% of people with multiple sclerosis [66]. Controlled trials in people with chronic incomplete SCI have not reported any significant effects [59].

10.4.5 Monoaminergic Agents for the Rehabilitation of Walking in SCI

Adrenergic agonists can aid in the recovery of walking following acute SCI in cats and rats when combined with treadmill training. The drug activates neurons involved in central pattern generation, leading to alternating rhythmic activation of muscles. Serotonergic agonists have been associated with improvements in stepping patterns in animals, but can also lead to spasms and clonus that interfere with walking [59].

Trials of adrenergic agonists (clonidine) and serotonergic antagonists (cyroheptadine) in isolation or in combination in humans with incomplete SCI suggest that they may also aid recovery of walking speed, muscle activation patterns, and antigravity activity. However, the effects are small in comparison to the effect sizes associated with locomotor retraining [59]. With the possibility of regenerative techniques in the future (e.g., olfactory ensheathing cells), it may be that combined therapies could lead to better functional improvements in people with SCI.

10.5 Surgical Treatment

10.5.1 Orthopaedic Management of Walking

Surgical procedures are often combined together in single-event, multilevel surgery. This makes the evaluation of individual techniques difficult. This is compounded by difficulties in finding an appropriate control list. In adults and children with cerebral palsy, retrospective review of cases of de-rotational femoral osteotomy indicates that it is associated with improved external hip rotation and foot progression angle while walking [67, 68]. Contracted two-joint muscles such as the hip flexors, hamstrings, rectus femoris, and gastrocnemius may be the target of muscle-lengthening techniques, and tendon transfers have been used to treat inappropriately timed muscle activity. Improvements in stiff knee gait, for example, are seen following a tendon transfer of the rectus femoris. However, this is only seen if there is demonstrable overactivity of the rectus femoris during swing phase as measured using EMG. People without increased EMG activation where stiff knee gait could be caused by weakness in muscle initiating swing phase did not improve [69]. This highlights an area where instrumented gait analysis could be important for patient selection.

10.5.2 Functional Neurosurgery

Deep brain stimulation (DBS) is covered in more detail elsewhere (see Chapter 12). DBS of the subthalamic (STN) nucleus for Parkinson's disease is effective in reducing many motor complications. However, although STN stimulation is effective in reducing L-dopa responsive freezing, its effects on symptoms such as freezing, festination, and poor balance are often not marked. More recently, DBS of the pedunculopontine (PPN) nucleus has been explored [10]. The PPN receives direct input from the basal ganglia and when stimulated in animals results in walking initiation. Stimulation of this in initial trials shows promising results, suggesting further research is required.

References

1. Winter DA. Human balance and posture control during standing and walking. *Gait and Posture* 1995; **3**: 193–214.

2. Lyon IN, Day BL. Control of frontal plane motion in human stepping. *Experimental Brain Research* 1997; **115**: 345–56.

3. Duysens J, Van de Crommert HAA. Neural control of locomotion. Part 1: The central pattern generator from cats to humans. *Gait and Posture* 1998; **7**: 131–41.

4. Dietz V, Sinkjaer T. Spastic movement disorder: Impaired reflex function and altered muscle mechanics. *Lancet Neurology* 2007; **6**: 725–33.

5. Duysens J, Pearson KG. From cat to man: Basic aspects of locomotion relevant to motor rehabilitation of SCI. *NeuroRehabilitation*. 1998; **10**(2): 107–18.

6. Lord SR. Visual risk factors for falls in older people. *Age Ageing* 2006; **35** Suppl. 2: ii42–ii5.

7. Allum JHJ, Bloem BR, Carpenter MB, Hulliger M, Hadders-Algra M. Proprioceptive control of posture: A review of new concepts. *Gait and Posture* 1998; **8**: 214–42.

8. Bronstein AM. Vision and vertigo: Some visual aspects of vestibular disorders. *Journal of Neurology* 2004; **251** (4): 381–7.

9. Bronstein AM, Lempert T. Management of the patient with chronic dizziness. *Restor. Neurol. Neurosci.* 2010; **28**(1): 83–90.

10. Collomb-Clerc A, Welter ML. Effects of deep brain stimulation on balance and gait in patients with Parkinson's disease: A systematic neurophysiological review. *Neurophysiol. Clin.* 2015; **45**(4–5): 371–88.

11. Mori S. Integration of posture and locomotion in acute decerebrate cats and in awake freely moving cats. *Progress in Neurobiology* 1987; **28**: 161–95.

12. Spildooren J, Vercruysse S, Meyns P, Vandenbossche J, Heremans E, Desloovere K, et al. Turning and unilateral cueing in Parkinson's disease patients with and without freezing of gait. *Neuroscience* 2012; **207**: 298–306.

13. Yarnall A, Rochester L, Burn DJ. The interplay of cholinergic function, attention, and falls in Parkinson's disease. *Mov. Disord.* 2011; **26**(14): 2496–2503.

14. Marsden J, Harris C. Cerebellar ataxia: Pathophysiology and rehabilitation. *Clin. Rehabil.* 2011; **25**(3): 195–216. LID – 10.1177/0269215510382495 [doi].

15. Christensen LOD, Petersen N, Andersen JB, Sinkjaer T, Nielsen JB. Evidence for transcortical reflex pathways in the lower limb of man. *Progress in Neurobiology* 2000; **62**: 251–72.

16. Dawes H, Enzinger C, Johansen-Berg H, Bogdanovic M, Guy C, Collett J, et al. Walking performance and its recovery in chronic stroke in relation to extent of lesion overlap with the descending motor tract. *Exp. Brain Res.* 2008; **186**(2): 325–33.

17. Nutt JG. Higher-level gait disorders: An open frontier. *Mov. Disord.* 2013; **28**(11): 1560–5.

18. Hafer-Macko CE, Ryan AS, Ivey FM, Macko RF. Skeletal muscle changes after hemiparetic stroke and potential beneficial effects of exercise intervention strategies. *Rehabil. Res. Dev.* 2008; **45**(2): 261–72.

19. Balaban CD. Neural substrates linking balance control and anxiety. *Physiol. Behav.* 2002; **77**(4–5): 469–75.

20. Teodoro T, Edwards MJ. Functional movement disorders. *Curr. Opin. Neurol.* 2016; **29**(4): 519–25.

21. Gor-Garcia-Fogeda MD, Cano de la Cuerda R, Carratala Tejada M, Alguacil-Diego IM, Molina-Rueda F. Observational gait assessments in people with neurological disorders: A systematic review. *Arch. Phys. Med. Rehabil.* 2016; **97**(1): 131–40.

22. Baker RW. *Measuring walking: A handbook of clinical gait analysis*. London, UK: Wiley, 2013.

23. Mudge SS, Stott, NS. Outcome measures to assess walking ability following stroke: A systematic review of the literature. *Physiotherapy* 2007; **93**(3): 189–200.

24. Taylor D, Stretton CM, Mudge S, Garrett N. Does clinic-measured gait speed differ from gait speed measured in the community in people with stroke? *Clin. Rehabil.* 2006; **20**(5): 438–44.

25. Stretton CM, Mudge S, Kayes NM, McPherson KM. Interventions to improve real-world walking after stroke: A systematic review and meta-analysis. *Clin Rehabil.* 2017; **31**(3): 310–18.

26. Martin L, Haskard-Zolnierek K, DiMatteo MR. *Health behaviour change and treatment adherence: Evidence based guidelines for improving healthcare*. Oxford, UK: Oxford University Press, 2010.

27. Mansfield A, Wong JS, Bryce J, Brunton K, Inness EL, Knorr S, et al. Use of accelerometer-based feedback of walking activity for appraising progress with walking-related goals in inpatient stroke rehabilitation:

A randomized controlled trial. *Neurorehabil. Neural Repair* 2015; **29**(9): 847–57.

28. Wahl HW, Fange A, Oswald F, Gitlin LN, Iwarsson S. The home environment and disability-related outcomes in aging individuals: What is the empirical evidence? *Gerontologist* 2009; **49**(3): 355–67.

29. Bohannon RW. Muscle strength and muscle training after stroke. *Journal of Rehabilitation Medicine* 2007; **39**: 14–20.

30. Pak S, Patten C. Strengthening to promote functional recovery poststroke: An evidence-based review. *Top Stroke Rehabil.* 2008; **15**(3): 177–99.

31. Howlett OA, Lannin NA, Ada L, McKinstry C. Functional electrical stimulation improves activity after stroke: A systematic review with meta-analysis. *Arch. Phys. Med. Rehabil.* 2015; **96**(5): 934–43.

32. Katalinic OM, Harvey LA, Herbert RD. Effectiveness of stretch for the treatment and prevention of contractures in people with neurological conditions: A systematic review. *Phys. Ther.* 2011; **91**(1): 11–24.

33. Carda S, Invernizzi M, Baricich A, Cisari C. Casting, taping or stretching after botulinum toxin type A for spastic equinus foot: A single-blind randomized trial on adult stroke patients. *Clin. Rehabil.* 2011; **25**(12): 1119–27.

34. Mead G, Van Wijck F. eds. *Exercise and fitness training after stroke.* London, UK: Churchill Livingstone, 2013.

35. Rochester L, Burn DJ, Woods G, Godwin J, Nieuwboer A. Does auditory rhythmical cueing improve gait in people with Parkinson's disease and cognitive impairment? A feasibility study. *Mov. Disord.* 2009; **24**(6): 839–45.

36. Brauer SG, Morris ME. Can people with Parkinson's disease improve dual tasking when walking? *Gait Posture* 2010; **31**(2): 229–33.

37. Tyson SF, Kent RM. Effects of an ankle-foot orthosis on balance and walking after stroke: A systematic review and pooled meta-analysis. *Arch. Phys. Med. Rehabil.* 2013; **94**(7): 1377–85.

38. Van der Wilk D, Dijkstra PU, Postema K, Verkerke GJ, Hijmans JM. Effects of ankle foot orthoses on body functions and activities in people with floppy paretic ankle muscles: A systematic review. *Clin. Biomech.* (Bristol, Avon). 2015; **30**(10): 1009–25.

39. Franceschini M, Baratta S, Zampolini M, Loria D, Lotta S. Reciprocating gait orthoses: A multicenter study of their use by spinal cord injured patients. *Arch. Phys. Med. Rehabil.* 1997; **78**(6): 582–6.

40. Arazpour M, Samadian M, Bahramizadeh M, Joghtaei M, Maleki M, Ahmadi Bani M, et al. The efficiency of orthotic interventions on energy consumption in paraplegic patients: A literature review. *Spinal Cord* 2015; doi:10.1038/sc.2014.227

41. Karimi MT. Functional walking ability of paraplegic patients: Comparison of functional electrical stimulation versus mechanical orthoses. *European Journal of Orthopaedic Surgery & Traumatology: Orthopedie Traumatologie* 2013; **23**(6): 631–8.

42. Ramdharry G, Marsden JF, Day BL, Thompson AJ. De-stabilizing and training effects of foot orthoses in multiple sclerosis. *Multiple Sclerosis* 2006; **12**: 219–26.

43. Alfuth M. Textured and stimulating insoles for balance and gait impairments in patients with multiple sclerosis and Parkinson's disease: A systematic review and meta-analysis. *Gait Posture* 2016; **51**: 132–41.

44. Hatton AL, Rome K, Dixon J, Martin DJ, McKeon PO. Footwear interventions: A review of their sensorimotor and mechanical effects on balance performance and gait in older adults. *J. Am. Podiatr. Med. Assoc.* 2013; **103**(6): 516–33.

45. Jeka JJ. Light touch as a balance aid. *Physical Therapy* 1997; **77**: 476–87.

46. Mehrholz J, Pohl M, Elsner B. Treadmill training and body weight support for walking after stroke. *Cochrane Database Syst. Rev.* 2014; **1**: CD002840.

47. States RA, Pappas E, Salem Y. Overground physical therapy gait training for chronic stroke patients with mobility deficits. *Cochrane Database Syst. Rev.* 2009; **3**: CD006075.

48. Ni X, Liu S, Lu F, Shi X, Guo X. Efficacy and safety of Tai Chi for Parkinson's disease: A systematic review and meta-analysis of randomized controlled trials. *PLoS One* 2014; **9**(6): e99377.

49. Synofzik M, Ilg W. Motor training in degenerative spinocerebellar disease: Ataxia-specific improvements by intensive physiotherapy *Biomed. Res. Int.* 2014; **2014**: 583507.

50. Mehrholz J, Pohl M. Electromechanical-assisted gait training after stroke: A systematic review comparing end-effector and exoskeleton devices. *J. Rehabil. Med.* 2012; **44**(3): 193–9.

51. Laver KE, George S, Thomas S, Deutsch JE, Crotty M. Virtual reality for stroke rehabilitation. *Cochrane Database Syst. Rev.* 2015; **2**: CD008349.

52. McDonnell MN, Hillier SL. Vestibular rehabilitation for unilateral peripheral vestibular dysfunction. *Cochrane Database Syst. Rev.* 2015; **1**: CD005397.

53. Bunn L, Marsden J, Giunti P, Day B. Training balance with optokinetic stimuli: Feasibility testing of a home based therapy and clinical trial design for use with people with pure cerebellar disease (SCA6). *Clinical Rehabilitation* 2014; **29**(2): 143–53.

54. Eftekhar-Sadat B, Azizi R, Aliasgharzadeh A, Toopchizadeh V, Ghojazadeh M. Effect of balance training with Biodex Stability System on balance in

diabetic neuropathy. *Therapeutic Advances in Endocrinology and Metabolism* 2015; **6**(5): 233–40.

55. Bleyenheuft C, Cockx S, Caty G, Stoquart G, Lejeune T, Detrembleur C. The effect of botulinum toxin injections on gait control in spastic stroke patients presenting with a stiff-knee gait. *Gait Posture* 2009; **30** (2): 168–72.

56. Roche N, Zory R, Sauthier A, Bonnyaud C, Pradon D, Bensmail D. Effect of rehabilitation and botulinum toxin injection on gait in chronic stroke patients: A randomized controlled study. *J. Rehabil. Med.* 2015; **47**(1): 31–7.

57. Pin TW, McCartney L, Lewis J, Waugh MC. Use of intrathecal baclofen therapy in ambulant children and adolescents with spasticity and dystonia of cerebral origin: A systematic review. *Dev. Med. Child Neurol.* 2011; **53**(10): 885–95.

58. Kofler M, Quirbach E, Schauer R, Singer M, Saltuari L. Limitations of intrathecal baclofen for spastic hemiparesis following stroke. *Neurorehabilitation and Neural Repair* 2009; **23**(1): 26–31.

59. Domingo A, Al-Yahya AA, Asiri Y, Eng JJ, Lam T. A systematic review of the effects of pharmacological agents on walking function in people with spinal cord injury. *J. Neurotrauma.* 2012; **29**(5): 865–79.

60. Kim SD, Allen NE, Canning CG, Fung VS. Postural instability in patients with Parkinson's disease. Epidemiology, pathophysiology and management. *CNS Drugs* 2013; **27**(2): 97–112.

61. Smulders K, Dale ML, Carlson-Kuhta P, Nutt JG, Horak FB. Pharmacological treatment in Parkinson's disease: Effects on gait. *Parkinsonism Relat. Disord.* 2016; **31**: 3–13.

62. Chung KA, Lobb BM, Nutt JG, Horak FB. Effects of a central cholinesterase inhibitor on reducing falls in Parkinson disease. *Neurology* 2010; **75**(14): 1263–9.

63. Moreau C, Delval A, Defebvre L, Dujardin K, Duhamel A, Petyt G, et al. Methylphenidate for gait hypokinesia and freezing in patients with Parkinson's disease undergoing subthalamic stimulation: A multicentre, parallel, randomised, placebo-controlled trial. *Lancet Neurol.* 2012; **11**(7): 589–96.

64. de Jong MR, Van der Elst M, Hartholt KA. Drug-related falls in older patients: Implicated drugs, consequences, and possible prevention strategies. *Therapeutic Advances in Drug Safety* 2013; **4**(4): 147–54.

65. Woolcott JC, Richardson KJ, Wiens MO, Patel B, Marin J, Khan KM, et al. Meta-analysis of the impact of 9 medication classes on falls in elderly persons. *Arch. Intern. Med.* 2009; **169**(21): 1952–60.

66. Lugaresi A. Pharmacology and clinical efficacy of dalfampridine for treating multiple sclerosis. *Expert Opinion on Drug Metabolism & Toxicology* 2015; **11**(2): 295–306.

67. Putz C, Wolf SI, Geisbusch A, Niklasch M, Doderlein L, Dreher T. Femoral derotation osteotomy in adults with cerebral palsy. *Gait Posture* 2016; **49**: 290–6.

68. Saglam Y, Ekin Akalan N, Temelli Y, Kuchimov S. Femoral derotation osteotomy with multi-level soft tissue procedures in children with cerebral palsy: Does it improve gait quality? *J. Child. Orthop.* 2016; **10**(1): 41–8.

69. Goldberg SR, Ounpuu S, Arnold AS, Gage JR, Delp SL. Kinematic and kinetic factors that correlate with improved knee flexion following treatment for stiff-knee gait. *J. Biomech.* 2006; **39**(4): 689–98.

Management of Spasticity in Neurorehabilitation

Valerie L. Stevenson

11.1 Introduction

Spasticity is a common feature in the neurorehabilitation setting and is seen in many neurological conditions, including single-insult events such as head injury, spinal cord injury, stroke, or cerebral palsy, as well as many chronic neurological conditions such as multiple sclerosis, hereditary spastic paraparesis, or motor neurone disease. It does impact individuals in wide-ranging ways. For some, it means pain, discomfort, and sleep disturbance, whilst others are more aware of the functional consequences of troublesome spasticity with negative impact on their ability to walk, self-propel a wheelchair, or transfer safely. Other activities of daily living, including washing, dressing, toileting, and sexual activity, can also be affected, which all lead to restriction of fulfilment of life roles, including those as an employee, parent, or partner. At its worst, spasticity can result in complete immobility with the loss of ability to be seated preventing access to the community and causing severe contractures and pressure sores. However, paradoxically for some, the presence of spasticity is extremely important, perhaps allowing them to stand or walk when their weakness would not otherwise permit or through utilizing spasms to become independent in transfers or bed mobility. When considering how best to manage a person's symptoms or prevent complications from poorly managed spasticity, it is important to consider all these aspects; however, it is also essential to remember that spasticity is only one component of upper motor neurone syndrome. Other symptoms such as muscle weakness, decreased postural responses, and reduced dexterity often coexist and also impact an individual's function.

11.2 Pathophysiology

'Spasticity' can be considered an umbrella term and is understood to include hypertonia, clonus, and spasms [1].

Hypertonia: this is the increase in tone or resistance to movement, felt when a limb is passively moved by another person. Resistance to movement can have both neural and non-neural components.

Neural (or reflexive) changes in resistance are caused by the triggering of enhanced stretch reflexes. Whilst non-neural changes reflect alterations in the viscoelastic properties of soft tissues (e.g., muscles and connective tissue) surrounding the joint and intrinsic muscle changes (alteration in muscle fibre composition and formation of cross-bridges within the muscle). It is important to distinguish between the different components of hypertonia as treatment options vary – the non-neural component may be more amenable to physical interventions such as splinting and stretching whilst pharmacological interventions only target the neural component.

The pathophysiology of neural hypertonia is complex, but includes an enhanced and prolonged response to muscle stretch, decreased task- and phase-dependent modulation of stretch reflexes due to a reduction in spinal cord inhibitory control, and intrinsic changes within the motor neuron. Prolonged plateau-like potentials of motor neuron discharges combined with reduced inhibitory spinal cord control mean that, once triggered, muscle contraction can continue unabated [2].

Clonus: this is a rhythmic pattern of contraction at a rate of several times per second, caused by alternate stretching and unloading of the muscle spindles. If the stretching force is sustained, there is continuous triggering of the phasic stretch reflex. This may be seen with the rhythmic contractions of the gastrocnemius and soleus muscles that occur in response to dorsiflexion of the ankle, commonly seen as a continuous tapping or shaking of the leg when feet are positioned on wheelchair footplates.

Spasms: these sudden involuntary (often painful) movements can be spontaneous or caused by muscle stretch or other stimuli. It is important to note that so-

Table 11.1 Trigger or aggravating factors which may exacerbate spasticity or spasms

Cutaneous stimuli	Visceral stimuli
• Inflamed/broken skin	• Any systemic or localized infection
• Pressure sores	• Bowel dysfunction, e.g., constipation, impaction, diarrhoea
• Skin or nail infections	• Bladder dysfunction, e.g., infections, retention, incomplete emptying, bladder stones
• Ingrown toenails	• Deep vein thrombosis
• Tight-fitting clothes or urinary leg bag straps	• Fractures
• Uncomfortable orthotics, splints or seating systems	

called spontaneous spasms may well be the result of as-yet-unidentified stimuli; it is therefore essential to search for any possible trigger factors, which may be cutaneous or visceral in nature (see Table 11.1). Spasms can also occur, as a result of disinhibited polysynaptic reflexes such as the flexor withdrawal reflex, or reflecting abnormal activity within spinal cord circuits that have the effect of synchronizing the discharge of motor neurons supplying multiple muscles.

A sound knowledge of the underlying pathophysiology of spasticity is extremely important for all members of the multidisciplinary team. This knowledge will not only guide the team in devising the most appropriate management plan for an individual, but will also allow them to provide clear and relevant education to the person with spasticity, and, if appropriate, their families and carers. This provision of education and promotion of self-management is instrumental in the overall success of any spasticity management programme.

11.3 Creating an Individualized Treatment Plan

The fact that spasticity is relevant to many neurological conditions, and that the absence of early identification and instigation of effective management can

result in progressive disability, makes it essential that a coordinated multidisciplinary treatment approach is used with successful liaison between secondary, primary, and social care. Treatment plans must always be individualized and function focused rather than simply aimed at reducing spasticity.

11.3.1 Assessment and Goal Setting

Before devising a treatment plan, it is essential to have an accurate understanding of the individual's hopes, concerns, level of function, and symptoms. This should include a detailed history comprising documentation of any potential trigger factors (see Table 11.1) and previous treatments trailed (including therapy, orthotics, and drugs – importantly with details on dose and duration). The examination documents physical changes such as resistance to movement, weakness, and contractures and considers the role of spasticity in the individual's function. The use of outcome measures quantitatively informs the assessment process, allowing effective communication between teams and providing a vital objective record that informs therapeutic decisions for that individual, facilitates monitoring over time, and aids in assessing the efficacy of interventions in the research or audit setting.

This process of understanding the individual's concerns and building up a picture of how spasticity impacts on their daily life – both positively and negatively – is vitally important and leads to goal identification (e.g., transferring independently, being able to sleep through the night). From this, an individualized management plan can be devised utilizing the following treatment options (see Figure 11.1 for an example of a treatment algorithm [3]). Tailoring successful treatment programmes to suit each individual is dependent on this understanding and requires detailed ongoing liaison between the person with spasticity, any carers or family members, and their treating teams [4]

11.3.2 Education and Self-Management

Educating people with long-term conditions to participate in the management and treatment of their symptoms has been central to UK health and social care policy over the past decade; it is recognized that by involving people in planning their own care (for

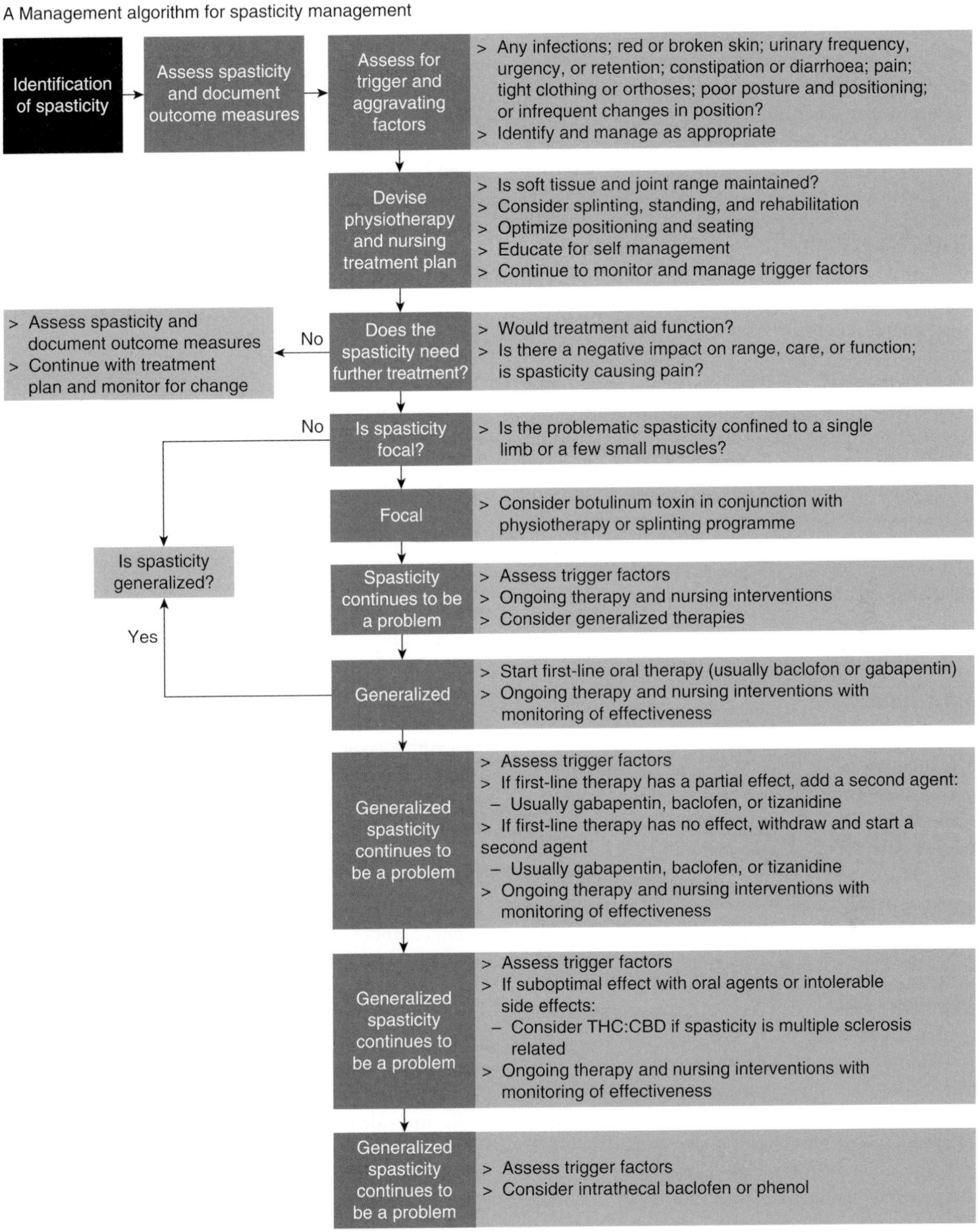

A Management algorithm for spasticity management

THC: CBD = delta-9-tetrahydrocannabinol/cannabidiol

Figure 11.1 An algorithm for spasticity management (Adapted with permission from Stevenson VL, Playford ED. Neurological rehabilitation and the management of spasticity. *Medicine* 2016;44(9): 530–6)

example, collaborative goal setting, shared decision-making), improvements in outcomes can be demonstrated and people feel more in control of their lives [5].

Education is therefore at the centre of any management plan. This includes knowledge about spasticity, its associated features (spasms, clonus) and what affects them, and how individuals can help themselves to manage and prevent symptoms. Awareness of the trigger and aggravating factors detailed in Table 11.1 is particularly important. Material should be presented in a format that suits the individual; this may be a combination of verbal, written, web-based, DVD content, or through user groups and discussions.

Self-management describes the strategies a person uses to control their symptoms and to promote wellness [6]. The role of the professional is to promote self-management through sharing knowledge and providing advice and support. To enable successful self-management access to the wider multidisciplinary team including nursing, physiotherapy, occupational therapy, continence advisors and orthotics is essential for the individual.

11.4 Physical and Postural Management

One key component of effective self-management is the instigation of a tailored realistic physical programme, including attention to posture and positioning that the person with spasticity or their family and carers is able to carry out at home, whatever the individual's level of function. The use of written material to reinforce verbal information can be useful as an aide memoire or to help with communication between carers.

Liaison between health and social care teams within both primary and secondary care will ensure that a consistent approach is maintained over time, with reinforcement to the individual, their family, and carers about the aims and benefits of continuing a physical management programme. For instance, daily exercises or stretches can be successfully factored into the morning regime of a person's care package. Open channels of communication between teams and services and mechanisms for review are essential to respond to changes in spasticity or functional levels.

The physiotherapist is key to devising the physical management programme; however, as previously explained, it is important for all members of the multidisciplinary team to have an understanding of the pathophysiology of spasticity ensuring they are able to support the individual in their self-management. The awareness of coexistence of non-neural and neural causes of hypertonia reinforces the need for a moving, stretching, and positioning programme aimed at minimizing changes in the viscoelastic properties of soft tissues (maintaining range and preventing contractures), preventing overuse of spasticity or spasms (whilst maintaining function when spasticity is necessary for this), and hopefully maintaining or improving function (strengthening and cardiovascular fitness) [7].

The specific makeup of a physical programme will be tailored to the individual, but usually includes a range of the following.

11.4.1 Active Exercise and Strengthening

Where possible, active exercise to increase strength, re-educate movement patterns, and improve cardiovascular fitness should be encouraged, as the effects are greater than those seen with passive exercise alone. Programmes need to be realistic and include when possible task-specific exercises such as sit-to-stand or step-ups as these are often more easily incorporated into daily routines. Historically strengthening muscles with spasticity was discouraged in the belief that this would exacerbate spasticity; however, it is now accepted that muscles with spasticity and their antagonists may all be weak, but there is invariably relative overactivity of one versus the other. This imbalance often impairs functional movement and in turn may lead to muscle atrophy, soft tissue changes, and, ultimately, joint deformity.

The value of strengthening muscles in individuals with significant spasticity has been highlighted in several research studies, including a systematic review of strength-training programmes for people with cerebral palsy which analysed the results of 11 studies and reported increased strength and motor function with no evidence of negative effects such as reduced range of motion or increasing spasticity [8].

A recent Cochrane review in people with stroke support that it is possible to improve strength, activity levels, walking speed, and balance without increasing spasticity. The Cochrane review recommended that there is sufficient evidence to incorporate cardiorespiratory and mixed training, involving walking, within post-stroke rehabilitation programmes [9].

Likewise a 2004 Cochrane systematic review confirmed there is good evidence that exercise can be beneficial for mobility, isometric muscle strength, physical fitness, and mood in people with MS [10].

The benefits of exercise have also been confirmed in relation to aerobic training, moderate progressive resistance exercise, and core stability training [7]. It is important to note that when devising strengthening programmes, it is essential that the trunk and pelvis are not neglected, as proximal control is crucial for limb function and a poorly aligned weak trunk can have a significant impact on both spasms and spasticity.

11.4.2 Standing

Assisted standing has been used as a neurorehabilitation technique since the 1970s, and its usefulness in multiple sclerosis was recently highlighted in the National Institute for Care Excellence (NICE) guidelines [11]. Research studies, predominantly of tilt table-assisted standing in patients with spinal cord injury, acquired brain injury, cerebral palsy, stroke, and multiple sclerosis, have demonstrated beneficial effects of standing, with changes in passive range of movement, spasticity bladder and bowel function, psychological well-being, and neurophysiological measures, although study numbers are small. The beneficial effects of standing are postulated to be secondary to promotion of antigravity muscle activity in the trunk and lower limbs, maintenance or improvement in soft tissue and joint flexibility, modulation of the neural component of spasticity through prolonged stretch and altered sensory input, reduction of lower limb spasms, and positive psychological effect [7]. There is no clear guidance regarding the optimum time and frequency for standing; in practice; advice on standing regimes is individualized to the person and their lifestyle. Self-report studies suggest that individuals chose to stand for an average of 30–40 minutes, three or four times a week. In a recent study in multiple sclerosis, beneficial effects were seen with 30 minutes three times weekly [12]. If achievable, half an hour most days would seem a reasonable target.

When considering the practicalities of standing, it is necessary to ensure optimal alignment of the trunk, pelvis, and legs is achieved. Household equipment (e.g., kitchen units, wall bar, armchair) or specialist equipment, including Oswestry standing frames, motorized standing frames, standing wheelchairs, tilt tables, or standing hoists, can be utilized. Careful assessment by a physiotherapist with trials of equipment is essential to ensure standing is both effective and safe.

11.4.3 Passive Movements

Passive movement is useful when active movement is not possible or induces severe spasticity or spasms; it relies upon assistance from a second person or a mechanical aid (passive cycling or continuous passive movement machines) to move the limb. By moving all affected body parts through their available range on a daily basis it is hoped secondary non-neural changes can be prevented; certainly passive movements before functional tasks such as washing and dressing can ease care and increase comfort. The evidence base to support this is, however, small [13].

11.4.4 Stretches, Positioning, and Seating

The aim of stretching is to combat the viscoelastic changes occurring in muscles and soft tissues around joints, thus ensuring muscle length is maintained or improved.

A systematic review on the use of stretching in people with muscle, central, and peripheral nervous system disorders reported a small, immediate effect on joint mobility, but little effect [14]. However, the studies varied significantly in methodology.

More recent studies have confirmed the short-term benefit of stretching in spasticity. These results suggest that stretching before functional tasks or before applying splints or positioning aids will ease care and improve comfort and function. This is reflected in the 2015 UK practice guidelines for the use of splinting for the prevention and correction of contractures. Further research is, however, needed to guide on the duration, intensity, and frequency of stretch application necessary [15]. On a pragmatic note, it is suggested to highlight to individuals, their families, and carers that stretching can be particularly beneficial prior to carrying out activities of daily living such as washing and dressing and also prior to exercise.

Periods of prolonged stretch can be achieved by positioning, including standing, sitting, and lying, and also via the use of splints or orthotics. Remember, however, that stretching one muscle puts the opposing muscle group in a position of relative shortening; it is therefore important that stretching regimes are balanced and aim for optimal alignment for function. In this way, the risk of skin breakdown can be reduced, comfort and sleep improved, and deformity prevented. Spasticity and spasms can be reduced by positioning in postures opposite to the pattern of the spasticity or spasms (e.g., if extensor spasms are problematic, then position in flexion over a T-roll or pillows). Equipment can be useful, including pillows and towels, wedges, T and E rolls, electrically powered profiling beds, and specialized sleep systems, as well as trays and tables to help position the upper limbs.

For individuals who are wheelchair users, posture and seating is of paramount importance. Spasticity can impact posture in positive (maintenance of sitting with severe truncal weakness) and negative ways (postural instability, reduced upper limb function). Optimal positioning of a person via the use of an appropriate seating system (e.g., a tilt-in-space system) can assist in reducing these problems and will help maximize function and comfort [16].

It is essential to remember that over the course of time, levels of function and spasticity may change; this is particularly evident after therapeutic interventions such as intrathecal baclofen (ITB) or phenol (see Section 11.7). It is therefore extremely important that seating needs are reviewed regularly and promptly, especially after any treatment interventions. Ideally, if intrathecal therapies are proposed, liaison should be established between the seating service and the multidisciplinary team before the treatment.

11.4.5 Splinting and Orthotics

Externally applied devices such as splints or casts made by therapists or off-the-shelf/custom-made orthotics are rarely used in isolation to manage spasticity, but are part of a comprehensive physical management programme. Their use requires careful assessment combined with goal setting and ongoing review of outcomes to ensure suitability of use and avoidance of complications. Goals of use may centre around providing control of the range of movement around a joint and thereby facilitating function, allowing a prolonged stretch to modulate the neural component of spasticity and/or prevent or correct contracture, compensation for deformity (e.g., a heel raise to correct a leg length discrepancy), or to increase comfort/reduce pain secondary to

malalignment. The evidence base for use of splints and orthotics is small as many studies use functional outcomes such as the impact of walking on ankle-foot orthoses, or combine splinting with other interventions such as physiotherapy or botulinum toxin. In 2015, the UK College of Occupational Therapists – Specialist Section Neurology Practice and the Chartered Society of Physiotherapists – Association of Physiotherapists Working in Neurology produced a practice guideline which provided specific recommendations to support best clinical practice in the prevention and correction of contractures [15].

On a practical level, it is important to consider the risk of skin breakdown. In at-risk individuals, splinting should be used with caution, and soft splints (such as foam, sheepskin, pillow wrapping, lycra) should be considered. Combining splinting with therapeutic interventions such as botulinum toxin, oral medication, or intrathecal therapies is often very valuable [17].

11.4.6 Functional Electrical Stimulation

Functional electrical stimulation (FES) may be used to improve specific functions such as walking, to help strengthen weak muscles, to facilitate stretching, to maintain range of movement, and potentially to reduce spasticity. The most frequently used is common peroneal nerve stimulation, resulting in dorsiflexion and eversion of the foot, thus correcting dropped foot. When this is timed to the gait cycle using foot switches placed in the shoe, walking performance can be significantly improved. The UK NICE guidance published in 2009 recommended the use of FES in people with foot drop of central neurological origin of any cause [18].

Neuromuscular electrical stimulation also has a role in the upper limb and has been shown to reduce shoulder pain in the stroke population, although this may be due to correction of subluxation rather than by reducing spasticity [19].

11.4.7 Other Physical Treatment Modalities

Other treatments aimed at reducing spasticity have been explored; these include hippotherapy, hydrotherapy, vibration therapy, electromagnetic field therapy, extracorporeal shock wave therapy, reflexology, acupuncture, and massage. However, levels of evidence remain low or effects anecdotal, so further studies are necessary before any such treatments can be recommended [11, 20].

11.5 Oral Medication

Despite optimization of trigger factors and instigation of a physical management programme, it may be necessary to escalate to the use of pharmacological agents (see Figure 11.1); these are usually in the form of oral medication, but for focal problems botulinum toxin (see Section 11.6) can be very effective, and for regional effects predominantly targeting the lower limbs, intrathecal therapies can be utilized (see Section 11.7).

No agreed evidence-based model is available to guide the choice of agent or dosing schedule. Identification of treatment goals will help to optimize drug therapy not only in terms of choice of agent but also in terms of timing and dose. For example, painful nocturnal spasms may best be managed with a long-acting agent taken at night-time that has sedative side effects. Alternatively, stiffness and spasms, which interfere with a person's morning transfers and personal care, may benefit from medication taken on waking prior to the person transferring out of bed. Dosages for individuals who are walking, and who may be relying on their spasticity to do so, are often lower than in those who use a wheelchair for mobility. If other features such as neuropathic pain or epilepsy are present, then this will also impact the choice of agent.

A general rule with all medication is to 'start low and go slow'; this approach limits any deleterious effects on function or troublesome side effects. The most commonly reported side effect is of increased weakness, although it is of course important to recognize that this may actually be as a result of unmasking the degree of underlying weakness by reducing stiffness or spasm that was functionally useful.

Sometimes, it is preferable to use a combination of drugs at low levels to enable effective treatment within the realm of tolerable side effects or when appropriate to combine oral therapy with focal or intrathecal treatments. All of the commonly used drugs – baclofen, tizanidine, benzodiazepines, dantrolene, gabapentin, pregabalin, and delta-9-tetrahydrocannabinol/cannabidiol spray (THC/CBD) – can be used alone as monotherapy or in combination with each other (not all have a license specifically for spasticity treatment or monotherapy). As a general rule, if the first-line drug proves to be partially effective but causes side effects at higher doses, then a second-line drug can be added in and titrated upwards. If spasticity becomes well managed on this regime, the first drug can be cautiously withdrawn to see if monotherapy with the second-line drug alone is sufficient to achieve the goal of treatment. Likewise, if necessary, a third drug can be introduced along the same principles. If a drug is trialled that is completely ineffective either as a first-line treatment or as an adjunct, it can be gradually withdrawn before the next agent is tried (see Figure 11.1).

Whichever drug is chosen, it is essential that effective processes are in place for monitoring of effect and timely review. This is usually best done by the individual (or their family and carers), the prescriber, and physiotherapist.

The evidence base for all agents is fairly limited, with few placebo-controlled trials and little attention paid to functional benefit. The commonly used agents are summarized in Table 11.2.

11.5.1 Baclofen

This is the most commonly prescribed medication for spasticity. It is an analogue of the inhibitory neurotransmitter gamma-aminobutyric acid (GABA) and binds to GABA-B receptors, found predominantly presynaptically in the Ia sensory afferent neurons, the interneurons and also postsynaptically in the motor neurons. The predominant effect appears to be inhibition of monosynaptic and polysynaptic reflexes at the spinal level.

Clinical trials of baclofen demonstrating positive effects on spasticity and spasms were first carried out in the 1970s and have involved patients with multiple sclerosis, spinal cord injury, cerebral palsy, and stroke. In comparison studies, no difference in efficacy has been shown between baclofen and tizanidine, or between baclofen and diazepam [21–23]. Baclofen should be used with caution in individuals with epilepsy, as the seizure threshold may be reduced. Sudden withdrawal should be avoided in all individuals, as it may precipitate seizures, confusion, anxiety, and hallucinations. The recommended dose range for baclofen is up to 100 mg daily, usually in three divided doses with a starting dose of 5–10 mg daily.

11.5.2 Tizanidine

Tizanidine is a selective α2-adrenergic receptor agonist; its main effect is on spinal polysynaptic reflexes

Table 11.2 Oral medications for spasticity

Drug	Starting dose	Maximum dose	Main adverse effects	Mechanism of action	Special considerations
Baclofen	5–10 mg daily	100 mg in three or four divided doses	Drowsiness, weakness	GABA analogue, binds to $GABA_B$ receptors	Use with caution in epilepsy. Avoid abrupt withdrawal (seizures).
Tizanidine	2 mg daily	36 mg in three or four divided doses	Drowsiness, weakness, dry mouth, postural hypotension	α_2-Adrenoceptor agonist	Monitoring of liver function required
Gabapentin	100–300 mg daily	3,600 mg daily in three divided doses	Drowsiness, dizziness	GABA-ergic: appears to act at the $\alpha_2\delta$ subunit of calcium channels	May be particularly useful for spasms and pain
Dantrolene	25 mg daily	400 mg in four divided doses	Anorexia, nausea, vomiting, drowsiness, weakness, paraesthesia, rare hepatic failure	Acts peripherally by suppressing calcium release from the sarcoplasmic reticulum of skeletal muscle	May be particularly useful for spasms. Monitoring of liver function essential.
Clonazepam	0.25–0.5 mg usually at night time	2 mg at night	Drowsiness, reduced attention, memory impairment	Stimulation of $GABA_A$ receptors	Useful for nocturnal spasms, sleep disturbance. Avoid abrupt withdrawal (dependency syndrome)
Diazepam	2 mg daily	40–60 mg daily in three or four divided doses	Drowsiness, reduced attention, memory impairment	Stimulation of $GABA_A$ receptors	Best avoided because of tolerance, dependency and withdrawal syndromes
Pregabalin	25–50 mg daily	600 mg in two divided doses	Drowsiness, dizziness	GABA-ergic: appears to act at the $\alpha_2\delta$ subunit of calcium channels	May be particularly useful for spasms and pain. Also licensed for anxiety
γ9-tetrahydrocannabinol (THC) and cannabidiol (CBD) – THC:CBD, nabiximols, Sativex®	One spray. Each 100 microlitre spray contains 2.7 mg THC and 2.5 mg CBD	12 sprays per day	Dizziness, fatigue, psychotropic effects (anxiety, mood disturbance, delusions, paranoia), oromucosal irritation	Partial agonist action at CB1 and CB2 receptors of the endocannabinoid system	Licensed as an add-on therapy in MS

GABA, γ-aminobutyric acid.

through a reduction in presynaptic excitatory inter-neuronal activity.

Placebo-controlled trials in people with multiple sclerosis, spinal cord injury, and acquired brain injury have demonstrated a reduction in muscle tone, frequency of spasms, and clonus. In addition, it has been shown to be effective in myofascial and low back pain [22, 24]. The side-effect profile of tizanidine is comparable to that of baclofen; however, changes in liver function tests have been noted in people taking tizanidine, so it is important that liver function is monitored during use. Tizanidine is usually started at a dose of 2 mg daily, with increments every few days to a maximum of 36 mg daily.

11.5.3 Benzodiazepines

Benzodiazepines exert their effect through stimulation of GABA-A receptors and consequent reduction of mono- and polysynaptic reflexes. Their use is limited by side effects, including drowsiness, reduced attention, and memory impairment. In addition, there are risks of toxicity, physiological dependency with withdrawal syndromes, and tolerance. Clinical trials have shown efficacy in reducing spasticity and spasms but an excess of side effects compared to other agents [21]. Due to sedation being a common feature, benzodiazepines are often preferred for night-time use only. The two most commonly used benzodiazepines are clonazepam and diazepam. Clonazepam appears to be particularly useful for nocturnal spasms and stiffness; it can be started at a dose of 0.25–0.5 mg at night.

11.5.4 Dantrolene

Unlike all other agents discussed, dantrolene works in a completely novel way – directly on skeletal muscle by suppressing calcium ion release from the sarcoplasmic reticulum. It is therefore a potentially useful adjunct to a centrally acting agent for combination therapy. Studies in multiple sclerosis, spinal cord injury, stroke, and cerebral palsy suggest benefit in spasticity, although no functional benefit was shown. Unfortunately, side effects such as drowsiness, fatigue, weakness, dizziness, and gastrointestinal effects are fairly common and there is a risk of hepatotoxicity, which necessitates careful monitoring of liver function tests. Treatment usually starts at a dose of 25 mg once daily and is increased gradually to a maximum of 100 mg four times a day [3].

11.5.5 Gabapentin

Gabapentin is another GABAergic drug, and although its specific mode of action is unknown, it has been shown to bind to the α^2 subunit of calcium channels, and thus may modulate cell function through alterations in calcium ion influx. Its main use is now neuropathic pain having been launched as an anti-epileptic agent; however, its use as an anti-spasticity agent is accepted and features in the UK NICE MS guidelines [11]. Four small double-blind, placebo-controlled randomized studies have been performed to date, all of which showed favourable tolerability and a beneficial effect on measures of spasticity [25]. Generally it is well tolerated; it appears to be particularly useful in the management of spasms or when pain coexists. Normal starting dose is 100–300 mg once a day, which is usually escalated up to a maximum total daily dose of 3,600 mg.

11.5.6 Pregabalin

Like gabapentin, pregabalin is not licensed for spasticity but for neuropathic pain, epilepsy, and generalized anxiety disorder. It is useful for spasms and when pain or anxiety compound symptoms. Pregabalin also acts on the α^2 subunit of calcium channels. Evidence of efficacy is limited with no placebo-controlled trials, but observational study supports its benefit [26]. Pregabalin is generally well tolerated; the usual starting dose is 50–75 mg daily, increasing to a maximum of 600 mg in two to three divided doses.

11.5.7 Canabinoids

The main active ingredient of the cannabis plant (Cannabis sativa) is D9-tetrahydrocannabinol (THC), which is available as a synthetic pharmaceutical product (Dronabinol, Marinol®) or through whole-plant extracts (available as THC/CBD oromucosal spray; nabiximols, Sativex®: GW Pharma Ltd, UK). THC/CBD exerts its neurological effect through CB1 (and possibly other) receptors. Several studies have suggested a beneficial effect of THC/CBD, although objective measures of spasticity failed to show a consistent difference. A 'definitive' placebo-controlled trial utilized an enriched design; 572 subjects were enrolled and given THC/CBD for four weeks; 272 achieved a ≥20% improvement (47% responder status). Intention-to-treat analysis showed a highly significant difference in favour of THC/CBD [27]. THC/CBD is generally well tolerated; side effects are usually mild and commonly consist of dizziness, disorientation, mood disturbance, and local oromucosal irritation. Open-label studies suggest that the effect is maintained over time without escalation in dose and with no detrimental effects on sudden withdrawal. It is important to counsel patients with regard to driving and international travel to check local laws regarding the use of cannabinoids. As less than 50% of patients are responders, it is important to define responder status as quickly as possible; this can be achieved by titrating THC/CBD up over 14 days to the maximum dose of 12 sprays/day and its efficacy and tolerability assessed.

11.6 Focal Treatment of Spasticity

Spasticity may present as a focal problem predominantly affecting one or two body areas; treatment strategies can therefore be targeted at the relevant muscle groups and potential side effects of oral drugs avoided. Some individuals, although they have a generalized spasticity that is for the most part being effectively managed with oral medication or intrathecal therapies, are still troubled by a focal problem such as a clenched fist that is interfering with function or care. Of the focal treatments available, botulinum toxin is the most widely used and the treatment of first choice as, unlike chemical neurolysis or surgical neurotomies, its clinical effects are entirely reversible. As with all interventions for spasticity, focal treatments must be given in the context of a multidisciplinary management plan with well-defined, realistic, and measurable goals. Therapy input and appropriate education for the individual (and if applicable their family or carers) to aid in goal formulation are essential to maximize the therapeutic effects.

11.6.1 Botulinum Toxin

Botulinum toxin is the most widely used treatment for focal spasticity. Of the seven serotypes, types A and B are currently licensed for therapeutic use; it is important to note that different serotypes and preparations have differing potencies and dosages are not transferrable. Botulinum toxin mediates its effect by interfering intracellularly with the process of calcium regulated synaptic vesicle exocytosis, thereby preventing release of acetylcholine into the synaptic cleft resulting in partial muscle paralysis. This effect begins immediately with clinically apparent effects seen between 4 and 14 days post injection and peak effect approximately three to six weeks after administration. Although this neuromuscular blockade is said to be permanent, the clinical effect is reversible – predominantly due to nerve sprouting and re-innervation in a few months. Thus injections may have to be repeated.

Trials in multiple sclerosis, stroke, cerebral palsy, spinal cord, and brain injury have demonstrated efficacy in reducing tone and improving passive function such as ease of hygiene or dressing [28]; however, there is little evidence to support benefits in active function [29]. Whether the lack of demonstration of functional improvement is real or related to inappropriate trial design, under-powering of studies, or the lack of responsive function-based outcome measures is difficult to ascertain.

Multidisciplinary involvement is essential throughout the assessment and goal-setting phase and in delivering botulinum toxin treatment. The weakening of targeted muscles allows a window of opportunity to enable establishment of a splinting or physical management programme which will hopefully allow the goal to be achieved and maintained long term without necessarily requiring repeat injections. UK and European guidelines have been developed which address this important area [15, 17, 30].

If a therapeutic effect is not seen following treatment, it is worth considering if the dose was insufficient, if the wrong muscle was injected, or whether anti-drug antibody production against the toxin has occurred. This is particularly relevant in so-called 'secondary non-responders' who initially had a good response to botulinum toxin injections but then failed to respond. In these individuals, switching to a different serotype may be helpful. To try to limit the development of neutralizing antibodies, it is advisable to use the lowest dose that is clinically effective and to avoid injections at intervals of less than three months [30]. Injection technique is also relevant with accuracy improved by the use of electromyography (EMG) or ultrasound. Botulinum toxin is usually well tolerated, though injections may be painful and this can be a limiting factor in children. Side effects are rare and transient; the main effects seen are due to the therapeutic effect of muscle weakness causing functional difficulties. Migration of the toxin can occur and is most relevant in the neck or facial muscles, where it can cause swallowing difficulties, ptosis, or diplopia. Rarely, generalized effects can occur with global weakness, fatigue, and cardiovascular changes [31].

11.6.2 Chemical Neurolysis

Local injection of phenol or alcohol is an alternative option for focal management. Chemical neurolysis results in destruction of neural tissue by protein coagulation and is said to be irreversible. It may therefore be an attractive option to avoid repeat injections of botulinum toxin. However, partial nerve regeneration and sprouting can occur so the clinical effect may 'wear off' after several weeks or months. Injections may be targeted at peripheral nerves or motor points. Most commonly applied are tibial (medial popliteal) blocks in the management of children with developing foot deformities and obturator nerve blocks in ambulatory patients with scissoring gait or for improving ease of perineal hygiene and aiding in seating posture [32].

11.7 Intrathecal Therapies

Usually spasticity and its functional consequences can be well controlled through multidisciplinary input with close attention to minimizing trigger or aggravating factors and a combination of physical measures, oral medication, and, if appropriate, focal therapies. However, occasionally this is not possible, and if the individual is predominantly troubled by lower limb spasticity, then ITB or phenol are further options to consider.

11.7.1 Intrathecal Baclofen

The concentration of GABA receptors in the lumbar spinal cord allows very small dosages of baclofen to be effective when delivered directly into the cerebrospinal fluid (CSF) without causing systemic side effects. The baclofen is delivered by a programmable pump which is usually implanted into the abdomen, although subfascial, infraclavicular, and gluteal placement may be considered in those with low body weight, complex postures, or limited abdominal space (for example, when used alongside a suprapubic catheter, colostomy, and/or gastrostomy). A catheter conveys the baclofen from the pump into the intrathecal space with the catheter tip sited at T11 or higher (see Figure 11.2). The pump is programmed via telemetry with options to vary the dose of baclofen throughout the day or deliver boluses at key times. Current models have a battery that

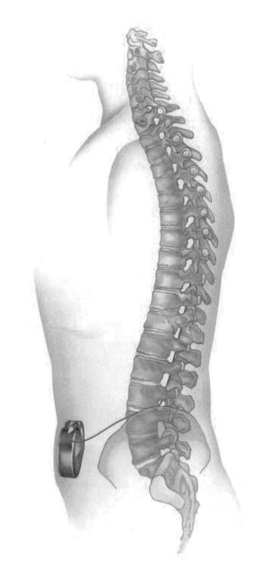

Figure 11.2 Position of intrathecal baclofen pump and catheter (Courtesy of Medtronic, Inc. [Minneapolis, MN, USA])

depletes within 6–10 years, necessitating further surgery to replace the pump.

ITB has been shown to be an effective treatment in the management of severe spasticity of either cerebral or spinal origin and for specific conditions such as brain or spinal cord injury, multiple sclerosis, cerebral palsy, hereditary spastic paraparesis, and stroke/hemiplegia [33]. Case series have also reported benefits in the stabilization of autonomic dysfunction early after brain injury and in disorders of consciousness, including persistent vegetative states, where reports have described effective control of spasticity and improvements in consciousness, although these effects need further investigation [34]. Historically, ITB was regarded as a last resort and reserved for people with significant levels of disability; more recently, it has been demonstrated to be effective in improving mobility in carefully selected individuals with spasticity from all causes, including cerebral palsy, multiple sclerosis, spinal cord injury, hereditary spastic paraparesis, and stroke, prompting ITB to be considered earlier to improve or maintain walking and limit the development of muscle shortening and contracture [35]. There is also the additional benefit of being able to reduce or withdraw oral medication which may be impacting fatigue, cognition, and bulbar function.

Careful selection and assessment of patients, education, and identification of clear treatment goals is essential before considering a trial of ITB. The trial can be done either as a lumbar puncture bolus injection of usually 25–100 mcg or via a temporary intrathecal catheter; the latter is often preferred in children when the catheter is sited under general anaesthesia. The trial dose is guided by functional level (ambulant individuals usually trialled with low levels ~25 mcg) and diagnosis (hypoxic or traumatic brain injury often requiring higher doses of 75–100 mcg). The peak effect of the trial dose is at four hours when the pre-trial assessment is repeated and outcome measures compared. Occasionally the trial may need to be repeated at a higher or lower dose to gain sufficient information to aid decision-making in whether to proceed to an implant. Following implantation, the individual's oral drugs are tapered and the intrathecal dose optimized. The pump then requires refilling at least every six months.

In long-term follow-up studies, the benefit of ITB has proved sustainable over time, with high levels of satisfaction from users. It must, however, be remembered that the use of ITB is not without risk of complications; abrupt withdrawal (through perhaps the pump reservoir emptying) or overdosing can result in death. Therefore services require a robust clinical governance framework and a coordinated approach by an experienced team including a neurologist/rehabilitation physician, neurosurgeon, physiotherapists, and nurses with access to the wider rehabilitation team [4].

When complications occur, or system dysfunction is suspected, investigation and treatment should be instigated promptly. Complications can be considered as mechanical (e.g., pump dysfunction, catheter disconnection or fracture, erosion of the skin over the pump), infection related, drug, or procedure related (e.g., baclofen overdose or deep vein thrombosis). For consenting purposes, a 1% per month annualized complication rate (of any kind) appears appropriate, although this is probably skewed with a higher rate in the first month following implantation [33, 36]. The most dangerous complications are those of baclofen overdose or withdrawal. Overdose is most likely to occur during the trial or following a programming or refill error; patients may present with drowsiness, flaccid weakness, nystagmus, diplopia, dizziness, cardiac abnormalities, delirium, respiratory depression, and coma. Emphasis should be on respiratory support and ITB dose reduction/cessation. For large overdoses, CSF drainage (30–50 mL) via lumbar puncture can be considered. Acute baclofen withdrawal can also be life threatening with the development of severe spasticity/spasms, goosebumps and pruritis, rhabdomyolysis, pyrexia, cardiac abnormalities, and seizures. Treatment with oral baclofen, benzodiazepines, tizanidine, or propofol should be initiated while the reason for withdrawal is established and rectified. In severe cases lumbar punctures or a temporary externalized catheter can be used to deliver ITB until long-term therapy is restored [37].

11.7.2 Intrathecal Phenol

There is a small group of patients with severe, troublesome, and often painful spasticity who cannot be effectively managed with simple measures and who are not appropriate for, or do not desire, ITB therapy. This group includes those nearing end of life, people in whom an ITB trial showed little benefit, or individuals who are not fit for, or do not want, surgery. If these individuals are carefully selected following thorough assessment and extensive education, intrathecal phenol has been found to be a highly effective and well-tolerated treatment [38, 39].

Phenol is a neurolytic chemical that causes coagulation of neural tissue and denaturing of proteins, which leads to cell damage, axonal degeneration, and indiscriminate destruction of motor and sensory nerves. Consequently, the potential impact on bladder, bowel, sexual, and sensory function needs to be carefully considered, and informed consent is vital with appropriate involvement of family members. This is especially important in view of new research strategies which are aimed at repair and regeneration of the nervous system through, for example, stem cell therapy. It is essential that patients and their families are clear that intrathecal phenol is about improving quality of life for individuals with severe spasticity *now*, and its use may compromise any future therapies aimed at neural repair [33].

Following careful patient assessment, selection, education, and consent a temporary block with intrathecal bupivacaine should be carried out to ascertain the potential benefits. This is particularly important when the goal of treatment is around seating as it allows the contribution of non-neural changes (contractures) to be demonstrated and informs on potential goal achievement. If the result is felt to be beneficial and the proposed goals achievable, then the individual will go on to have two phenol injections, each targeting one leg, 24 hours apart. Injecting 2 mL of 5% phenol in glycerol limits the dispersal into CSF and nerve tissue, resulting in a relatively neuro-selective effect, which can be further enhanced by specific positioning of the patient during and after the intrathecal injection (30 degrees prone), enabling motor nerve roots to be targeted while limiting the effect on sensory nerves. Like focal phenol blocks, although intrathecal phenol is considered permanent, the effects can wear off over time and injections may need to be repeated after six to nine months. The wearing off is thought to be due to regenerating axons eventually re-innervating the motor endplates of the nerves.

As phenol can significantly affect bladder, bowel, and sexual dysfunction, careful management plans need to be in place prior to treatment, including urinary catheterization. Although the sensory nerves are hopefully spared, it is important to inform individuals that there may be a change in sensation or pain. In practice, though, most individuals considering intrathecal phenol already have significant sensory and sphincter disturbance.

Spasticity, spasms, and associated pain can be dramatically reduced or eradicated by intrathecal phenol. This can lead to improved positioning, comfort, and ease of carrying out personal care either for the individual or for their carers. In addition, oral medication can often be withdrawn, which may be impacting arousal, cognitive, and bulbar function. As the effect is immediate with often considerable impact on an individual's posture in sitting and lying, it is imperative that treating services liaise with the relevant seating specialists or community therapists during the assessment phase to allow for prompt reassessment following treatment.

11.8 Selective Dorsal Rhizotomy

Selective dorsal rhizotomies (SDR) involve sectioning some of the rootlets of each targeted dorsal root to reduce the afferent input while preserving sensory and sphincter function. To date, SDR has mainly been used in ambulant children with cerebral palsy with good efficacy and sustained improvement in both spasticity and function [40], but it has recently been proposed as an alternative to ITB in non-ambulant children with cerebral palsy [41].

11.9 Conclusion

Spasticity is a common feature in the neurorehabilitation setting and is seen in many neurological conditions. However, by utilizing the basic principles of rehabilitation, including careful assessment and realistic goal setting, an individualized treatment plan can be formulated which will optimize function, reduce symptoms, and prevent long-term complications of poorly managed spasticity. A wide range of physical and pharmacological treatments is available to the multidisciplinary team which when used timely and appropriately, can be effective at reducing pain and discomfort without compromising function, whilst preventing secondary complications such as contractures or pressure sores. As with any area of rehabilitation, keeping the individual central to this process and ensuring close liaison between primary, secondary, and social care teams is essential for optimal management.

References

1. Kheder A, Nair KPS. Spasticity: Pathophysiology, evaluation and management. *Practical Neurology* 2012; **12**(5): 289–98.

2. Marsden JF. What is spasticity? In Stevenson VL, Jarrett L eds. *Spasticity management: A practical multidisciplinary guide* (2nd edn.). Boca Raton, FL: Taylor and Francis, 2016; 3–28.

3. Stevenson VL. Oral medication. In Stevenson VL, Jarrett L eds. *Spasticity management: A practical multidisciplinary guide* (2nd edn.). Boca Raton, FL: Taylor and Francis, 2016; 83–101.

4. Stevenson VL, Playford ED. Neurological rehabilitation and the management of spasticity. *Medicine* 2016; **44**(9): 530–6.

5. NHS Outcomes Framework England. 2014. www .england.nhs.uk/resources/resources-for-ccgs/out-frwrk/dom-2/.

6. Koch T, Jenkin P, Kralik D. Chronic illness self-management: Locating the 'self'. *J. Adv. Nurs.* 2004; **48**: 484–92.

7. Buchanan K, Hourihan S. Physical and postural management of spasticity. In Stevenson VL, Jarrett L eds. *Spasticity management: A practical multidisciplinary guide* (2nd edn.). Boca Raton, FL: Taylor and Francis, 2016; 57–82.

8. Andersson C, Grooten W, Hellsten M, Kaping K, Mattsson E. Adults with cerebral palsy: Walking ability after progressive strength training. *Dev. Med. Child. Neurol.* 2003; **45**: 220–8.

9. Saunders DH, Sanderson M, Brazzelli M, Greig CA, Mead GE. Physical fitness training for stroke patients. *Cochrane Database Syst. Rev.* 2013; **10**: CD003316.

10. Rietberg M, Brooks D, Uitdehaag B, Kwakkel G. Exercise therapy for multiple sclerosis. *Cochrane Database Syst. Rev.* 2004; **3**: CD003980.

11. National Institute for Health and Care Excellence. *Guideline for the management of MS in primary and secondary care.* London, UK: National Institute for Health and Care Excellence, 2014. www.nice.org.uk/g uidance/cg186.

12. Hendrie, WA, Watson, MJ, McArthur MA. A pilot mixed methods investigation of the use of Oswestry standing frames in the homes of nine people with severe multiple sclerosis. *Disabil. Rehab.* 2015; **37**(13): 1178–85.

13. Chang YJ, Liang JN, Hsu MJ et al. Effects of continuous passive motion on reversing the adapted spinal circuit in humans with chronic spinal cord injury. *Arch. Phys. Med. Rehabil.* 2013; **94**: 822–8.

14. Katalinic OM, Harvey LA, Herbert RD. Effectiveness of stretch for the treatment and prevention of contractures in people with neurological conditions: A systematic review. *Phys. Ther. J.* 2011; **91**(1): 11–24.

15. College of Occupational Therapists. Splinting for the prevention and correction of contractures in adults with neurological dysfunction, 2015. www.cot.co.uk/p ublication/cot-publications/splinting-prevention-and-correction-contracturesadults-neurological-dy.

16. Pope P. *Posture management and special seating: Neurological physiotherapy. A problem solving approach.* London, UK: Churchill Livingstone, 2002.

17. Intercollegiate Stroke Working Party. *National clinical guideline for stroke* (4th edn.). London, UK: Royal College of Physicians, 2012.

18. National Institute for Health and Care Excellence. *IPG278 functional electrical stimulation for drop foot of central neurological origin: Public information.* London,

UK: National Institute for Health and Care Excellence, 2009.

19. Price CI, Pandyan AD. Electrical stimulation for preventing and treating post-stroke shoulder pain: A systematic Cochrane review. *Clin. Rehabil.* 2001; **15** (1): 5–19.

20. Mills PB, Finlayson H, Sudol M, O'Connor R. Systematic review of adjunct therapies to improve outcomes following botulinum toxin injection for treatment of limb spasticity. *Clin. Rehabil.* 2016 Jun; **30** (6): 537–48.

21. Montane E, Vallano A, Laporte JR. Oral antispastic drugs in nonprogressive neurologic diseases: A systematic review. *Neurology* 2004; **63**: 1357–63.

22. Beard S, Hunn A, Wight J. Treatments for spasticity and pain in multiple sclerosis: A systematic review. *Health Technol. Assess.* 2003; **7**(40): iii, ix–x, 1–111, 24.

23. Paisley S, Beard S, Hunn A, Wight J. Clinical effectiveness of oral treatments for spasticity in multiple sclerosis: A systematic review. *Mult. Scler.* 2002; **8**: 319–29.

24. Malanga G, Reiter RD, Garay E. Update on tizanidine for muscle spasticity and emerging indications. *Expert Opin. Pharmacother.* 2008; **9**(12): 2209–15.

25. Formica A, Verger K, Sol JM, Morralla C. Gabapentin for spasticity: A randomized, double-blind, placebo controlled trial. *Med. Clin. (Barc.)* 2005; **124**: 81–5.

26. Bradley LJ, Kirker SGB. Pregabalin in the treatment of spasticity: A retrospective case series. *Disabil. Rehabil.* 2008; **30**(16): 1230–2.

27. Novotna A, Mares J, Ratcliffe S et al. A randomized, double-blind, placebo-controlled, parallel-group, enriched-design study of nabiximols (Sativex®), as add-on therapy, in subjects with refractory spasticity caused by multiple sclerosis. *Eur. J. Neurol.* 2011; **18**(9): 1122–31.

28. Baker JA, Pereira G. The efficacy of botulinum toxin A on improving ease of care in the upper and lower limbs: A systematic review and meta-analysis using the Grades of Recommendation, Assessment, Development and Evaluation approach. *Clin. Rehabil.* 2015; **29**(8): 731–40.

29. Foley N, Pereira S, Salter K et al. Treatment with botulinum toxin improves upper extremity function post stroke: A systematic review and meta-analysis. *Arch. Phys. Med. Rehabil.* 2013; **94**(5): 977–89.

30. Wissel J, Ward AB, Erztgaard P et al. European consensus table on the use of botulinum toxin type A in adult spasticity. *J. Rehabil. Med.* 2009; **41**(1): 13–25.

31. Farrell R, Buchanan K. Focal treatments, including botulinum toxin. In Stevenson VL, Jarrett L eds. *Spasticity management: A practical multidisciplinary*

guide (2nd edn.). Boca Raton, FL: Taylor and Francis, 2016; 103–27.

32. Barnes MP. Local treatment of spasticity. *Baillieres Clin. Neurol.* 1993; **2**(1): 55–71.

33. Stevenson VL. Intrathecal baclofen and phenol. In Stevenson VL, Jarrett L eds. *Spasticity management: A practical multidisciplinary guide* (2nd edn.). Boca Raton, FL: Taylor and Francis, 2016; 129–60.

34. Hoarau X, Richer E, Dehail P, Cuny E. A 10-year follow-up study of patients with severe traumatic brain injury and dysautonomia treated with intrathecal baclofen therapy. *Brain Injury* 2012; **26**(7–8): 927–40.

35. Sadiq SA, Wang GC. Long-term intrathecal baclofen therapy in ambulatory patients with spasticity. *J. Neurol* 2006; **253**(5): 563–9.

36. Borrini L, Bensmail D, Thiebaut JB, Hugeron C, Rech C, Jourdan C. Occurrence of adverse events in long-term intrathecal baclofen infusion: A 1-year follow-up study of 158 adults. *Arch. Phys. Med. Rehabil.* 2014; **95**(6): 1032–8.

37. Watve SV, Sivan M, Raza WA, Jamil FF. Management of acute overdose or withdrawal state in intrathecal baclofen therapy. *Spinal Cord* 2012; **50**(2): 107–11.

38. Jarrett L, Nandi P, Thompson AJ. Managing severe lower limb spasticity in multiple sclerosis: Does intrathecal phenol have a role? *J. Neurol. Neurosurg. Psychiatry* 2002; **73**: 705–9.

39. Pinder C, Bhakta B, Kodavali K. Intrathecal phenol: An old treatment revisited. *Disability and Rehabilitation* 2008; **30**(5): 381–6.

40. McLaughlin J, Bjornson K, Temkin N et al. Selective dorsal rhizotomy: Meta-analysis of three randomized controlled trials. *Dev. Med. Child. Neurol.* 2002; **44**(1): 17–25.

41. Ingale H, Ughratdar I, Muquit S, Moussa AA, Vloeberghs MH. Selective dorsal rhizotomy as an alternative to intrathecal baclofen pump replacement in GMFCS grades 4 and 5 children. *Childs Nerv. Syst.* 2016; **32**(2): 321–5.

Neurorehabilitation in Parkinson's Disease and Parkinsonism

Amit Batla and Fiona Lindop

12.1 Introduction

Parkinson's disease (PD) is a progressive, neurodegenerative disorder, which is characterized by both motor and non-motor symptoms. Rehabilitation plays an important role in managing all movement disorders, and each movement disorder requires a specific individualized neurorehabilitation approach with an understanding of aspects of presentation that might be ameliorated by intervention.

'Kinesis', or movement, is one of the most important functions of the human body. A useful definition of movement disorders is:

Either an excess of movement or a paucity of voluntary and automatic movements, unrelated to weakness or spasticity. [1]

Movement disorders can be classified as hypokinetic, e.g., PD and Parkinsonism, or hyperkinetic, comprising a broad and heterogeneous group which includes tremor, dystonia, chorea, tics, and myoclonus.

12.1.1 Understanding PD from a Rehabilitation Perspective

12.1.1.1 Parkinsonism

Parkinsonism is characterized by bradykinesia, tremor at rest, rigidity, flexed posture, gait, and balance disturbance, including freezing of gait. The aetiology of Parkinsonism can be degenerative, as in PD or in atypical Parkinsonism (also called Parkinson's plus), or secondary to stroke (vascular Parkinsonism), medication (such as haloperidol or valproate), infections, or encephalitis (postencephalitic Parkinsonism), among other causes. Parkinsonism can also be seen as an additional clinical feature in other movement disorders such as spinocerebellar ataxias and dystonia, or in systemic diseases or metabolic that manifest with multiple neurological features and movement disorders

(e.g., Wilson's disease). Typically, PD responds well to dopaminergic medication, but atypical Parkinsonism – progressive supranuclear palsy (PSP), multiple system atrophy (MSA), dementia with Lewy bodies (DLB), and corticobasal degeneration (CBD) – shows little or no response. Table 12.1 lists 'red flag' signs that should alert the clinician to the possibility of another diagnosis which could be MSA, PSP, CBD, or DLB. Although atypical Parkinsonian disorders are life-limiting conditions with no cure, early multidisciplinary team involvement is vital and should be directed at both quality of life and symptom management.

A detailed discussion of the pathophysiological process is beyond the scope of this chapter, but, essentially, in PD the lack of uptake of dopamine in the striatum secondary to loss of dopaminergic projections of cells based in substantia nigra contributes to motor and, to an extent, non-motor symptoms.

12.1.1.2 Motor Symptoms of PD

Resting symptoms of PD include:

- Bradykinesia or slowness of movement
- Resting tremor
- Rigidity
- Postural instability.

These symptoms, as well as dopamine-induced dystonia and dyskinesia, can impact both function and quality of life. In addition, fluency, coordination, efficiency, and speed of composite and fine motor movements are affected.

12.1.1.3 Non-Motor Symptoms

Non-motor symptoms of PD may sometimes manifest even prior to the onset of motor signs, and include changes in cognition (depression, anxiety, lack of motivation, cognitive impairment, hallucinations, psychosis), bowel, bladder, and sexual functions (constipation, delayed gastric emptying, nocturia, erectile dysfunction), sleep (including REM sleep disorder),

Table 12.1 Red flags for atypical Parkinsonism

Multiple system atrophy [13]	Progressive supranuclear palsy [12]	Corticobasal degeneration	Dementia with Lewy bodies
Poor response to dopaminergic treatment			
Early falls	Personality and cognitive changes	Personality and cognitive changes	Early onset of cognitive decline (within one year of motor symptoms)
Ataxic gait or cerebellar features (MSA-C)	Early falls (usually backwards)	Dystonia (asymmetric)	Fluctuating cognition
Orthostatic hypotension	Reduced eye movements (especially downward gaze)	Myoclonus	Hallucinations
Early bladder disturbance, impotence	Motor recklessness	Apraxia	Autonomic features
Inspiratory stridor	Dysarthria (pseudobulbar)	Alien limb	Falls
Anterocollis (forward flexed posture of neck)			

and pain (musculoskeletal, dystonic, central, radicular, akathisia [an inner restlessness]).

12.1.1.4 Atypical Parkinson's

Atypical Parkinson's (also known as Parkinson's plus syndromes) can have similar features to PD.

12.2 Management: An Overview

12.2.1 Multidisciplinary Team (MDT)

Individuals will experience differing problems according to their particular combination of symptoms with a resulting impact on activities and quality of life. The multidisciplinary team (MDT) approach is the optimal model for intervention in PD [2]. Team membership may differ from one health provider to another, but the disciplines work together to provide support and advice, optimizing the individual's function and mobility. Core professional disciplines represented in any MDT are likely to include a neurologist or geriatrician, PD nurse specialist (PDNS), physiotherapist, occupational therapist (OT), speech and language therapist (SLT), and dietician.

12.2.2 Medication

The timing of medication is an important factor in PD management and any intervention from members of the MDT should take this into account. For example, where possible treatment is timed for when the patient is in an 'on' state (when the medicine is

working at its optimal and enhancing movement quality), but assessment should also include during the 'off' state (when the medication levels are below an effective range) to enable a full understanding of the problems encountered.

12.2.3 Parkinson's Disease Nurse Specialist (PDNS)

The PDNS provides expert knowledge, advice, and support to patients and their families. They can undertake regular reviews in clinic, at home, or over the telephone advising on symptom management, medication, and side effects, and many are independent prescribers. They work closely with other professionals, including neurologists, general practitioners (GPs), and members of the MDT and are often the first point of contact for patients if they are experiencing problems.

12.2.4 Physiotherapy

The role of the physiotherapist focuses on maintaining or improving quality of life and independence. This will include maintaining and improving activity and function for the individual, as well as maximizing muscle power and flexibility. In order to achieve these aims, exercise and movement strategies may be taught, with intervention targeting gait, transfers, posture and balance, and falls prevention, and offering advice, education, and support to the patient and their family.

Basal ganglia dysfunction affects complex, well-learned activities and, combined with bradykinesia and rigidity, can make activities including walking and transfers difficult. Walking commonly becomes slower, with reduced stride length, although some patients find their speed increases involuntarily and they have difficulty coming to a safe halt. Transfer difficulties include standing up from a low chair or getting in and out of bed, or turning over. There is mounting evidence of the physical and physiological benefits of exercise in PD; therefore early referral to physiotherapy is recommended.

12.2.5 Occupational Therapy

The OT role includes assessment and intervention for activities of daily living (ADL) as well as cognition and mood. Non-motor symptoms such as depression, mild cognitive impairment, apathy, sleep problems (including difficulty falling asleep, fragmented sleep, or early waking), and fatigue all impact quality of life and can be addressed by the OT. A home visit may be conducted to assess ADL and transfers in the individual's own environment (both indoors and outdoors). Advice and equipment can also be offered to combat problems with mobility in bed.

12.2.6 Speech and Language Therapy

The SLT can assess and address problems with both communication and swallowing.

12.2.6.1

Speech can be affected by reduced volume, a flat or monotone pitch, a weak or hoarse voice, palilalia (a phrase or word repeated increasingly quickly), fast/mumbled speech, and word-finding difficulties. Following assessment, SLT intervention may include breathing and relaxation strategies, voice and pitch exercises, auditory feedback, and techniques to control over-fast speech. Communication aids or devices may be beneficial, particularly in the complex and palliative phases.

12.2.6.2 Swallowing

Problems may be experienced by up to 82% of people with PD [3], and an essential SLT role is to assess swallowing function in order to reduce risk of choking or aspiration. Advice can be given on diet-texture to reduce risk of aspiration. Techniques and aids can be considered for management of drooling.

12.2.7 Dietician

The dietician can provide advice regarding weight gain or loss, nutrition, and dietary management of constipation. In the palliative stages, advice on nutrition and percutaneous endoscopic gastrostomy (PEG) feeding may also be necessary.

12.2.8 Other Disciplines and Services

Referral to other disciplines and services may become necessary as the condition progresses. These may include:

- Psychology: for assistance in understanding change in life circumstances, roles, and vocation as a result of symptoms, diagnosis, or progression
- Psychiatry: to help in managing side effects of medication or progression such as psychosis, dementia
- Orthotics: for provision of specialist footwear, splints, or other supports
- Gait laboratory: for assessment of specific gait issues
- Urology: to help in managing bladder and sexual complaints
- Gastroenterology: to help in managing constipation and other bowel-related problems.

12.3 Treatment: Non-Pharmacological

Each individual will experience different problems from their particular combination of symptoms with an impact on activities and quality of life; therefore, as already suggested, an MDT approach is the optimal model for non-pharmaceutical management. This may be delivered through an inpatient, outpatient, or community setting signposting individuals to essential external support and information, such as Parkinson's UK. There is some overlap in the areas each discipline might address, and therefore an integrated, holistic approach is recommended. It is vital that the whole team communicates effectively, and applies common principles of management such as cues and strategies based on the premise of bypassing the defective basal ganglia and using other brain pathways to overcome the resulting problems in automaticity.

Table 12.2 Strategies to help with movement [30, 31]

Type of strategy	Examples	Application
Attentional	Mental rehearsal	Prior to attempting the task, the individual imagines themselves carrying out the intended action with good-quality movements, e.g., walking with big steps to the other side of the room.
Auditory	Vocal	Carer says 'BIG STEPS' or counts 'One, Two')
	Metronome	Patient walks to the preset metronome beat.
	Music	MP3 player and headphones (with appropriate selected music)
Visual	'Post-it' note	*Freezing in Doorway*: Patient focuses on post-it note placed beyond doorway.
		Freezing or festination when turning near toilet or sink: Patient steps onto post-its to enable a 360-degree turn.
	Laser	*Gait initiation failure*: Patient points pen at floor and steps onto the light.
Proprioceptive	Weight transfer	*Gait initiation failure*: Patient stands with feet apart, then rocks weight between feet, then takes step forward.

12.3.1 Application of Movement Strategies (External Cues and Attentional Strategies)

Strategy training can be a useful therapeutic adjunct to the overall management of gait disturbance in PD [4]. External movement triggers, such as auditory, visual, or proprioceptive cues, or attentional strategies (internally driven) can be taught. Strategies which break complex activities into component parts can reduce problems with transfers. Examples of cue application are listed in Table 12.2.

12.3.2 Physiotherapy Intervention

There is mounting evidence of the physical and physiological benefits of exercise in PD; therefore, early referral to physiotherapy is recommended [5]. It is important to encourage the patient to engage in exercise, which may include sporting activities, high-intensity exercise (HIT), progressive resistance exercise, treadmill training [6], dance, Tai Chi, or Nordic walking. Prevention of deconditioning is important. Some class II–III studies suggest that physiotherapy, especially exercise, can improve motor impairments or disabilities in PD. Several review articles also highlight the positive effects of physiotherapy [7].

12.3.2.1

The combination of symptoms affects gait in many ways, and gait dysfunction in PD can be categorized as continuous (slow, reduced stride length) or episodic (freezing or festination), and patients may experience both at different times. Heel-strike is often impaired and the patient walks with a flat-footed pattern, affecting the whole anti-gravity and propulsion system. Variation in gait, combined with cognitive decline, increases the risk of falls [8]. Falls are also more likely in PD when turning or reaching above the head or below the knees.

A detailed assessment of both gait and balance, using appropriate measures, ensures the physiotherapist can determine postural stability and falls risk factors, ready to implement a programme of gait and balance re-education. Treatment will depend on the assessment findings, e.g., encouraging conscious attention to stride length or avoidance of dual-tasking (not walking and talking at the same time) may improve gait quality and safety, as can use of an appropriate cue. Freezing of gait (often described as 'feet feel glued to the floor') occurs in up to 80% of people with PD [9]. It can occur when trying to initiate gait, passing through doorways, turning, arriving at a destination, and performing dual tasks [10]. When turning, cues such as consciously lifting the feet higher (marching) while turning, counting steps, or a using wider turning arc can be effective in improving movement quality. Other cues are suggested in Table 12.2. Further intervention may include the provision of aids[11, 12]. The European Physiotherapy Guidelines for Parkinson's Disease [13] provide evidence-based guidance on assessment, intervention, and outcome measurement. Although cueing helps with freezing in most patients, it is worth noting that it may reduce walking speed and be ineffective for ON-freezing in others [14].

12.3.2.2

Physiotherapy assessment and interventions consider the impact of altering posture. Early subtle changes in posture often go unnoticed by the patient (e.g., reduced hip extension), and it is important to assess this early, and, where required, teach exercises to strengthen anti-gravity musculature and stretches to maintain flexibility. Posture can be measured with the patient standing with their back against a wall, head held level, and the distance between measuring the tragus of the ear to the wall is taken. This can provide a baseline, indicate deterioration, and give the incentive to engage in daily exercises to improve posture.

12.3.2.3

Transfers can become increasingly difficult in PD. Lower limb weakness and inflexibility contribute to this. Specific strengthening exercises can be taught, and strategies breaking the action down into component parts can enable the transfer to be carried out more easily. Examples of these are in Table 12.3. A cue card with key words can be supplied as a reminder, or a carer, where available and able, can also be taught.

12.3.3 Occupational Therapy Intervention (OT)

The OT will address activities of daily living (ADL) in relation to the patient's cognition, mood, fatigue, and motor symptoms (particularly in the upper limb) [15]. A combination of tremor, bradykinesia, and reduced dexterity can impact activities such as eating, drinking, and dressing. The asymmetric tremor can increase with stress or anxiety. Fatigable bradykinesia will impact many activities such as tying shoelaces, handwriting, and fastening clothes, as well as affecting actions which require larger alternating or rotating movements such as buttering and cutting bread, washing hair, and brushing teeth. Activities requiring balance, such as reaching and bending, can also be difficult.

12.3.3.1

Advice and equipment can be offered to combat bed mobility problems such as providing a bed lever, suggesting a satin sheet on the middle third of the mattress to make turning over easier, or teaching strategies for transfers (Table 12.3). Cognitive strategies may also be advised to address freezing of thought (bradyphrenia), freezing during ADL, and the accompanying frustration which further impedes

Table 12.3 Strategies for transfers

Problem	Strategy instructions
Getting up from a chair	1. Bottom forward on chair 2. Feet placed correctly 3. Hands placed correctly 4. Chin forward over knees and push up
Turning in bed	1. Turn head in direction of movement 2. Bend knees 3. Reach opposite arm across body 4. Roll

Table 12.4 Cognitive strategy

	Action	Detail of action
1.	STOP	Stop attempting the activity
2	THINK	Think about what it is that you are trying to do
3.	PLAN	Plan how you are going to do it
4.	DO	Do it!

successfully restarting the action. This can be further complicated by reduced ability to manage several subconscious activities whilst attending to one task. A cognitive strategy can improve the situation and give the patient greater sense of control (Table 12.4). Upper limb function and dexterity will also be assessed and a targeted treatment plan can be devised for arising issues. Relaxation techniques may be taught which can help manage anxiety and fatigue. Sleep hygiene advice, such as not using computer or phone screens at bedtime, ensuring the room is neither too hot nor cold, having a regular bedtime routine, and no daytime siesta after 3 PM, can all help. Fatigue can be improved by working out a routine that includes daytime rests. Anxiety may be addressed with cognitive behavioural interventions. In some teams, these areas may be covered by the psychologist. Vocational support and/or participation in leisure activities will also be addressed, and assessment of fitness to drive can be conducted with referral to a driving assessment centre as required.

12.3.4 Speech and Language Therapy Intervention (SLT)

Following assessment, SLT intervention may include breathing and relaxation strategies, voice and pitch exercises, voice projection with auditory feedback, and pacing (using tapping or pointing to dots on a card) to control over-fast speech [16]. There is evidence that Lee Silverman Voice Treatment (LSVT/LOUD) (an intensive intervention delivered in 16 hour-long sessions over four weeks) can give long-term improvement in vocal loudness [9, 30]. Provision of devices such as amplifiers and light writers or tablet pads with communication apps downloaded can also help.

To address swallowing issues, advice on food or liquid texture, swallow strategies (e.g., head turn, chin tuck), and swallowing exercises may be included. Avoiding different textures in the same mouthful (e.g., mixing liquid and solid food) may be helpful, and patients struggling to swallow tablets may be advised to swallow the medication with yogurt instead of water. Expiratory muscle strength training may also be taught to reduce aspiration risk [17]. Aids may be considered such as a swallow reminder, a brooch to cue swallowing and thus reduce drooling [18].

No scientific evidence supports or refutes the efficacy of non-pharmacological swallowing therapy for dysphagia in PD [19]. However, patients report benefits from advice and education regarding swallowing difficulties and how to manage them.

12.3.5 Dietetic Intervention

Dietary protein can affect effectiveness of levodopa medication, leading to motor fluctuations, and the dietician can offer advice on protein redistribution. It is important for patients to maintain their daily protein intake; however, they should avoid taking levodopa with large amounts of protein-containing foods, as this may interfere with gut absorption of the medication. Dietary manipulation may also be helpful in management of orthostatic hypotension, which can occur as a non-motor symptom, as well as a side effect of medication in PD.

12.4 Pharmacological Treatment

12.4.1

Although dopaminergic therapy is usually effective in the management of PD, experience of symptoms varies from individual to individual, and therefore medication management will also differ from person to another. Prescribing is also likely to become more complex as the condition progresses, and over time

patients may be started on multiple medications at frequent intervals. Timing of medication becomes particularly important as symptoms progress, and it is important to ensure that PD patients admitted to hospital are either self-medicating or given their medication at the correct time. Failure in achieving this can lead to a longer length of stay and poorer outcomes. It is important to remember that the diagnosis may need to be reviewed if there is little or no effectiveness to dopaminergic medications.

12.4.1.1 Drugs Used for Managing PD
Levodopa
Dopaminergic therapy is the mainstay of pharmacological management. The Levo-isomer of dopamine is combined with either beserazide (co-beneldopa) or carbidopa (co-careldopa) to prevent peripheral decarboxylation and increase bioavailability. In addition to the standard (normal release) tablet, it is also available in a dispersible form and controlled (or slow) release. The most common short-term side effects include vomiting. Long-term complications include fluctuations of motor response and dyskinesia.

Dopamine Agonists
Ropinirole, pramipexole, and apomorphine can be used as initial therapy or as an add-on to levodopa to help reduce the complications. In addition to normal-release tablets, both ropinirole and pramipexole are available as prolonged-release tablets. Another dopamine agonist is rotigotine, which is available as skin patches (which can be particularly useful for inpatients who report dysphagia). Apomorphine is mainly used as subcutaneous injections or apomorphine pump for managing advanced PD. Dopamine agonists can have behavioural side effects and predispose to impulse control disorders such as compulsive shopping, gambling, and hypersexuality. These must be carefully monitored in all patients taking dopamine agonists.

MAO-B Inhibitors
Monoamine oxidase type B is an enzyme which breaks down dopamine. The most commonly used drugs in this class are selegiline and rasagiline. Treatment with selegiline in otherwise untreated Parkinsonian patients has been shown to postpone treatment with levodopa, or to keep the levodopa dosage at a lower level [20]. Side effects are uncommon.

COMT Inhibitors

Entacapone and more recently marketed tolcapone block the enzyme catechol-O methyl-transferase and can prolong the action of levodopa. They do not have any anti-Parkinsonian property of their own. The common problem with their use is that intense staining of urine and staining of clothes can be a problem in patients with poor bladder control.

Amantadine

Amantadine is a glutamate agonist but has possible other mechanisms of helping PD, including mild anticholinergic properties. It can be quite useful in selected cases with PD.

Anticholinergics

Trihexiphenidyl was very commonly prescribed in younger patients with PD reporting tremor before the advent of dopamine agonists. It is still useful in selected cases with tremor-predominant PD, but must be used cautiously in the elderly because of adverse effects and the increasing anticholinergic burden, which is associated with adverse outcomes among individuals with PD [21].

12.4.2 Useful Considerations from the Rehabilitation Perspective

12.4.2.1

Motor fluctuations may include 'on' and 'off' phases. At this stage, adjustments in the frequency of levodopa dosing during the day, tending to achieve four to six daily doses, might attenuate the wearing off. Switching from standard levodopa to CR formulation can also help. Adding dopamine agonists, amantadine, and anticholinergics may help reduce fluctuations [7]. Advanced therapies with deep brain stimulation, apomorphine, and duodopa should be considered at this stage [7, 22].

12.4.2.2

Peak-dose dyskinesia can be managed by adding amantadine or clozapine. Reducing the individual dose of levodopa and stopping entacapone should be considered. Dopamine agonists and long-acting preparations should be avoided in patients with hallucinations and psychoses. Advanced therapies with deep brain stimulation, apomorphine, and duodopa should be considered at this stage. Bi-phasic dyskinesia (dyskinesia

during on and off periods), can be reduced by increasing the dose and frequency of levodopa, but at the risk of increasing peak-dose dyskinesia [7].

12.4.2.3

Additional doses of levodopa or dopamine agonist at night may be effective in controlling night-time or early-morning dystonia [7].

12.4.2.4

Amantadine may be helpful in reducing freezing and can also be prescribed for atypical Parkinsonism; however, hallucinations and ankle oedema may increase with its use. Freezing should also be addressed by physiotherapy intervention as it increases the risk of falls [22].

12.4.2.5

Management of dementia in PD may include discontinuation of potential aggravators such as anticholinergics, amantadine, tricyclic antidepressants, tolterodine, oxybutynin, and benzodiazepines. Adding cholinesterase inhibitors such as rivastigmine, donepezil, and galantamine can help the cognitive functions; rivastigmine has been shown to help with gait and balance as well [8]. In patients with psychosis, dopaminergic therapy, potential aggravators (review of prescription), and using clozapine, quetiapine, or olanzapine may help [7].

12.4.2.6

Depression may be best managed by serotonin selective reuptake inhibitors as they are less likely to result in adverse effects than tricyclic antidepressants [7, 22].

12.4.2.7

Autonomic dysfunction may be addressed with midodrine and fludrocortisone in patients with orthostatic hypotension. Solifenacin is useful for managing overactive bladder symptoms [23]. A bladder diary can be helpful in detecting nocturnal polyuria [24] and intranasal desmopressin [25] may improve this.

12.4.2.8

Botulinum toxin may be considered for dystonia. Injections can reduce foot dystonia that may be painful or impairing gait in both patients with PD patients and those with generalized dystonia. Injections in finger flexors can help relax muscles and open the hand, which benefits maintaining hand hygiene. The toxin can also be used to help with blepharospasm.

Table 12.5 Common side effects of medications used to manage PD

Side effect	Drugs that commonly cause this	Examples
Nausea/vomiting	Levodopa	Nausea
	Dopamine agonists	Vomiting
Sleepiness	Dopamine agonists	Excessive daytime sleepiness
		Sudden sleep onset.
Dyskinesia	Levodopa	Involuntary choreiform movements
Dystonia	Levodopa	Abnormal posturing of affected part, usually limbs
Leg oedema	Amantadine	Swelling of ankles and feet
Orthostatic hypotension	Levodopa	Dizziness on standing due to fall in blood pressure. May lead to recurrent falls.
Hallucinations	Levodopa	Commonly hallucinations of animals, spiders, or small children.
	Dopamine agonists	Usually visual or tactile.
	Amantadine	
	Anticholinergics	
Psychosis	Levodopa	Hallucinations, delusions, and agitation.
	Dopamine agonists	
	Amantadine	
	Anticholinergics	
Impulse control behaviour	Dopamine agonists	Compulsive shopping, eating, gambling, Hypersexuality
		Punding (purposeless repetitive behaviour)

12.4.2.9

Management of drooling in PD: oral medications, botulinum toxin injections, surgical interventions, radiotherapy, speech therapy, and trials of devices may be used to treat sialorrhea in PD, but few controlled trials have been published [26]. Anticholinergic drugs, e.g., a scopolamine patch applied below the ear or one drop of atropine solution (containing 0.5 mg of drug from a 1% wt./vol. solution) sublingually can reduce the formation of saliva. Botulinum toxin injections in salivary glands also reduce the formation of saliva and improve sialorrhea [27]. Referral to speech therapy may also help.

12.4.2.10

As with any medication, side effects are a potential risk with management of PD. Some of the common side effects are listed in Table 12.5.

12.5 Surgical Intervention and Advanced Therapies

12.5.1 Deep Brain Stimulation

Deep brain stimulation (DBS) has revolutionized the care of patients with advanced PD. Consideration of DBS should be undertaken by an MDT that includes a movement disorder neurologist, neurosurgeon, and neuro-psychiatrist. A detailed description of the surgical techniques and patient selection is beyond the scope of this chapter. Some rehabilitative considerations are highlighted next.

1. DBS may worsen speech and therefore all prospective candidates undergo speech assessment.
2. DBS can help with tremor, bradykinesia, and rigidity. However, this treatment is not effective for freezing and falls and gait instability may sometimes worsen after DBS.

3. Previous dopamine responsiveness is predictive of good outcome and most patients continue to need dopaminergic medication after DBS, although the dosages required reduce in most cases.

4. Poor cognitive function, hallucinations or psychosis, and severe depression are associated with poor outcome after DBS and hence most patients with these features are not suitable for surgical therapy.

12.5.2 Duodopa

Continuous dopamine release matches physiological states much more than intermittent peaks of plasma concentration as it is delivered by oral medication. To overcome this limitation, a levodopa/carbidopa intestinal gel (LCIG) has been developed which can be delivered directly to the intestines via a percutaneous endoscopic jejunostomy (PEJ) tube for a more predictable absorption that results in a constant level of dopamine in the blood of patients with PD. This requires a surgery for insertion of the PEJ tube and the dopamine gel is filled into a pump that constantly delivers it to the tube at a planned rate. The gel needs to be refilled periodically. The use of a trial period of LCIG via nasojejunal administration allows objective evaluation of improvement in PD symptom control in advance of the placement of the more invasive PEJ procedure. This technique may be suitable in some patients with advanced PD who are not suitable for DBS, but all therapy options must be evaluated before undertaking this surgery [28].

12.5.3 Apomorphine Pump

A surgical implantation of a subcutaneous pump follows similar principles as duodopa in terms of constant delivery of dopaminergic therapy. In this case a dopamine agonist apomorphine is used. This technique may be used in advanced PD patients who are not suitable for DBS and can significantly improve quality of life in some carefully selected patients [29].

References

1. Fahn S. Classification of movement disorders. *Movement Disorders* 2011; **26**(6): 947–57.

2. Skelly R, Lindop F, Johnson C. Multidisciplinary care of patients with Parkinson's disease. *Progress in Neurology and Psychiatry* 2012; **16**(2): 10–14.

3. Kalf JG, de Swart BJ, Bloem BR, Munneke M. Prevalence of oropharyngeal dysphagia in Parkinson's disease: a meta-analysis. *Parkinsonism & Related Disorders* 2012; **18**(4): 311–15.

4. Nieuwboer A, Kwakkel G, Rochester L, Jones D, Van Wegen E, Willems AM, et al. Cueing training in the home improves gait-related mobility in Parkinson's disease: The RESCUE trial. *Journal of Neurology, Neurosurgery, and Psychiatry* 2007; **78**(2): 134–40.

5. Tomlinson CL, Herd CP, Clarke CE, Meek C, Patel S, Stowe R, et al. Physiotherapy for Parkinson's disease: A comparison of techniques. *Cochrane Database of Systematic Reviews* 2014; **6**: CD002815.

6. Mehrholz J, Kugler J, Storch A, Pohl M, Hirsch K, Elsner B. Treadmill training for patients with Parkinson's disease. *Cochrane Database of Systematic Reviews* 2015; **9**: CD007830.

7. Horstink M, Tolosa E, Bonuccelli U, Deuschl G, Friedman A, Kanovsky P, et al. Review of the therapeutic management of Parkinson's disease. Report of a joint task force of the European Federation of Neurological Societies and the Movement Disorder Society-European Section. Part I: Early (uncomplicated) Parkinson's disease. *European Journal of Neurology: Official Journal of the European Federation of Neurological Societies* 2006; **13**(11): 1170–85.

8. Henderson EJ, Lord SR, Brodie MA, Gaunt DM, Lawrence AD, Close JC, et al. Rivastigmine for gait stability in patients with Parkinson's disease (ReSPonD): A randomised, double-blind, placebo-controlled, phase 2 trial. *Lancet Neurology* 2016; **15**(3): 249–58.

9. Hely MA, Reid WG, Adena MA, Halliday GM, Morris JG. The Sydney multicenter study of Parkinson's disease: The inevitability of dementia at 20 years. *Movement Disorders: Official Journal of the Movement Disorder Society* 2008; **23**(6): 837–44.

10. Fahn S. The freezing phenomenon in Parkinsonism. *Advances in Neurology* 1995; **67**: 53–63.

11. Canning CG, Allen NE, Bloem BR, Keus SHJ, Munneke M, Nieuwboer A, et al. Interventions for preventing falls in Parkinson's disease. *Cochrane Database of Systematic Reviews* 2015; **3**.

12. Van der Marck MA, Klok MP, Okun MS, Giladi N, Munneke M, Bloem BR, et al. Consensus-based clinical practice recommendations for the examination and management of falls in patients with Parkinson's disease. *Parkinsonism & Related Disorders* 2014; **20**(4): 360–9.

13. Keus SHJM, Graziano, M; et al. *European physiotherapy guideline for Parkinson's disease*. Netherlands: ParkinsonNet K, 2014.

14. Kompoliti K, Goetz CG, Leurgans S, Morrissey M, Siegel IM. 'On' freezing in Parkinson's disease: Resistance to visual cue walking devices. *Movement Disorders: Official Journal of the Movement Disorder Society* 2000; **15**(2): 309–12.

15. Jansa J, Aragon A. Living with Parkinson's and the emerging role of occupational therapy. *Parkinson's Disease* 2015; **2015**: 196303.

16. Herd CP, Tomlinson CL, Deane KH, Brady MC, Smith CH, Sackley CM, et al. Comparison of speech and language therapy techniques for speech problems in Parkinson's disease. *Cochrane Database of Systematic Reviews* 2012; (**8**): CD002814.

17. Pitts T, Bolser D, Rosenbek J, Troche M, Okun MS, Sapienza C. Impact of expiratory muscle strength training on voluntary cough and swallow function in Parkinson disease. *Chest* 2009; **135**(5): 1301–8.

18. Marks L, Turner K, O'Sullivan J, Deighton B, Lees A. Drooling in Parkinson's disease: a novel speech and language therapy intervention. *International Journal of Language & Communication Disorders/Royal College of Speech & Language Therapists.* 2001; **36** Suppl.: 282–7.

19. Deane KH, Ellis-Hill C, Jones D, Whurr R, Ben-Shlomo Y, Playford ED, et al. Systematic review of paramedical therapies for Parkinson's disease. *Movement Disorders: Official Journal of the Movement Disorder Society* 2002; **17**(5): 984–91.

20. Parkinson Study Group. DATATOP: A multicenter controlled clinical trial in early Parkinson's disease. *Archives of Neurology* 1989; **46**(10): 1052–60.

21. Crispo JAG, Willis AW, Thibault DP, Fortin Y, Hays HD, McNair DS, et al. Associations between anticholinergic burden and adverse health outcomes in Parkinson disease. *PLoS One* 2016; **11**(3). e0150621. doi:10.1371/journal.pone.0150621

22. Fox SH, Katzenschlager R, Lim SY, Ravina B, Seppi K, Coelho M, et al. The Movement Disorder Society evidence-based medicine review update: Treatments for the motor symptoms of Parkinson's disease. *Movement Disorders: Official Journal of the Movement Disorder Society* 2011; **26** Suppl. 3: S2–41.

23. Zesiewicz TA, Evatt M, Vaughan CP, Jahan I, Singer C, Ordorica R, et al. Randomized, controlled pilot trial of solifenacin succinate for overactive bladder in Parkinson's disease. *Parkinsonism & Related Disorders* 2015; **21**(5): 514–20.

24. Batla A, Phé V, De Min L, Panicker JN. Nocturia in Parkinson's disease: Why does it occur and how to manage? *Movement Disorders: Clinical Practice* 2016; **3**(5): 443–51.

25. Suchowersky O, Furtado S, Rohs G. Beneficial effect of intranasal desmopressin for nocturnal polyuria in Parkinson's disease. *Movement Disorders: Official Journal of the Movement Disorder Society* 1995; **10**(3): 337–40.

26. Chou KL, Evatt M, Hinson V, Kompoliti K. Sialorrhea in Parkinson's disease: A review. *Movement Disorders: Official Journal of the Movement Disorder Society* 2007; **22**(16): 2306–13.

27. Petracca M, Guidubaldi A, Ricciardi L, Ialongo T, Del Grande A, Mulas D, et al. Botulinum toxin A and B in sialorrhea: Long-term data and literature overview. *Toxicon: Official Journal of the International Society on Toxinology* 2015; **107**(Pt. A): 129–40.

28. Foltynie T, Magee C, James C, Webster GJ, Lees AJ, Limousin P. Impact of duodopa on quality of life in advanced Parkinson's disease: A UK case series. *Parkinsons Disease* 2013; **2013**: 362908.

29. Drapier S, Eusebio A, Degos B, Verin M, Durif F, Azulay JP, et al. Quality of life in Parkinson's disease improved by apomorphine pump: The OPTIPUMP cohort study. *Journal of Neurology* 2016; **263**(6): 1111–19.

30. Orgeta V, McDonald KR, Poliakoff E, Hindle JV, Clare L, Leroi I. Cognitive training interventions for dementia and mild cognitive impairment in Parkinson's Disease. *Cochrane Database of Systematic Reviews* 2015; **11**.

31. Bloem BR, de Vries NM, Ebersbach G. Nonpharmacological treatments for patients with Parkinson's disease. *Movement Disorders: Official Journal of the Movement Disorder Society* 2015; **30**(11): 1504–20.

Chapter 13

Neuropathic Pain

Elina Zakin and David M. Simpson

13.1 Introduction

Neuropathic pain is defined by the International Association for the Study of Pain as a 'pain initiated or caused by a primary lesion or dysfunction in the nervous system' [1]. It refers to a range of conditions that can differ in their anatomic localization and aetiology. The aetiologies range from degenerative to post-traumatic to toxic-metabolic [2]. Neuropathic pain is a manifestation of several different disorders that affect the peripheral nervous system, including polyneuropathies (i.e., due to diabetes, alcoholism, amyloidosis, small-fibre neuropathies), hereditary neuropathies, mononeuropathies (i.e., trigeminal, glossopharyngeal, post-herpetic), entrapment neuropathies, and post-traumatic nerve injuries (i.e., complex regional pain syndrome type II). Additionally, pain syndromes can result from abnormalities in the central nervous system, such as spinal cord injury, multiple sclerosis, or cerebrovascular events [3].

13.2 Aetiology of Neuropathic Pain

The aetiology of neuropathic pain may be [1] primary nerve damage or [2] secondary to non-neural tissue compressing or infiltrating the nerve, or [3] occlusion of blood supply to the nerves [4]. The mechanisms of neuropathic pain include: ectopic activity, peripheral sensitization, central sensitization, impaired inhibitory modulation, and activation of microglia. A patient's neuropathic pain can often have multiple mechanisms. This is important to remember when selecting therapies for neuropathic pain control.

Ectopic activity occurs as a result of nerve injury, which leads to nerve hyperexcitability and subsequent generation of ectopic action potentials in afferent neurons. This can result in stimulus independent paresthesias, dysesthesias, and pain [5]. Post-lesional changes in voltage-gated sodium and potassium channels along with hyperpolarization of persistently activated cyclic

nucleotide gated channels are implicated in the molecular aetiology of this ectopic activity [6]. Peripheral sensitization is defined as post-nerve injury hyperexcitability with the concomitant reduction in the threshold for primary afferent neuron activation, which results in hyperalgesia and allodynia [7]. The transient receptor potential TRPV1 ion channel family plays an important role in peripheral sensitization, and we discuss the role of a particular TRPV1 agonist, capsaicin, later in this chapter [7].

Central sensitization is defined as the 'prolonged but reversible increase in the excitability and synaptic efficacy of neurons in central nociceptive pathways' that results in various pain phenotypes [8]. Examples include: allodynia, defined as touch-evoked pain; hyperalgesia, the exaggeration of pain experience relative to intensity of noxious stimuli; and pain extending beyond the distribution of the injured nerve (secondary hyperalgesia). The aetiology of central sensitization is thought to be due to changes in $A\beta$ fibre phenotype, which results in increased excitatory neuropeptides such as CGRP (calcitonin gene-related peptide) and substance P, and neurotransmitter activity. Currently, work is ongoing on the antagonist for excitatory neuropeptides as therapy for neuropathic pain [9].

Impaired inhibitory modulation is another proposed mechanism of neuropathic pain, which suggests that nerve injury results in the impairment of the endogenous inhibitory mechanisms of nociception. This hypothesis proposes that pain results from the nerve injury-mediated apoptosis of GABAergic spinal inhibitory interneurons which subsequently results in post-nerve injury increased sensitivity to pain [10]. Post-injury activation of micro glia and other non-neuronal cells in the central nervous system can result in pain. The proposed mechanisms include phosphorylation of mitogen-activated protein kinase, upregulation of chemokine receptors, and release of glial cytokines and growth factors [11].

13.3 Diagnosis of Neuropathic Pain

The diagnosis of neuropathic pain requires a careful history and a physical examination, with special attention to sensory testing [12]. The patient's description of the sensation is very important. For example, a patient who has mononeuropathy due to trauma may have pain that often exceeds the distribution of the injured nerve or severity of the injury (i.e., complex regional pain syndrome can occur after very minor skin or joint injury). The neuropathic pain is often stimulus-independent. Commonly used terms to describe neuropathic pain are burning, lancinating, electric shock-like, jabbing, and cramping. It can also be described as a 'pins-and-needles sensation' (positive phenomenon) or numbness/loss of sensation (negative phenomenon). The pains may not adhere to a particular dermatomal distribution. The pain due to peripheral neuropathy often begins most distally in the extremities and progresses to involve the proximal portions in a length-dependent, bilaterally symmetric fashion. It may also evolve even more centripetally to the intercostal nerve distributions, affecting the lateral extensions of the flank. The pain may be worsened by cold, damp weather and movement of the involved extremity. Patients may also report worsening of the pain at night [3]. Autonomic symptoms, including abnormal sweating, impotence, orthostatic hypotension, and gastrointestinal motility disorders, may also occur.

Specific serologic testing includes serum thyroid-stimulating hormone (TSH), vitamin B12, haemoglobin A1c, HIV, hepatitis serology, and serum immunofixation to help in the evaluation of a systemic derangement that could result in painful peripheral nerve injury. The focus on the evaluation for reversible conditions (such as spinal cord compression, neoplasm, vitamin deficiency) is also important [13]. It is also important to identify co-morbid conditions that influence pain (i.e., sleep difficulties, autonomic neuropathy, co-morbid substance abuse).

Other diagnostic tests include neurophysiologic evaluation with nerve conduction studies, electromyography, quantitative sensory testing, autonomic function testing, and skin biopsy. Nerve conduction studies do not evaluate the smaller A δ and C-fibre activities, and may be normal in small-fibre neuropathy. Autonomic function testing may be informative in individuals with normal nerve conduction studies [3]. Quantitative sensory testing evaluates a larger spectrum of nerve fibres. For example, it can test A δ nerve fibres by evaluating the cold and cold/pin detection thresholds. C-fibres can be evaluated with heat and heat-pain detection thresholds. The larger A $\alpha\beta$ nerve fibres can be evaluated with vibration detection thresholds. Elevated sensory thresholds correspond to sensory loss and lowered thresholds are seen in allodynia and hyperalgesia [14].

Punch biopsy of the skin is used to evaluate the epidermal nerve fibre density and morphology, to look for evidence of nerve tortuosity, complex branching, clustering, and swelling of axons. Patients with small-fibre neuropathy, diabetic neuropathy, and impaired glucose tolerance neuropathy commonly have reduced epidermal nerve fibre density. Additionally, skin biopsy is thought to be more sensitive than the Quantitative Sudomotor Axonal Reflex (QSART) test in patients with normal nerve conduction studies for the evaluation of small-fibre neuropathy [3].

13.4 Non-Pharmacologic Therapy for Neuropathic Pain

There is evidence for the role of physical therapy in diabetic peripheral neuropathy, phantom limb pain, HIV sensory neuropathy, post-herpetic neuralgia, central post-stroke pain, low back and neck pain with neuropathic origin, complex regional pain syndrome, carpal tunnel syndrome, and pain from multiple sclerosis. Endurance training with a target heart rate of 60–80% of an individual's maximum heart rate and daily aerobic conditioning routines were found to be helpful. Isometric and isotonic strengthening can also be beneficial to prevent disuse atrophy of muscles. Stabilization exercises improve balance and proprioception and can be helpful to restore spinal joint motion and prevent further injury in radiculopathy. It is most helpful when combined with strengthening exercises [4].

Movement therapies, including Tai Chi, aquatic therapy, and the McKenzie and Feldenkrais techniques, have also been shown to be helpful in management of neuropathic pain. The Feldenkrais therapy was initially described by the physicist Dr Moshe Feldenkrais. In this therapy, patients are retrained to do their activities of daily living. This form of therapy uses specific body movements for various tasks and decreases the severity and frequency of neck and shoulder pain in patients with radiculopathies. The Chinese relaxation technique Tai Chi uses low-impact, low-velocity smooth movements to improve balance, prevent falls, enhance cardiovascular health, and reduce stress [15]. Aquatic therapy uses the buoyancy of warm water as a means to block nociception via thermal receptors and mechanoreceptors. It is thought to enhance blood flow and facilitate flexibility and muscle relaxation. The ease of movements performed under water may activate supraspinal pathways that decrease pain intensity [16]. In McKenzie techniques, commonly used for patients with back pain, the physical therapist creates a specific exercise plan for an individual patient. These techniques focus on patient education and active patient involvement for pain control. These skills and behaviours are thought to reduce the symptom recurrence, and give the patient the capability to manage their symptoms independently [16].

Posture training focuses on the importance of teaching the patient specific techniques for self-adjustment in body posture so as to decrease pain in daily activities, such as adjusting one's workstation or seat angle. Randomized controlled trials showed intervention at work to be more effective at pain reduction than physical therapy or no intervention at all [16]. The occupational therapist works with the patient to identify safe ways to use the body during activities. This trains the patient to use larger muscle groups during heavy tasks and reduce energy spent on lighter, more repetitive tasks. The occupational therapist also teaches the patient how to use adaptive equipment to perform certain tasks without causing or increasing pain [17].

Cognitive behavioural therapy (CBT) incorporates the environment, behaviour, and cognition to provide a session-based, structured, goal-oriented, and problem-driven therapy. It functions to incorporate patient education, behavioural skill training, and cognitive skill training. CBT utilizes reinforcement and attentional training along with relaxation and controlled breathing exercises to help patients monitor situation-specific triggers for pain. It can be performed in various settings, including individual, group, phone, and computer, thus making it a more accessible form of therapy for an individual patient. In a study of 442 patients with chronic pain, comparing the use of telephone

CBT, exercise, or a combination of both showed significantly better outcomes for the combined intervention group, at six and nine months [18].

Transcutaneous electrical stimulation (TENS) delivers low-voltage electrical current from a small devise to skin via surface electrodes. These devices have variable frequencies, pulse durations, intensities, and output types (i.e., burst or continuous), but lack rigorous randomized controlled trial data about the efficacy in management of chronic pain [19].

Acupuncture involves stimulation of anatomical points through solid metallic needle penetration, which is subsequently manually or electrically manipulated. This is a form of therapy based on the traditional Chinese medicine belief that stimulating the body's energy-carrying channels improves imbalances of *Qi* (vital energy) and restores health. Biochemically, it is thought that the benefits are derived from modulation of intracellular calcium ions of nerves in proximity of each acu-point. Additionally, it has been suggested that acupuncture enhances action of endogenous opiates, such as dynorphin, endorphin, and encephalin, and also releases corticosteroids, thus relieving pain [20]. Hypnotherapy has been studied in patients with painful HIV distal sensory polyneuropathy. The use of brief self-treatment sessions, which can be done by patients whenever necessary for pain control, was evaluated in a group of 36 patients with painful HIV distal sensory polyneuropathy. This study did note improvement in quality of life in addition to pain scores, with effects lasting for at least seven weeks following intervention [21].

13.5 Pharmacologic Therapy for Neuropathic Pain

The current guidelines for the treatment of neuropathic pain by the International Association for the Study of Pain and Neuropathic Pain Special Interest Group (NeuPSIG) recommend a combination of medications with efficacy for neuropathic pain over the use of monotherapy. The guidelines also recommend a stepwise increase in medication [22] (see Table 13.1).

Antidepressant drugs are not appropriate for treatment of acute analgesia and require long-term administration to relieve neuropathic pain, thus implicating a secondary mechanism of pain control, like longer-term molecular and neuronal plasticity

Table 13.1 Pharmacologic therapies for neuropathic pain

Drug Class	Agent	Route	Initial Dose	Dose Increment	Typical Effective Dose	Adverse Side Effects
Tricyclic antidepressants	Amitriptyline	PO	10–20 mg daily	Increase by 25 mg every three to seven days	25–100 mg daily	–anticholinergic effects: dry mouth, orthostatic hypotension, urinary retention –use with caution in patients with cardiac disease –obtain EKG if > 40 years old and receiving > 100 mg/day
Serotonin-norepinephrine reuptake inhibitors	Duloxetine	PO	20–60 mg daily	Increase from 30 to 60 mg after seven days	60 mg daily	–nausea –gastrointestinal upset
	Venlafaxine	PO	37.5 mg daily	37.5–75 mg every four days	150–225 mg taken daily (extended release) or three times daily (immediate release)	–cardiac conduction derangements in patients with cardiac disease –should be tapered on discontinuation due to concern for withdrawal syndrome
Calcium channel α2-δ ligands	Gabapentin	PO	100–300 mg daily to three times/day	100–300 mg every one to five days	300–1,200 mg three times daily	–administer in reduced doses for patients with renal insufficiency –dose-related dizziness and sedation, therefore recommended to start at low dose and titrate with caution
	Pregabalin	PO	25–75 mg daily to three times/day	25–50 mg every three days	50–200 mg three times daily or 75–300 mg twice daily	–oedema, weight gain –delayed onset to analgesic effect
Molecular drug targets (TRPV)	Capsaicin (0.025–0.075%)	Topical	Apply three to four times daily			–local erythema, oedema, and swelling –sensory complaints of burning/stinging pain
	Capsaicin (8%)	Topical	Apply up to four patches every three months for 60 minutes			–if aerosolized, may cause mucous membrane irritation and tearing

Table 13.1 (cont.)

Drug Class	Agent	Route	Initial Dose	Dose Increment	Typical Effective Dose	Adverse Side Effects
Sodium channel antagonists	Lidocaine	Topical	– 5 g/day ointment – up to three patches/day		17–20 g per day	
	Lamotrigine	PO	25 mg daily or every other day for two weeks	Increase by 25–50 mg per week	100–200 mg once or twice daily	– rash (Steven-Johnson syndrome involving oral mucosa) – gastrointestinal symptoms – headache – somnolence – dizziness
	Topiramate	PO	25–50 mg daily	Increase by 25–50 mg every week	50–200 mg twice daily	– weight loss – nausea – somnolence – dizziness – paraesthesias (due to carbonic anhydrase inhibitor activity)
	Oxcarbazepine	PO	300 mg twice daily	300 mg every Week	1,200–1,800 mg daily	– somnolence – ataxia – nausea/vomiting – up to 23% of patients may develop hyponatremia
	Carbamazepine	PO	100–200 mg daily	100–200 mg every week.	200–400 mg three times per day	– drowsiness – difficulties with balance – skin rash – dizziness – rarely, can cause leukopenia, thrombocytopenia, and liver damage

Opioid analgesics	Tramadol	PO	25–50 mg every six hours prn	– gastrointestinal symptoms: constipation, nausea, dyspepsia, abdominal pain
	Codeine	PO	30 mg every three to four hours prn	– headache
	Methadone	PO	2.5–5 mg every 8–12 hours	– mental status changes: sedation, fatigue, lethargy, somnolence
	Morphine Immediate-release (IR)	PO	10 mg every three to four hours prn	– dry mouth
	morphine Sustained-release (SR)	PO	15 mg every 12 hours prn	– urinary hesitancy and retention
	oxycodone IR	PO	5 mg every four to six hours prn	– abuse, dependence, addiction
	Oxycodone ER	PO	10–40 mg every 12 hours prn	
	Fentanyl patch	transdermal	25–100 mic/hr every 72 hours prn	

[23–24]. Some mechanistic explanations have implied the recruitment of noradrenergic descending pathways as well as the peripheral recruitment of noradrenaline from sympathetic fibres sprouting into the dorsal root ganglia. Monoamine reuptake inhibitors may have an indirect effect on pro-inflammatory cytokines with some effect on the mu-opioid and delta-opioid receptors.

13.5.1 Tricyclic Antidepressants

Based on the current guidelines, the first-line medications are the antidepressant class of medications, which have both norepinephrine and serotonin reuptake inhibition. Tricyclic antidepressants (TCAs) are cost-effective, are administered once daily, and treat co-morbid depression. It is advisable to initiate amitriptyline at a low dose (i.e., 10–20 mg) and increase by 25 mg every three to seven days as tolerated. An adequate trial of amitriptyline can usually take six to eight weeks for efficacy. Adverse side effects include the anticholinergic effects of dry mouth, orthostatic hypotension, constipation, and urinary retention. The provider should prescribe TCAs with caution to patients with cardiac disease or ventricular conduction abnormalities. It is advised to obtain an electrocardiogram (EKG) for patients over the age of 40 and for those individuals who are receiving more than 100 mg per day [25]. NeuPSIG guidelines recommend the use of tricyclic antidepressants in the management of central post-stroke pain.

13.5.2 Serotonin-Norepinephrine Reuptake Inhibitors

Serotonin-norepinephrine reuptake inhibitors (SNRIs), such as duloxetine and venlafaxine, are effective in maintaining sustained pain relief for one year in an open-label trial in diabetic neuropathy [25]. Duloxetine can be used as treatment of co-morbid major depression and generalized anxiety disorder at a dose of 60 mg twice daily. The efficacy in the management of other neuropathic pain subtypes has not been adequately studied. Duloxetine is safe in patients with co-morbid cardiac conditions, but can cause nausea as an adverse side effect. Venlafaxine, another SNRI, has demonstrated efficacy at higher dosages for painful diabetic peripheral neuropathy and various polyneuropathies, but not in post-herpetic neuralgia [26]. Venlafaxine is available in both short- and long-acting formulations and requires two to four weeks to titrate to the efficacious dose. The adverse side effects have been associated with cardiac conduction derangements in patients with cardiac disease [27]. Venlafaxine can also result in a withdrawal syndrome and therefore should be tapered instead of rapidly discontinued [26].

13.5.3 Calcium Channel α2-δ Ligands

Another first-line class of medications in the treatment of neuropathic pain are gabapentin and pregabalin, which bind to the voltage-gated calcium channels at the α2-δ subunit and produce changes in neurotransmitter release. The presumed mechanism of action of gabapentin and pregabalin is by way of inhibiting the calcium channel activation of excitatory transmitter release and spinal sensitization [23]. This class of drugs also activates the descending noradrenergic pain inhibitory system that is coupled to the spinal α2 adrenoreceptors. Additionally, these drugs may have an effect on pro-inflammatory cytokines and are effective when compared to placebo in various neuropathic pain conditions. The adverse side effects include dose-related dizziness and sedation; therefore, it is recommended that these drugs are started at a low dose and titrated with caution. Gabapentin and pregabalin have few drug interactions, but should be administered in reduced dosage to patients with renal insufficiency. Gabapentin is administered three times daily given the drug's complex, non-linear pharmacokinetics (to a maximum dose of 3,600 mg/day). Gabapentin may have a delayed onset to reach analgesic effect with the adequate therapeutic dose, taking up to two months to reach analgesic effect, which may be difficult for some patients suffering from neuropathic pain. Pregabalin has more predictable pharmaco-kinetics, with dosing starting at 150 mg/day divided in two to three doses with titration every one to two weeks to a maximum dose of 300 mg/day. Pregabalin has a shorter titration schedule, and thus a faster onset of efficacy compared to gabapentin at providing analgesia.

13.5.4 Molecular Drug Targets

Molecular drug targets are an important class of drugs in the management of neuropathic pain. The transient receptor potential channel (TRPV) family of proteins plays a role in transducing physical stress. The TRPV1 family of proteins functions in nociceptive pain transmission as an integrator of noxious chemical and physical stimuli [4]. It is thought that TRPV1 is expressed in the visceral sensory neurons in the bladder, bronchopulmonary, colonic, and cardiac afferents, where they are thought to play a role in visceral sensation and tissue homeostasis via the release of chemokines, tachykinin, and CGRP (calcitonin gene-related peptide) [28]. TRPV1 activation occurs by ligands such as capsaicin and resiniferatoxin, noxious heat (>42°C), protons, and endogenous ligands including lipid anandamide, which results in the opening of nonselective cation channels with a subsequent influx of sodium and calcium ions, and subsequent depolarization of nociceptor afferent neurons.

Capsaicin is a vanilloid, TRPV1 agonist that is used as a topical agent in neuropathic pain. The mechanism of action is unknown, but it is thought that it is a neurotoxin that activates but then depletes substance P from the nerve terminals of unmyelinated C-fibres, with the suspected mechanism thought to involve TRPV1-mediated calcium influx, with subsequent glutamate release. This glutamate release results in desensitization with repeated application of the drug. With repeated administration of topical capsaicin, there is impairment of heat perception and other sensory stimuli, due to the loss of intraepidermal nerve fibre immunoreactivity [4]. Topical capsaicin comes in two formulations: low concentration (0.075%) and high concentration (8%), with evidence showing that low-concentration application four to five times daily for eight weeks is effective in the treatment of painful diabetic neuropathy, post-herpetic neuralgia, and post-surgical pain [29]. Most of the evidence for the high-concentration capsaicin comes from post-herpetic neuralgia, HIV neuropathy, and diabetic neuropathic pain studies, where a single application for 30–60 minutes was shown to be effective, though it does require pretreatment with topical lidocaine or oral analgesia due to the intense pain with initial application [30, 31]. Some adverse side effects include local erythema, oedema, and swelling, along with sensory complaints of burning/stinging pain. Capsaicin may cause mucous membrane irritation, tearing, and potential respiratory complications; therefore, it must be handled carefully [30].

13.5.5 Sodium Channel Antagonists

The sodium channel antagonists, including topical lidocaine, lamotrigine, topiramate, oxcarbazepine, and carbamazepine, are another class of drugs that can be used in the management of neuropathic pain. Randomized controlled trials using 5% lidocaine patch have shown efficacy in post-herpetic neuralgia, as well as in patients with allodynia from other types of peripheral neuropathic pain [32].

Lamotrigine is a voltage-dependent sodium channel antagonist that helps suppress repetitive firing of sodium-dependent action potentials and is thought to inhibit the release of excitatory neurotransmitters, such as glutamate and aspartate [32]. This agent has been studied in painful diabetic neuropathy, chemotherapy-induced neuropathic pain, spinal cord injury-related pain, HIV-associated neuropathic pain, and post-stroke pain. It is administered orally with its time to peak concentration 1.4–4.8 hours with a 98% bioavailability. Lamotrigine is metabolized by the liver, with a half-life of 25–70 hours. On initiation, it should be titrated slowly to doses between 200 and 400 mg daily [4]. Adverse side effects include rash, gastrointestinal symptoms, headache, somnolence, and dizziness. A serious and potential fatal side effect of lamotrigine is Stevens-Johnson syndrome, which can spread to involve the oral mucosa.

Topiramate is used as an anticonvulsant and migraine prophylactic agent, but has also been shown in one study to significantly reduce pain compared to placebo in a population of patients with painful diabetic neuropathy [33]. This agent has several mechanisms of action, including the blockage of voltage-activated sodium channels, along with kainite and alpha-amino-3-hydroxy-5-methyisoxazole-4-propionic acid (AMPA) glutamate receptors. It also acts to enhance GABA-mediated inhibition, as well as the inhibition of the carbonic anhydrase enzyme, which subsequently inhibits calcium currents [34]. Topiramate is administered orally with a time to peak concentration 1.5–4 hours after ingestion and 80% bioavailability. Most of the drug is excreted through the urine, though a small amount undergoes hepatic metabolism with an elimination half-life of 21 hours [35]. This agent should be slowly titrated to a goal dose of between 50 and 200 mg twice daily. Common side effects include weight loss, nausea, somnolence, dizziness, and paraesthesias, which are thought to be due to the inhibition of carbonic acid anhydrase enzymes, along with cognitive dysfunction [4].

Oxcarbazepine is another agent whose mechanism of action is thought to be mediated by the 10-

monohydroxy metabolite (MHD) blocking voltage-gated sodium channels which stabilize the hyper-excited neuronal membranes, thus allowing for the inhibition of repetitive neuronal discharges and diminishing further synaptic impulse propagation. Though limited data exist, a single randomized, placebo-controlled trial showed the maximum titrated dose of oxcarbazepine of 1,800 mg per day to be effective in the treatment of painful diabetic neuropathy [36]. Oxcarbazepine is orally administered with 100% bioavailability. It undergoes hepatic metabolism to the active form MHD with renal excretion and has an elimination half-life of two hours [37]. The medication should be titrated slowly to doses between 1,200 and 2,400 mg per day. Common side effects include somnolence, ataxia, nausea, and vomiting. Up to 23% of patients may develop hyponatremia.

Lastly, carbamazepine is an agent approved by the Food and Drug Administration (FDA) for the treatment of trigeminal neuralgia, but has been shown to have modest clinical success in small trials for the treatment of painful diabetic neuropathy [38]. The mechanism of action works to slow the recovery rate of voltage-gated sodium channels. The drug is orally administered. The side effects include drowsiness, difficulties with balance, skin rash, and dizziness, with more rare side effects, including leukopenia, thrombocytopenia, and liver damage [39].

13.5.6 The Opioid Analgesics and Tramadol

According to the NeuPSIG guidelines, second-line medications are deemed appropriate in certain circumstances, such as for the treatment of acute neuropathic pain, exacerbations of severe neuropathic pain episodes, neuropathic cancer pain, or during a titration of a first-line medication, when immediate pain relief is required. These second-line agents are, namely, opioid analgesics. Opioids provide rapid relief of pain and thus are commonly used in the community as a first line for pain control. In patients with neuropathic pain, opioid analgesics may be used to achieve quick relief of pain while a first-line medication is being titrated to effect. Additionally, in some patients with chronic neuropathic pain, opioid analgesia may be useful for exacerbations of pain (i.e., during certain activities which provoke their pain), though patients must be advised to take short-acting opioids immediately at onset of

pain for best relief. Neuropathic pain from cancer may be managed with the addition of opioid analgesia for optimal pain control.

There are significant concerns for safety of use with this class of drugs. Opioid use could have many deleterious consequences, including opioid-associated hyperalgesia, although extrapolation of animal to human data is controversial. Additionally, there are concerns for opioid abuse and addiction in patients who suffer from chronic pain, thus opioids should be reserved for patients who fail to respond to first-line therapy. When prescribing opioid analgesia, clinicians should use the lowest effective dose and monitor the patient closely for evidence of drug misuse or abuse. Some common side effects of opioid use are constipation, nausea, and sedation, thus promptly starting a bowel regimen at drug initiation is advised. A slow taper of opioid analgesia is important when discontinuing the medication. In April 2015, the FDA published the *Abuse-Deterrent Opioids: Evaluation and Labeling* guidance, which described seven categories of abuse-deterrent technologies, including physical/chemical barriers, agonist/antagonist combinations, various aversion, delivery system, new molecular entities and prodrugs, combinations, and various novel approaches. The aim of this guidance was to 'meaningfully deter abuse' [42].

Evidence for the use of opioid analgesia in the management of neuropathic pain comes from randomized controlled trials (extending from one to eight weeks), which show that opioid analgesics have better efficacy at pain relief as compared to tricyclic antidepressants and gabapentin, though more side effects are seen in opioid use compared to the use of TCAs and gabapentin in these head-to-head trials [43]. Prescribing long-acting opioid analgesics at fixed dosage/interval is preferred to the administration of short-acting agents. Clinicians can start with short-acting opioid analgesics while titrating long-acting preparations to the desired effect, with the practitioner evaluating the effective total daily short-acting opioid analgesic requirement in this titration period.

Tramadol is an agonist of the opioid μ-receptor but also works to inhibit the reuptake of serotonin and norepinephrine. It is similar to other opioid analgesics as it is effective in achieving quick analgesic efficacy and has the same recommendations by the NeuPSIG as for opioids for appropriateness in treatment of neuropathic pain. The side effect profile of tramadol is similar to that of other opioid analgesics. It lowers seizure threshold and can precipitate serotonin syndrome when combined with other SNRIs and SSRIs. Serotonin syndrome is an often fatal reaction to serotonergic medications, which can result in cognitive impairment, autonomic derangements, and neuromuscular hyperactivity [44]. Dosing of tramadol can start at 50 mg once daily or twice daily with a titration to a maximum dose of 400 mg/day, or 300 mg/day in older patients.

The combination of opioids with non-opioid agents has been studied extensively. One study trial randomized patients to three groups to examine the efficacy of nortriptyline-morphine combination to either agent as monotherapy alone during a six-week period. Pain Inventory scores were used as a primary end point, with data showing significant lower pain scores for the drug combination as compared to either agent as monotherapy [45].

13.5.7 Other Agents

Due to inconsistent results in randomized controlled trials, several medications have Grade B recommendations. Several antidepressants can be administered for patients with co-morbid neuropathic pain and depression, such as buproprion, citalopram, and paroxetine.

Cannabinoids have been shown to have efficacy in pain associated with multiple sclerosis, though they are limited by availability, long-term tolerability, abuse potential, and the risk to precipitate psychosis [46]. A randomized, double-blinded, placebo controlled crossover study was done in 16 patients with painful diabetic peripheral neuropathy to study the short-term efficacy and tolerability of inhaled cannabis. Subjects were given aerosolized cannabis or placebo, with subsequent measure of pain intensity and subjective 'highness' scores measured at 5, 15, 30, 45, and 60 minutes, then every 30 minutes for an additional 3 hours with concomitant cognitive testing. The study revealed a dose-dependent reduction in diabetic peripheral neuropathic pain [47].

13.6 Interventional Therapy for Neuropathic Pain

Interventional therapies are defined as 'invasive procedures that involve the delivery of drugs into targeted areas, or ablation/modulation of targeted nerves' for the treatment of neuropathic pain [48]. Several pain syndromes, including post-herpetic neuralgia, herpes zoster, painful diabetic neuropathy, peripheral nerve injury, and brachial plexus avulsion, have underlying data to suggest interventional techniques for the management of neuropathic pain.

In neuropathic pain due to herpes zoster, two randomized controlled trials have suggested that epidural blocks with local anaesthetics combined with steroids just after the onset of herpes zoster can result in diminished pain and allodynia [49]. Randomized controlled trials show that neural blockade (both repeated epidural injection and paravertebral injections of local anaesthetics with steroids) early in herpes zoster may prevent post-herpetic neuralgia (PHN), though results are difficult to replicate given the variable frequency, duration, and number of blocks from various studies [50].

Several non-randomized trials have shown no benefit of sympathetic blockade in the treatment of PHN [48]. Other trials have attempted to study the efficacy of intrathecal methylprednisolone with mixed results, with the most recent independent research group finding an increase in pain at eight weeks with intrathecal methylprednisolone as compared to placebo [52]. Also of note, the use of pulsed radiofrequency (PRF) treatment in thoracic dermatomes was compared to sham and showed some decreased pain scores and decreased need for tramadol use in the PRF group at three weeks as compared to the sham group. These groups were followed for six months and data suggest improved pain scores, improved quality of life domain scores, and decreased use of tramadol in the PRF-treated group [53]. Though the data are encouraging, the current recommendation for the role of PRF for the treatment of PHN is deemed 'inconclusive' given the need to replicate these data [54].

For the management of painful diabetic and other peripheral neuropathies (DPN), there have been no studies on neural blockade. Small, prospective trials, which do demonstrate benefit, have evaluated the efficacy of spinal cord stimulation on pain in patients with pharmacologically refractory diabetic neuropathy, though procedure-related complications occur in 33% of cases [55]. Spinal cord stimulators (SCS) are a form of invasive therapy that can be permanently implanted after an initial temporary screen trial with an external pulse generator. They are commonly used in therapy of radiculopathy, failed spinal surgery, chronic low back pain, complex regional pain syndrome, and even in peripheral vascular disease. They are also known as dorsal column stimulators, which are devices that are implanted subcutaneously and through which a small electrical current is applied via a wire that carries the impulse from the pulse generator to the nerve fibres of the cord [56].

The Current European Federation of Neurologic Societies (EFNS) Task Force classified the evidence from various trials conducted between 1968 and 2006 as level B for efficacy of SCS in failed back surgery syndrome and complex regional pain syndrome type I, level B for repetitive transcranial magnetic stimulation for transient efficacy in central and peripheral neuropathic pains, and level C for motor cortex stimulation efficacy in the treatment of central post-stroke and facial pain. Additionally, limited data exist for the use of SCS in neuropathic pain aside from evidence in CRPS and failed back surgery syndrome [57].

Another systematic review of 11 case series evaluated the use of surgical decompression in patients with Diabetic Peripheral Neuropathy (DPN), of which 8 studies reported improved pain scores in patients undergoing decompression, though the data could not be reproduced and no recommended surgical intervention currently exists for DPN [58]. In patients with peripheral nerve injury and brachial plexus avulsion, ablative procedures of a peripheral nerve may be considered in certain circumstances (i.e., neuroma, peripheral nerve lesion resulting in pain in that particular nerve's sensory distribution) [59]. Lesioning of the dorsal root entry zone (DREZ) may be performed as treatment for neuropathic pain due to brachial or lumbosacral plexus nerve root avulsion [60]. More than a dozen case series have been published with success rates of between 54% and 100%, though no rigorous clinical trials exist [61].

In summary, evidence is limited for interventional treatments for the management of chronic neuropathic pain. It is difficult to standardize approaches given difficulty of randomization across groups. Due to the lack of high-quality clinical trials, no strong recommendations can be made. The NeuPSIG recommendations for the interventional management of neuropathic pain are:

1. Epidural injections for herpes zoster
2. Steroid injections for radiculopathy
3. Spinal cord stimulators for failed back surgery syndrome
4. Spinal cord stimulators for chronic regional pain syndrome type 1 [54].

13.7 Botulinum Toxin in Neuropathic Pain

Botulinum toxin is produced by the gram-positive anaerobic bacteria *Clostridium botulinum*. The toxin functions to block the release of acetylcholine from the nerve terminals by binding to the soluble NSF attachment protein receptor (SNARE) proteins, which disrupts the ability of acetylcholine vesicles from fusing at the axon terminal, and thus prevents the release of the vesicle contents. This in turn results in chemical denervation, which then causes muscle relaxation for extended periods of time. Initial data suggested that botulinum toxin provided relief from pain by muscle relaxation and subsequent decreased compression on surrounding blood vessels and nerves, though more recent studies suggest that the toxin may also affect the release of pro-inflammatory substances such as substance P [62–63]. Currently, onabotulinum toxin Type A (Botox) is FDA approved for the treatment of chronic migraine, with the proposed mechanism of pain reduction thought to be decrease in the release of pain-mediating substance P, calcitonin gene-related peptide (CGRP) and glutamate, afferent signalling in trigeminal vascular pathways, mediating migraine [64]. In a rat formalin model, onabotulinum toxin was shown to have direct action on sensory neurons. In the same series of experiments, microdialysis of tissue homogenate from a rat hind paw revealed an inhibition of glutamate release and a dose-dependent reduction in the number of formalin-induced immunoreactive cells in the dorsal horn of the rat spinal cord [65]. These data suggest that onabotulinum toxin inhibits excitation of a large range of neurons of the dorsal horn, and by way of this inhibition of neurotransmitter release, acts to inhibit peripheral sensitization, which can lead to an indirect reduction in central sensitization [65].

Botulinum toxin has shown efficacy in the treatment of post-herpetic neuralgia in two class I studies, where the toxin was injected intradermally into the painful area with doses ranging from 20 to 190 units, and improvement from pain was noted at days 3 to 5 after the injection [66]. Additional literature exists to support the use of botulinum toxin in the treatment of trigeminal neuralgia, with toxin administration either intradermally or submucosally into the painful area. Data from these studies suggest a 50% reduction in pain frequency and intensity after toxin injection

[67]. Some reduction in pain and allodynia after botulinum toxin injection in post-traumatic and post-surgical neuralgia has been noted about two weeks post injection. In a randomized, double-blind, placebo-controlled study investigating the effect of onabotulinum toxin on focal painful neuropathies and mechanical allodynia, a single injection into a painful area was done, and patients were evaluated at 4, 12, and 24 weeks. The outcomes measured were average pain intensity, quantified testing of thermal and mechanical perception/pain, allodynia to brushing, neuropathic symptoms, clinical global impression, and quality of life. Data showed persistent effects of onabotulinum toxin on pain intensity (up to 14 weeks after injection), with improved allodynia to brush and decreased pain thresholds [68].

Botulinum toxin can be used alone or as adjunct therapy, as it targets different receptors than the oral agents, and if it is successful, this can diminish the amount of oral medications administered along with fewer drug interactions, and fewer visits to pain specialists. The toxin is costly, though the effect can last for several weeks to even months. Studies continue for the use of botulinum toxin in the management of neuropathic pain.

13.8 Conclusion

Neuropathic pain can involve various anatomic localizations and vary in its aetiology. This chapter summarizes the various pathophysiologic mechanisms that are implicated in neuropathic pain, including ectopic activity, peripheral sensitization, central sensitization, impaired inhibitory modulation, and activation of microglia. The various pharmacologic and non-pharmacologic therapies are introduced and evidence, for these therapies is discussed. It is important for the practitioner to remember that no single individual suffering from neuropathic pain will have a single pain phenotype, and as a result, each patient's pain will not be explained by a single mechanism, which is crucial in the selection of therapies for pain control. In fact, adequate pain control may be achieved with a single oral agent for some individuals, whereas a majority of patients may require a combination of both pharmacologic and various non-pharmacologic therapies to obtain adequate relief from pain.

References

1. Treede R, Jensen T, et al. Neuropathic pain: Redefinition and a grading system for clinical and research purposes. *Neurology* 2008; **70**(18): 1630–5.

2. Woolf CJ, American College of Physicians, American Physiological Society. Pain: Moving from symptom control toward mechanism-specific pharmacologic management. *Ann. Intern. Med.* 2004; **140**(6): 441–51.

3. Horowitz SH. The Diagnostic Workup of Patients with Neuropathic Pain. *Med. Clin. N. Am.* 2007; **91**: 21–30.

4. Simpson DM, McArthur JC, Dworkin RH. *Neuropathic pain: Mechanisms, diagnosis and treatment.* Oxford, UK: Oxford University Press, 2012.

5. von Hehn CA, Baron R, Woolf CJ. Deconstructing the neuropathic pain phenotype to reveal neural mechanisms. *Neuron.* 2012; **73**(4): 638–52.

6. Chaplan SR, Guo HQ, Lee DH, et al. Neuronal hyperpolarization-activated pacemaker channels drive neuropathic pain. *J. Neurosci.* 2003; **23**(4): 1169–78.

7. Simpson DM, Brown S, Tobias J. NGX-4010 C107 Study Group. Controlled trial of high-concentration capsaicin patch for treatment of painful HIV neuropathy. *Neurology* 2008; **70**(24): 2305–13.

8. Woolf CJ. Central sensitization: Implications for the diagnosis and treatment of pain. *Pain* 2011; **152**(3 Suppl.): S2–S15.

9. Nitzan-Luques A, Devor M, Tal M. Genotype-selective phenotypic switch in primary afferent neurons contributes to neuropathic pain. *Pain* 2011; **152**(10): 2413–26.

10. Scholz J, Broom DC, Youn DH, et al. Blocking caspase activity prevents transsynaptic neuronal apoptosis and the loss of inhibition in lamina II of the dorsal horn after peripheral nerve injury. *J. Neurosci.* 2005; **25**(32): 7317–23.

11. Ji RR, Berta T, Nedergaard M. Glia and pain: Is chronic pain a gliopathy? *Pain* 2013; **154**(Suppl. 1): S10–S28.

12. Bouhassira D, Attal N. Diagnosis and assessment of neuropathic pain: The saga of clinical tools. *Pain* 2011; **152**(Suppl. 3): S74–S83.

13. Backonja MM, Galer BS. Pain assessment and evaluation of patients who have neuropathic pain. *Neurol. Clin.* 1998; **16**(4): 775–90.

14. Suarez, GA, Dyck PJ. Quantitative sensory assessment. In Dyck PJ, Thomas PK eds. *Diabetic neuropathy* (2nd edn.). Philadelphia, PA: W. B. Saunders, 1999.

15. Galantino ML, Lucci SL. Living with chronic pain: Exploration of complementary therapies and impact on quality of life. In Wittnick, H, Michel TH eds. *Chronic pain management for physical therapists* (2nd

edn.). Boston, MA: Butterworth-Heinemann, 2002; 279–91.

16. Hall, J, et al. Does aquatic exercise relieve pain in adults with neurologic or musculoskeletal disease? A systematic review and meta-analysis of randomized controlled trials. *Arch. Phys. Med. Rehabil.* 2008; **89**(5): 873–83.

17. Bernaards CM, et al. The effective of a work style intervention and a lifestyle physical activity intervention on the recovery from neck and upper limb symptoms in computer workers. *Pain* 2007; **132**(1–2): 142–53.

18. McBeth J, et al. Cognitive behavior therapy, exercise or both for treating chronic widespread pain. *Arch. Intern. Med.* 2012; **172**(1): 48.

19. Walsh DM, Basford JR. Transcutaneous electrical nerve stimulation, chapter 47. In Smith HS. ed. *Current therapy in pain*. Philadelphia, PA: Saunders/Elsevier, 2009; 541–6.

20. Patil, S., et al. The role of acupuncture in pain management. *Curr. Pain Headache Rep.* 2016; **20**(4): 22.

21. Dorfman D, George MC, Schnir J, Simpson DM, Davidson G, Montgomery G. Hypnosis for treatment of HIV neuropathic pain: A preliminary report. *Pain Med.* 2013; **14**(7): 1048–56.

22. Dworkin, et al. Recommendations for the pharmacological management of neuropathic pain: An overview and literature update. *Mayo Clin. Proc.* 2010; **85**(3): S3–14.

23. Kremer M, et al. Antidepressants and gabapentinoids in neuropathic pain: Mechanistic insights. *Neuroscience* 2016; **S0306**-4522(16): 30296–2.

24. Gilron, et al. Morphine, gabapentin, or their combination for neuropathic pain. *N. Engl. J. Med.* 2005; **352**: 1324–34.

25. Dworkin, et al. Pharmacological management of neuropathic pain: Evidence-based recommendations. *Pain* 2007; **132**(3): 237–51.

26. Rowbotham, MC, et al. Venlafaxine extended release in the treatment of painful diabetic neuropathy: A double-blind, placebo-controlled study. *Pain* 2004; **100**: 697–706.

27. Fava, et al. Emergency of adverse events following discontinuation of treatment with extended-release venlafaxine. *Am. J. Psychiatry* 1997; **154**: 1760–2.

28. Caterina MJ. Vanilloid receptors take a TRP beyond the sensory afferent. *Pain* 2003; **105**: 5–9.

29. Capsaicin Study Group. Effect of treatment with capsaicin on daily activities of patients with painful diabetic neuropathy. *Diabetes Care* 1992; **15**: 159–65.

30. Gibbons, CH, et al. Capsaicin induces degeneration of cutaneous autonomic nerve fibers. *Ann. Neurol.* 2010; **68**(6): 888–98.

31. Simpson DM, Robinson-Papp J, Van J, et al. Capsaicin 8% patch in painful diabetic peripheral neuropathy: A randomized, double-blind, placebo-controlled study. *J Pain.* 2017; **18**(1): 42–53.

32. Cheung H, Kamp D, Harris E. An in vitro investigation of the action of lamotrigine on neuronal voltage-activated sodium channels. *Epilepsy Res.* 1992; **13**: 309–24.

33. Raskin P, Donofrio PD, Rosenthal NR, et al. Topiramate vs placebo in painful diabetic neuropathy: Analgesic and metabolic effects. *Neurology* 2004; **63**: 865–73.

34. Shank RP, Gardocki JF, Streeter AJ, et al. An overview of the preclinical aspects of topiramate pharmacology, pharmacokinetics, and mechanism of action. *Epilepsia* 2000; **41**(Suppl.): S3–9.

35. Perucca E, Bialer M. The clinical pharmacokinetics of the newer antiepileptic drugs. Focus on topiramate, zonisamide and tiagabine. *Clin. Pharmacokinet.* 1996; **31**: 29–46.

36. Dogra S, Beydoun S, Mazzola J, et al. Oxcarbazepine in painful diabetic neuropathy: A randomized, placebo-controlled study. *Eur. J. Pain.* 2005; **9**: 543–54.

37. McLean MJ, Schmutz M, Wamil AW, et al. Oxcarbazepine: Mechanism of action. *Epilepsia* 1994; **35**(Suppl. 3): S5–9.

38. Rull JA, Quibrera R, Gonzalez-Millan H, et al. Symptomatic treatment of peripheral diabetic neuropathy with carbamazepine (Tegretol): Double blind crossover trial. *Diabetologia* 1969; **5**: 215–18.

39. Wiffen PJ, McQuay HJ, Moore RA. Carbamazepine for acute and chronic pain. *Cochrane Database Syst. Rev.* 2005; CD005451.

40. Gilron I, et al. Morphine, gabapentin, or their combination for neuropathic pain. *N. Engl. J. Med.* 2005; **352**: 1324–34.

41. Jones D, Story DA. Serotonin syndrome and the anesthetist. *Aneasth. Intensive Care* 2005; **33**: 181–7.

42. Lionberger R. *General principles for evaluating the abuse deterrence of generic solid oral opioid drug products: Guidance for industry*. Food and Drug Administration Center for Drug Evaluation and Research (CDER). www.federalregister.gov/documents/2017/11/22/2017-25248/general-principles-for-evaluating-the-abuse-deterrence-of-generic-solid-oral-opioid-drug-products.

43. Finnerup NB, et al. Algorithm for neuropathic pain treatment: An evidence based proposal. *Pain* 2005; **188**: 289–305.

44. Vranken JH, et al. Pregabalin in patients with central neuropathic pain: A randomized, double-blind, placebo-controlled trial of a flexible-dose regimen. *Pain* 2008; **136**: 150–7.

45. Gilron I, Tu D, et al. Combination of morphine with notriptyline for neuropathic pain. *Pain* 2015; **156**(8): 1440–8.

46. O'Connor AB, et al. Pain associated with multiple sclerosis: Systematic review and proposed classification. *Pain* 2008; **137**: 96–111.

47. Wallace MS, Marcotte TD, Umlauf A, Gouaux B, Atkinson JH. Efficacy of inhaled cannabis on painful diabetic neuropathy. *J. Pain.* 2015; **16**(7): 616–27.

48. Accident Compensation Corporation. Interventional guidelines for pain management. www.acc.co.nz/for-providers/clinical-best-practice/interventional-pain-management/interventions/intervention-index/WC M1.034233.

49. Pasqualucci A, Pasqualucci V, Galla F, et al. Prevention of post-herpetic neuralgia: Acyclovir and prednisolone versus epidural local anesthetic and methylprednisolone. *Acta Anaesthesiol. Scand.* 2000; **44**: 910–18.

50. Ji G, Niu J, Hou L, Lu Y, Xiong L. The effectiveness of repetitive paravertebral injections with local anesthetics and steroids for the prevention of postherpetic neuralgia in patients with acute herpes zoster. *Anesth. Analg.* 2009; **109**: 1651–5.

51. Van Wijck AJ, Opstelten W, et al. The PINE study of epidural steroids and local anaesthetics to prevent postherpetic neuralgia: A randomized controlled trial. *Lancet* 2006; **367**: 219–24.

52. Rijsdijk M, Van Wijck AJ, et al. No beneficial effect of intrathecal methylprednisolone acetate in postherpetic neuralgia patients. *Eur. J. Pain.* 2013; **17**: 714–23.

53. Kim YH, Lee CJ, et al. Effect of pulsed radiofrequency for postherpetic neuralgia. *Acta Anaesthesiol. Scand.* 2008; **52**: 1140–3.

54. Dworkin R, O'Connor A, et al. Interventional management of neuropathic pain: NeuPSIG Recommendations. *Pain* 2013; **154**: 2249–61.

55. de Vos CC, Rajan V, et al. Effect and safety of spinal cord stimulation for treatment of chronic pain caused by diabetic neuropathy. *J. Diabetes Complications* 2009; **23**: 40–5.

56. Papuc E, Rejdak K. The role of neurostimulation in the treatment of neuropathic pain. *Ann. Agric. Environ. Med.* 2013; **1**: 14–17.

57. Cruccu G, et al. EFNS guidelines on neurostimulation therapy for neuropathic pain. *Eur. J. Neurol.* 2007; **14** (9): 952–70.

58. Lee CH, Delton AL. Prognostic ability of Tinel Sign in determining outcome for decompression surgery in diabetic and nondiabetic neuropathy. *Ann. Plast. Sug.* 2004; **53**: 523–7.

59. Stokvis A, Van der Avoort DJ, et al. Surgical management of neuroma pain: A prospective follow-up study. *Pain* 2010; **151**: 862–9.

60. Anderson VC, Burchiel KJ. A prospective study of long-term intrathecal morphine in the management of chronic nonmalignant pain. *Neurosurgery* 1999; **44**: 289–300.

61. Cetas JS, Saedi T, Burchiel KJ. Destructive procedures for the treatment of nonmalignant pain: A structured literature review. *J. Neurosurg.* 2008; **109**: 389–404.

62. Rivera Dia RC, Lotero MAA, et al. Botulinum toxin for the treatment of chronic pain: Review of evidence. *Colomb. J. Anesthesiol.* 2014; **42**(3): 205–13.

63. Sim WS. Application of botulinum toxin in pain management. *Korean J. Pain.* 2011; **24**(1): 1–6.

64. Yin S, Stucker FJ, Nathan CA. Clinical application of botulinum toxin in otolaryngology, head and neck practice (brief review). *J. La. State Med. Soc.* 2001; **153** (2): 92–7.

65. Aoki KR. Review of a proposed mechanism for the antinociceptive action of botulinum toxin type A. *NeuroToxicology* 2005; **26**(5): 785–93.

66. Emad MR, Emad M, Taheri P. The efficacy of intradermal injection of botulinum toxin in patients with post-herpetic neuralgia. *Iran Red Crescent Med. J.* 2011; **13**(5): 323–7.

67. Ngeow WC, Nair R. Injection of botulinum toxin type A (BOTOX) into trigger zone of trigeminal neuralgia as a means to control pain. *Oral Surg. Med. Oral Pathol. Oral Radiol. Endod.* 2010; **109**(3): e47–50.

68. Ranoux D, Attal N, et al. Botulinum toxin type A induces direct analgesic effects in chronic neuropathic pain. *Ann. Neurol.* 2008; **64**(3): 274–83.

Management of Phantom Limb in Neurorehabilitation

Rohit Bhide and Apurba Barman

14.1 Introduction

The phenomena of phantom limb sensation (PLS) and phantom limb pain (PLP) occur commonly in patients with limb amputations. PLS refers to the persistent perception that the amputated limb or a part of it continues to exist, whereas PLP is the subjective experience of painful symptoms in the area of the amputated limb or the organ. Although first described in the sixteenth century by Ambrose Pare, it was only in the nineteenth century that the term 'phantom limb pain' was coined by Silas Weir Mitchell. PLP can manifest in the form of neuropathic sensations like burning, tingling, throbbing, piercing, and pins-and-needles sensations. This pain can vary in intensity, frequency, duration, and location [1, 2].

PLP is a poorly understood condition and hence, reportedly difficult to treat. Studies show varying prevalence rates ranging between 50% and 80%, implying that at least one in two amputees experiences these distressing symptoms [3]. It is also likely that the overall prevalence is under-reported due to the lack of awareness amongst physicians and other healthcare professionals regarding the difference between PLP and PLS [4].

The phantom phenomenon consists of three distinct elements: (a) PLP, which refers to the painful sensations that arise from the phantom limb; (b) PLS, which refers to any sensations other than pain arising from the phantom limb; and (c) stump pain (SP) or residual limb pain, which is indicative of pain localized to the amputated stump [3]. These are commonly noted to be coexistent in a single patient and difficult to distinguish due to the subjective nature of the overall pain experience [5].

PLP is not the same as stump or residual limb pain. While PLP is classified as neuropathic pain, the residual limb pain is primarily nociceptive in nature [6]. Stump or residual pain usually occurs due to local causes like skin issues, poor healing, painful neuromas, vascular deficits, excess soft tissue, and bony

prominences [1]. Another point to highlight is that PLS and PLP are not limited to amputations of the extremities. They have been reported following removal of different body parts, including facial structures (eyes, teeth, tongue, nose) and other organs like breast, penis, bowel, and bladder [7].

14.2 Mechanisms

Although the phantom phenomenon is widely described in literature, exact knowledge regarding its mechanisms and the pathophysiology behind it remains elusive. New findings suggest that there is more to PLP than a psychogenic experience. It is likely that peripheral and central nervous system plasticity play a key role in its genesis [8]. Various studies have demonstrated the brain's capability to undergo plastic changes within the primary somatosensory cortex in response to neuropathic and nociceptive pain [9]. These complex mechanisms involve different elements along the different pathways, including somatic pain generators, peripheral neural factors, and the central nervous system. However, none of these mechanisms is in a position to explain the phenomenon of PLP independently, and it is likely that multiple mechanisms are at play simultaneously.

1. Peripheral neural and structural mechanisms

   Following amputation, regenerative sprouting of the injured axons leads to neuroma formation in the residual limb. Ectopic discharges from these neuromas lead to abnormal afferent nerve input to the spinal cord [10]. The resultant upregulation of sodium (Na^+) channels leads to hyper excitability and spontaneous discharges. This theory makes a good case for residual limb pain and the subsequent PLP experience [2]. Other factors such as neuroma formation, increased axonal excitability, and myofascial dysfunction also contribute to further augment the symptoms [11].

2. Central neural postulates

Spinal cord changes. Axonal sprouting in the amputated peripheral nerve forms connections and produces changes in the dorsal horn of the spinal cord, which is responsible for the transmission of nociceptive stimuli [12]. This results in central sensitization, and an increase in the N-methyl-D-aspartate (NMDA) receptor-mediated neurotransmitters such as substance P, tachykinins, and neurokinins at that site [13]. The resultant 'windup phenomenon' causes upregulation of these receptors, and a change in the firing pattern of the central nociceptive neurons. Similarly, there is a reduction in the descending inhibitory signals from the supraspinal centres, and the local intersegmental inhibitory mechanisms. These result in spinal disinhibition, causing nociceptive inputs to reach the supraspinal centres. Such changes happening at the level of the spinal cord have been proposed to result in the generation of PLP.

Changes at the level of the brain. Cortical reorganization remains one of commonest reasons suggested as a cause of PLP in recent years. It is proposed that following amputation, the cortical areas that represent the amputated extremity are taken over by the neighbouring representational zones in the primary somatosensory and the motor cortex [18, 25, 26]. This process also helps to shed a light on the way stimulation of afferent nociceptive neurons within the stump produces the phantom sensation in the amputated limb. Evidence shows that the extent of cortical reorganization is directly proportional to the degree of pain, and the phantom limb experience. Functional MRI studies have demonstrated a direct relationship between the severity of PLP with the area of cortical reorganization [14].

Another model is the 'body schema' concept proposed by Head and Holmes in 1912. It is postulated that a template of the entire body exists in the brain and procedures like amputation result in a change to the template, which leads to the phantom limb perception [9]. An expansion of this concept was suggested in 1989 involving the neuromatrix. It is a widely distributed network of neurons integrating numerous inputs from various areas. Following any insult or stress to the body, the output patterns of the body–self neuromatrix are responsible for activating perceptual and behavioural programmes. Pain perception results from the changes in the neuromatrix, rather than directly from sensory input secondary to noxious stimuli. The lack of actual inputs from the amputated limbs to the neuromatrix causes an abnormal neurosignature, which refers to the activity patterns generated within the brain undergoing constant updates based upon an individual's experiences and body perception. These abnormal neurosignatures are thought to cause PLP [15].

Psychogenic mechanisms. The assumption that PLP is of psychogenic origin has not been supported in the recent literature, even though stress, anxiety, exhaustion, and depression are believed to exacerbate PLP [16]. In fact, there is no evidence to suggest that major personality disorders are more common amongst patients with phantom limb pain [16].

A single theory which takes into account all these is the progressive sensitization theory. It suggests that the peripheral factors may dominate at the time of amputation. However, if the symptoms continue, the central factors may predominate the overall pain experience. Changes within the primary somatosensory cortex are in response to ongoing nociceptive stimuli or the lack of stimuli altogether. It is likely that central adaptation and peripheral sensitization both contribute towards the presence of PLP [17, 18].

14.3 Presentation

Patients who experience PLP describe positive sensory symptoms like sharp, burning, electric, crushing, cramping feelings [4]. Particular movements or positions of the phantom limb are also known to aggravate the PLP experience [19].

Phantom limbs sometimes undergo a 'telescoping' phenomenon, which refers to the retraction of the phantom limb into the stump [18]. It is considered to be a feature of central adaptation. Some phantom limbs are 'movable' while some are 'paralysed'. Patients with paralysed phantom limbs are more likely to have experienced actual paralysis of the limb prior to the amputation [20]. The reported mobility of the phantom limb by the patient may play a key role in determining the type of therapy offered and its success.

Phantom limb pain episodes are known to vary in intensity, frequency, duration, location, and character

[3]. They are usually unique to every individual. Studies suggest that in patients with PLP, the current or 'at-the-moment' state of pain is a better indicator than the general reporting of the pain experience [9]. The greater the shift of the surrounding organs into the deafferented cortical zone (as a result of amputation), the greater the PLP [9].

14.4 Factors Affecting Phantom Limb Sensation and Pain

Various factors have been shown to exacerbate phantom limb pain. Amongst them, psychological factors like stress, anxiety, and depression, and physical factors like pressure, temperature change, autonomous reflexes, pain from other sources, and prosthesis fitting are the common contributors [18]. The prevalence of PLP is reportedly more common amongst upper limb amputees than their lower limb counterparts. It is also more common amongst females than males. The presence of pre-amputation pain has been shown to increase the risks of developing PLP [2].

14.5 Assessment

A detailed assessment based on the history, examination, and appropriate investigations helps to identify the source of pain. The assessor should identify answers to three questions: (a) the origin of the pain – whether the pain is due to residual limb pain, phantom limb sensation, or phantom limb pain; (b) whether the pain is a result of ongoing nociceptive input or loss of input to the cortical zone of amputation or both; and, lastly, (c) the dominant factor responsible for the patient's PLP experience – central, peripheral, or psychological [6].

The most widely used rating scales are the visual analogue scale (VAS), the numerical rating scale (NRS), and the McGill pain questionnaire (MPQ). The Brief Pain Inventory, which gives an idea of the impact of the pain on everyday life, can be used in PLP. The prosthesis evaluation questionnaire also covers phantom limb sensations. Measures of PLP intensity should be scored and recorded for at least one week [8].

Assessing the fitness of the prosthesis, management of the referred pain, and other aggravating factors play a key role in keeping things under check. Distant pain syndromes, such as hip or lower back pain, which may not have a direct connection with the stump, can also aggravate PLP and should be managed by improving posture and biomechanical alignment to provide optimal pain relief.

14.6 Management

No single therapy is proven to eliminate PLP completely. A number of different therapies and strategies relying on varying principles have been proposed (Table 14.1). However, specific treatment guidelines are yet to evolve. Most successful measures employ multidisciplinary and multipronged approaches in the management of pain and rehabilitation. Conservative, pharmacologic, and adjuvant therapies are usually employed, either in isolation or simultaneously.

Early emphasis should be on managing and controlling the residual limb pain. This can be achieved by using appropriate analgesics and various measures to prevent stump oedema like limb positioning, semi-rigid dressings, or stump socks. Similarly, ensuring that the intrinsic and extrinsic factors related to the residual limb are adequately addressed contributes to the overall success. Extrinsic factors are usually a result of impaired wound healing, infection, inappropriate prosthetic fit, and poor scar formation. Appropriate skin care, including scar management and local massage for desensitization have been shown to help reduce the residual limb pain [6, 21]. Intrinsic factors like ischaemia, joint dysfunction, and neuroma need to be assessed with suitable investigations. Use of arterial and venous Doppler studies, appropriate imaging, and a detailed sensory assessment help determine treatment regimens for these factors.

More than 38 different treatments are described in the literature for the management of PLP, albeit with limited success [22]. Over the years, due to the lack of adequate response with any one type of treatment, emphasis has been on exploring newer strategies and options for management. Recent initiatives are increasingly focusing on prevention or prophylactic management of PLP, with the hope that this will prevent central neural sensitization. As with other ideas, these studies have yielded equivocal results.

14.6.1 Non-Pharmacological Treatment

Various non-pharmacological treatment regimens are aimed to equip the patients and provide them with tools and strategies to manage their pain. Common self-management strategies such as the use of an elastic stump sock, stump and scar massage, mental

Table 14.1 Treatment options for phantom limb pain

Non-pharmacological	**Residual limb care** • Prevent stump oedema Manage extrinsic factors – wound healing, scar, infection, prosthesis fit Manage intrinsic factors – vascular, joint dysfunction, neuroma **Desensitization techniques** • Transcutaneous electrical nerve stimulation (TENS) • Mirror therapy • Repetitive transcranial magnetic stimulation • Massage • Percussion **Biofeedback** • Visual, electromyographic, thermal **Biomechanics** • Appropriate prosthetic fit and alignment • Proximal joint range maintenance, posture and gait pattern normalization, proprioceptive exercises **Integrative** • Virtual reality interventions • Eye movement desensitization and reprocessing therapy (EMDR) • Guided imagery, relaxation techniques, acupuncture, hypnosis Ultrasound Sensory discrimination training Cognitive behavioural therapy
Pharmacological	**Analgesics** • Acetaminophen, NSAIDs **Antidepressants** • Tricyclic – amitriptyline, nortriptyline, desipramine • SNRIs – duloxetine, milnacipran **Anticonvulsants** • gabapentin, pregabalin, carbamazepine

Table 14.1 (cont.)

	Opioids • Morphine, tramadol • Synthetic – methadone **Anaesthetics** • Lidocaine, bupivacaine, mexiletine **NMDA receptor antagonists** • Ketamine, memantine **Other medications** • Calcitonin • Botulinum toxin A • Doxepin, topiramate, clonazepam, ropivicaine, propranolol
Surgical	**Ablative** • Cordotomy, rhizotomy, dorsal root entry zone lesion, thalamotomy Spinal cord stimulation Intrathecal drug delivery systems • Clonidine, local anaesthetic, opioids

imagery of the phantom limb, and continuing physical exercise go a long way in reducing the PLP experience. Maintaining range in the proximal joint, ensuring appropriate prosthetic fit and alignment, normalizing posture and gait pattern, and proprioceptive exercises ensure an optimal outcome [6, 23]. Prosthesis use has been shown to reduce PLP and is thought to normalize visual, sensory, and motor feedback and reverse cortical reorganization [24].

14.6.1.1 Desensitizing Technique

There is enough evidence in multiple placebo-controlled trials and epidemiologic surveys about the effectiveness of the desensitization technique, using transcutaneous electrical nerve (TENS) stimulation to reduce PLP [21]. Low-frequency and high-intensity TENS has been found to be more effective than other doses [25]. TENS devices are recommended due to their portability, ease of use, non-invasiveness, and relatively low cost. Some studies recommend TENS as a first-line therapy due to minimal side effects or contraindications [2]. However, its long-term effectiveness remains questionable [22]. Percussion and massage are some of the other forms of desensitization with limited benefits in patients with peripheral sensitization [6]. Repetitive transcranial magnetic stimulation has demonstrated some short-term relief in one high-quality study [22].

14.6.1.2 Mirror Therapy

The mirror therapy concept was introduced in 1996. The amputated limb is inserted in a mirror box placed along the midline of the body. The reflection of the intact moving limb overlapping the phantom hand or foot creates a visual illusion of non-painful movements in the phantom limb. This helps restore the projection of the amputated limb in the corresponding cortical motor and sensory areas [5]. The resultant reorganization and integration of the proprioceptive signals and visual feedback of the amputated limb help reduce the PLP [26]. This concept has been further explored by investigating the presence of mirror neurons in the brain and their activation, which creates a perception of tactile sensation [27]. Although this theory sounds convincing based on its hypothesis, there is only limited evidence to suggest that it is actually useful in patients with PLP [2, 5, 28]. A recent study comparing mirror therapy and TENS found that both tools were effective in reducing pain, but only for a short period of time [29].

14.6.1.3 Biofeedback, Integrative, and Behavioural Methods

Biofeedback techniques, specifically temperature and visual biofeedback, are helpful for the burning sensation of PLP [28, 30]. Use of immersive virtual reality interventions and eye movement desensitization and reprocessing therapy (EMDR) have been explored with reasonable success. Other tools like guided imagery, relaxation techniques, acupuncture, and hypnosis have been trialled in the treatment of PLP, although their effectiveness remains doubtful. Likewise, benefits of cognitive behavioural therapy (CBT) in neuropathic pain syndromes have been reported in a few case studies [31]. Persistent and intense PLP is known to affect quality of life, and it can cause depression. Various non-pharmacological strategies to address the depressive symptoms also help in alleviating the overall PLP experience. Some

recent initiatives have focussed on the use of myo-electric pattern recognition for virtual and augmented reality environments [32]. Although the evidence at this stage is relatively low, there is potential for these treatments to become more widespread due to the immersive experience, customizable environments, and decreasing costs [33]. Progressive muscle relaxation, mental imagery, and modified phantom exercises are also recommended as a valuable technique to reduce phantom limb pain and sensation [34].

14.6.2 Pharmacological Treatment

Pharmacological management of PLP is based on a combination of drugs which have proven effective for neuropathic pain management. Anticonvulsants, antidepressants, local anaesthetics, opioids, and other drugs in different doses and combinations are commonly employed with varying success. Most studies have failed to demonstrate noticeable difference in secondary outcomes like function, sleep, and quality of life. Given the limited evidence, clinicians should continue to rely on other modalities and plan treatment regimens based on patients' response and symptom management.

14.6.2.1 Acetaminophen and Nonsteroidal Anti-Inflammatory Drugs (NSAIDs)

Acetaminophen and NSAIDs are commonly used to address PLP [35]. Acetaminophen may act via multiple central nervous system pathways, whereas NSAIDs inhibit prostaglandin synthesis and reduce peripheral and central nociception. The ease of availability, the lack of need for a prescription, and the widespread knowledge about these drugs make them some of the most popular drugs in the initial stages for management of PLP. While acetaminophen is used primarily as an analgesic, it is hoped that the NSAIDs will help address the local inflammatory reactions and the swelling in the residual limb. While these drugs have been identified as good options for management of residual limb pain, they have not been effective for PLP reduction. Recent comprehensive reviews have failed to identify any studies on the use of acetaminophen and NSAIDs for PLP [22, 36]. The lack of studies is likely due to the logistical difficulties in designing a study in which the medication is so readily available.

14.6.2.2 Antidepressants

Tricyclic antidepressants (TCAs) are widely used for various neuropathic pain syndromes, including

PLP. These drugs act by inhibiting serotonin-nor-epinephrine uptake, NMDA receptor antagonism, and blockade of sodium channels. Amitriptyline, nortriptyline, and desipramine have been found to be effective in some reports. Few other reports advocating the benefits of mirtazapine and duloxetine exist, but are contradicted by the Cochrane review by Saarto [2, 37]. Dryness of mouth, daytime drowsiness, blurred vision, constipation, and dizziness are commonly reported side effects. These are more common with amitriptyline and are reportedly less seen with nortriptyline and desipramine.

14.6.2.3 Anticonvulsants

Gabapentin has shown mixed results in the control of PLP with some studies showing positive results while others report the opposite. The recent revised Cochrane review found conflicting results for pain-relieving properties of gabapentin with only short-term relief noted when compared to the placebo. Furthermore, it was found not to improve function, depression, or sleep quality. Noticeable side effects reported were somnolence, dizziness, headache, and nausea [22, 36]. Pregabalin has been shown to be effective in other neuropathic syndromes, but does not have any substantive study to back its use for management of PLP. Carbamazepine has been used to address the stabbing and lancinating pain associated with PLP [2].

14.6.2.4 Opioids

Opioids bind to the peripheral and central opioid receptors and provide analgesia without affecting touch and proprioception. Like gabapentin, opioids have been proven to provide short-term relief from PLP [22, 36]. Two studies have demonstrated the efficacy of opioids with significant reduction in VAS scores, lower pain intensities, and self-reported percentage pain relief [38, 39]. Amongst the available pharmacological treatment options, opioids have shown the most promising results [35]. It is possible to achieve synergistic treatment effects by combining opioids with other agents, such as TCAs or gabapentinoids for neuropathic pain modulation [40]. However, their use is limited by the reported adverse events, which include constipation, sedation, tiredness, dizziness, vertigo, itching, and respiratory problems [36]. Moreover, their habit-forming properties and development of

tolerance, along with their use for recreational purposes, make them unpopular amongst physicians.

14.6.2.5 NMDA Receptor Antagonist

Although six studies have been done to assess the effectiveness of NMDA receptor antagonists in established PLP, the results have demonstrated only short-term relief with the use of ketamine and dextromethorphan. Intravenous infusion of ketamine has demonstrated significant reduction in pain intensity in patients with chronic phantom pain of malignant aetiology [41]. The adverse events with ketamine are more common and include loss of consciousness, sedation, hallucinations, hearing and position impairment, and insobriety [22, 36].

14.6.2.6 Other Medications

Use of calcitonin for management of PLP has been explored in various studies involving small sample sizes with variable results. The potential for Botulinum toxin A to help manage PLP has been explored. However, a small study which investigated it against lidocaine/methylprednisolone did not find either treatment to be beneficial [36, 42]. The use of local anaesthetics for PLP has revealed some interesting findings. While lidocaine infusion is not effective, its long-acting counterpart, bupivacaine injection to the contralateral myofascial hyperalgesic area, is known to reduce phantom pain intensity [39, 43]. A recent review from Manchester identified various other medications that have been used for PLP. These low-quality studies separately explored the use of doxepin, topiramate, clonazepam, methadone, mexiletine, ropivicaine, propranolol, duloxetine, and milnacipran. Most of the studies reported reduced intensity of PLP [22].

14.6.3 Surgical Interventions

Surgical interventions are usually tried as a last resort. All other available tools and options need to be explored and trialled before undertaking any interventional procedures, which currently do not have great evidence to back them up. The evidence for these procedures only exists in the form of case reports and series, which report them to be partly beneficial. Surgical ablative therapy consists of cordotomy, rhizotomy, dorsal root entry zone lesion, spinal cord stimulation, or thalamotomy. Modalities like dorsal column stimulation and intrathecal drug delivery systems to infuse clonidine, local anaesthetic, or opioids have also been suggested. For refractory pain, implantable intrathecal pumps can be resorted to as a potential option [44–48]. This line of treatment certainly warrants a further investigation into the definitive management of PLP, especially in cases with refractory pain.

14.7 Conclusion

Phantom limb pain and other related pain syndromes remain one of the difficult symptoms to manage. Ongoing research initiatives to understand its mechanisms and various treatments will go a long way in making it easier to manage this condition. Based on the current evidence, a multipronged and multimodal treatment approach is necessary to help patients with phantom limb pain. The emphasis should be on empowering the patient with available tools and strategies to manage these symptoms and improve quality of life.

References

1. Padovani MT, Martins MRI, Venâncio A, Forni JEN. Anxiety, depression and quality of life in individuals with phantom limb pain. *Acta Ortop. Bras.* 2015; **23**: 107–10.

2. Subedi B, Grossberg GT. Phantom limb pain: Mechanisms and treatment approaches. *Pain Research and Treatment* 2011; **2011**: 864605.

3. Ahmed A, Bhatnagar S, Mishra S, et al. Prevalence of phantom limb pain, stump pain, and phantom limb sensation among the amputated cancer patients in India: A prospective, observational study. *Indian J. Palliat. Care* 2017; **23**: 24–35.

4. Ketz AK. The experience of phantom limb pain in patients with combat-related traumatic amputations. *Arch. Phys. Med. Rehabil.* 2008; **89**: 1127–32.

5. Barbin J, Seetha V, Casillas JM, et al. The effects of mirror therapy on pain and motor control of phantom limb in amputees: A systematic review. *Ann. Phys. Rehabil. Med.* 2016; **59**: 270–5.

6. Le Feuvre P, Aldington D. Know pain know gain: Proposing a treatment approach for phantom limb pain. *J. R. Army Med. Corps* 2014; **160**: 16–21.

7. Weeks SR, Anderson-Barnes VC, Tsao JW. Phantom limb pain: Theories and therapies. *Neurologist* 2010; **16**: 277–86.

8. Ferraro F, Jacopetti M, Spallone V, et al. Diagnosis and treatment of pain in plexopathy, radiculopathy, peripheral neuropathy and phantom limb pain. Evidence and recommendations from the Italian Consensus Conference on Pain on Neurorehabilitation. *Eur. J. Phys. Rehabil. Med.* 2016; **52**: 855–66.

9. MacIver K, Lloyd DM, Kelly S, et al. Phantom limb pain, cortical reorganization and the therapeutic effect of mental imagery. *Brain J. Neurol.* 2008; **131**: 2181–91.

10. Flor H, Nikolajsen L, Jensen TS. Phantom limb pain: A case of maladaptive CNS plasticity? *Nat. Rev. Neurosci.* 2006; **7**: nrn1991.

11. Kern U, Busch V, Müller R, et al. Phantom limb pain in daily practice: Still a lot of work to do! *Pain Med. Malden Mass.* 2012; **13**: 1611–26.

12. Dickinson BD, Head CA, Gitlow S, Osbahr AJ. Maldynia: Pathophysiology and management of neuropathic and maladaptive pain: A Report of the AMA Council on Science and Public Health. *Pain Med.* 2010; **11**: 1635–53.

13. Baron R. Mechanisms of disease: Neuropathic pain: A clinical perspective. *Nat. Rev. Neurol.* 2006; **2**: 95–106.

14. Diers M, Christmann C, Koeppe C, et al. Mirrored, imagined and executed movements differentially activate sensorimotor cortex in amputees with and without phantom limb pain. *Pain* 2010; **149**: 296–304.

15. Melzack R. Pain and the neuromatrix in the brain. *J. Dent. Educ.* 2001; **65**: 1378–82.

16. Sherman RA, Sherman CJ, Bruno GM. Psychological factors influencing chronic phantom limb pain: An analysis of the literature. *Pain* 1987; **28**: 285–95.

17. Birbaumer N, Lutzenberger W, Montoya P, et al. Effects of regional anesthesia on phantom limb pain are mirrored in changes in cortical reorganization. *J. Neurosci. Off. J. Soc. Neurosci.* 1997; **17**: 5503–8.

18. Flor H. Cortical reorganisation and chronic pain: Implications for rehabilitation. *J. Rehabil. Med.* 2003; (**41** Suppl.): 66–72.

19. Kooijman CM, Dijkstra PU, Geertzen JH, et al. Phantom pain and phantom sensations in upper limb amputees: An epidemiological study. *Pain* 2000; **87**: 33–41.

20. Ramachandran VS, Blakeslee S. *Phantoms in the brain: Human nature and the architecture of the mind* (new edn.). London, UK: Fourth Estate, 1999.

21. Black LM, Persons RK, Jamieson B. Clinical inquiries. What is the best way to manage phantom limb pain? *J. Fam. Pract.* 2009; **58**: 155–8.

22. Richardson C, Kulkarni J. A review of the management of phantom limb pain: Challenges and solutions. *J. Pain. Res.* 2017; **10**: 1861–70.

23. Comerford MJ, Mottram SL. Functional stability re-training: Principles and strategies for managing mechanical dysfunction. *Man. Ther.* 2001; **6**: 3–14.

24. Lotze M, Flor H, Grodd W, et al. Phantom movements and pain: An fMRI study in upper limb amputees. *Brain J. Neurol.* 2001; **124**: 2268–77.

25. Cruccu G, Aziz TZ, Garcia-Larrea L, et al. EFNS guidelines on neurostimulation therapy for neuropathic pain. *Eur. J. Neurol.* 2007; **14**: 952–70.

26. Kim SY, Kim YY. Mirror therapy for phantom limb pain. *Korean J. Pain* 2012; **25**: 272–4.

27. Ramachandran VS, Rogers-Ramachandran D. Sensations referred to a patient's phantom arm from another subject's intact arm: Perceptual correlates of mirror neurons. *Med. Hypotheses* 2008; **70**: 1233–4.

28. Chan BL, Witt R, Charrow AP, et al. Mirror therapy for phantom limb pain. *N. Engl. J. Med.* 2007; **357**: 2206–7.

29. Tilak M, Isaac SA, Fletcher J, et al. Mirror therapy and transcutaneous electrical nerve stimulation for management of phantom limb pain in amputees: A single blinded randomized controlled trial. *Physiother. Res. Int. J. Res. Clin. Phys. Ther.* 2016; **21**: 109–15.

30. Harden RN, Houle TT, Green S, et al. Biofeedback in the treatment of phantom limb pain: A time-series analysis. *Appl. Psychophysiol. Biofeedback* 2005; **30**: 83–93.

31. Castelnuovo G, Giusti EM, Manzoni GM, et al. Psychological treatments and psychotherapies in the neurorehabilitation of pain: Evidences and recommendations from the Italian Consensus Conference on Pain in Neurorehabilitation. *Frontiers in Psychology* 2016; **7**: 115.

32. Ortiz-Catalan M, Sander N, Kristoffersen MB, et al. Treatment of phantom limb pain (PLP) based on augmented reality and gaming controlled by myoelectric pattern recognition: A case study of a chronic PLP patient. *Frontiers in Neuroscience* 2014; **8**: 24.

33. Dunn J, Yeo E, Moghaddampour P, et al. Virtual and augmented reality in the treatment of phantom limb pain: A literature review. *NeuroRehabilitation* 2017; **40**: 595–601.

34. Brunelli S, Morone G, Iosa M, et al. Efficacy of progressive muscle relaxation, mental imagery, and phantom exercise training on phantom limb: A randomized controlled trial. *Arch. Phys. Med. Rehabil.* 2015; **96**: 181–7.

35. Hanley MA, Ehde DM, Campbell KM, et al. Self-reported treatments used for lower-limb phantom pain: Descriptive findings. *Arch. Phys. Med. Rehabil.* 2006; **87**: 270–7.

36. Alviar MJM, Hale T, Dungca M. Pharmacologic interventions for treating phantom limb pain. *Cochrane Database Syst. Rev.* 2016; **10**: CD006380.

37. Saarto T, Wiffen PJ. Antidepressants for neuropathic pain. *Cochrane Database Syst. Rev.* 2007; **4**: CD005454.

38. Huse E, Larbig W, Flor H, Birbaumer N. The effect of opioids on phantom limb pain and cortical reorganization. *Pain* 2001; **90**: 47–55.

39. Wu CL, Tella P, Staats PS, et al. Analgesic effects of intravenous lidocaine and morphine on postamputation pain: A randomized double-blind, active placebo-controlled, crossover trial. *Anesthesiology* 2002; **96**: 841–8.

40. Moulin D, Boulanger A, Clark AJ, et al. Pharmacological management of chronic neuropathic pain: Revised consensus statement from the Canadian Pain Society. *Pain Res. Manag.* 2014; **19**: 328–35.

41. Eichenberger U, Neff F, Sveticic G, et al. Chronic phantom limb pain: The effects of calcitonin, ketamine, and their combination on pain and sensory thresholds. *Anesth. Analg.* 2008; **10**: 1265–73.

42. Wu H, Sultana R, Taylor KB, Szabo A. A prospective randomized double-blinded pilot study to examine the effect of botulinum toxin type A injection versus lidocaine/depomedrol injection on residual and phantom limb pain: Initial report. *Clin. J. Pain* 2012; **28**: 108–12.

43. Casale R, Ceccherelli F, Labeeb AAEM, Biella GEM. Phantom limb pain relief by contralateral myofascial injection with local anaesthetic in a placebo-controlled study: Preliminary results. *J. Rehabil. Med.* 2009; **41**: 418–22.

44. Zheng Z, Hu Y, Tao W, Zhang X, Li Y. Dorsal root entry zone lesions for phantom limb pain with brachial plexus avulsion: A study of pain and phantom limb sensation. *Stereotact. Funct. Neurosurg.* 2009; **87**: 249–55.

45. Viswanathan A, Phan PC, Burton AW. Use of spinal cord stimulation in the treatment of phantom limb pain: Case series and review of the literature. *Pain Pract. Off. J. World Inst. Pain* 2010; **10**: 479–84.

46. Raslan AM, McCartney S, Burchiel KJ. Management of chronic severe pain: Spinal neuromodulatory and neuroablative approaches. *Acta Neurochir. Suppl.* 2007; **97**: 33–41.

47. Danshaw CB. An anesthetic approach to amputation and pain syndromes. *Phys. Med. Rehabil. Clin. N. Am.* 2000; **11**: 553–7.

48. Saris SC, Iacono RP, Nashold BS. Dorsal root entry zone lesions for post-amputation pain. *J. Neurosurg.* 1985; **62**: 72–6.

Chapter 15

Management of Neuro-Ophthalmologic Disorders in Neurorehabilitation

Simon J. Hickman and Martin J. Rhodes

15.1 Introduction

Chronic visual impairment is a major cause of limitation of participation. Its presence also leads to an increased risk of depression, injury, and decline in general health [1]. It is important when assessing people with visual impairment to work out their visual needs and priorities. The vision required may be close up or near, at intermediate or far distances. At each of these distances, the visual requirement may be for a short or long time period [2]. During the assessment, it is important to set a realistic set of goals; for example, it may prove impossible to restore vision to a standard required for driving; however, visual function may be improved such that it may be possible for the person to access public transportation independently.

Firstly, it is important to get an accurate refraction for both near and far vision [1]. With that in place, visual acuity can then be measured. It is important to offer sight impairment registration if the person is eligible, since that can help the person access services [3]. Also, the registration process usually includes the cause of the visual impairment. Knowledge of within-country data on causes of visual impairment can help in priority setting and resource allocation [4].

This chapter deals with three main areas of visual need: reading, general participation, and driving. The rehabilitation possibilities in these three areas are discussed for the principal neurological causes of visual impairment, which are reduced visual acuity, hemianopia, diplopia, and nystagmus.

15.1.1 Reading

Reading has now become central to life in modern society, both in the increasingly information-based working environment, and in the online world of the Internet and associated social media. To read standard newsprint (N8) at a distance of 25 cm, a visual acuity of at least 20/50 (0.4) is necessary. However, visual acuity is tested one letter (optotype) at a time,

whereas reading is a more complex activity and involves viewing groups of letters at a time [5]. This therefore requires an intact visual field of approximately $2°$ either side of fixation. In addition, intact vision in the parafoveal area is needed, out to $5°$ to the right in left-to-right readers. This provides information about word length and is used to plan the saccadic eye movement to the next group of letters. The whole viewing area is termed the 'perceptual window for reading' [6]. The duration of each fixation is about 250 ms when the letter information is captured and processed. If the eye movements of a normal subject are recorded during reading, then this shows a staircase pattern of fixations (the horizontals) and saccades (the verticals). At the end of each line of script, a large saccade is made to the start of the next line. Reading speed is used as a measure of reading because it integrates vision, comprehension, and eye movements.

15.1.2 General Participation

Vision assists in virtually all aspects of day-to-day life. In a survey of the impact of visual impairment on everyday life the areas of greatest restriction of participation were associated with reading, outdoor mobility, participation in leisure activities, and shopping [7].

Visual impairment also significantly impacts employment opportunities. In a telephone survey of 559 participants of working age with visual impairment, only 33% were in current employment. The key factors associated with being in work were the level of educational attainment, housing tenure, the degree of visual impairment, and the presence of additional disabilities [8]. For a child, vision impairment may lead to delays in reaching intellectual and physical milestones, as well as difficulties in social interaction with other children [9].

In addition, visual impairment is an independent risk factor for falls. In the Blue Mountains Eye Study, the factors associated with two or more falls were visual acuity (prevalence ratio [PR] 1.9 for visual acuity worse than 20/30), contrast sensitivity (PR 1.2 for a one-unit decrease at six cycles per degree), and suprathreshold visual field testing (PR 1.5 for five or more points missing) [10]. Visual field defects secondary to stroke and glaucoma also increase the risk of falling. In a retrospective study of 56 falls over a period of five years in 41 stroke patients undergoing rehabilitation, incremental risk factors included hemianopia or blindness in one eye in 25% of falls and visuospatial agnosia in 18% of falls [11]. In a study of people with glaucoma, high rates of visual field loss correlated with fall rate (rate ratio, 2.28 per 0.5 dB/year faster visual field loss, $p = 0.02$) [12]. Falls often occur due to failing to perceive obstacles. Additional factors that contribute to this are the level of illumination, obstacle location, and the contrast of the obstacle with its environment [13].

From a survey of 54 people with hemianopia or quadrantanopia, in addition to expected difficulties with reading, orientation, and mobility, a high proportion reported problems with impaired light sensitivity, colour vision, and depth perception [14].

From a regression analysis the strongest independent predictors of who would benefit most from vision rehabilitation services were found to be the visual acuity, the presence of co-morbidities, and the degree of dependence on others [15].

15.1.3 Driving

Driving allows independence for both work and leisure activities. An inability to drive vastly limits participation and increases the risk of depression [16]. Vision is the most important sensory input for driving. However, the correlation between visual acuity and motor vehicle accidents is weak. This probably reflects the importance of other factors in vision but also the need of drivers to react quickly and appropriately to what is seen [17]. Each driving licensing authority has its own laws regarding minimum vision standards. A comprehensive list of vision requirements for different countries has been published [18–24].

Driving commercial vehicles requires a much greater ability to see, and usually without the assistance of devices. Assessing people for returning to commercial vehicle work requires specific adherence to local licensing laws and is outside the scope of this chapter.

Driving should be viewed as a privilege, not a right, and the primary responsibility of those who assess potential drivers is to the public, not to the applicant, although ultimately it is up to the licensing authority who should be allowed to drive [18]. That said, there are a number of ways of assisting a person with visual impairment back to driving. The use of devices may not be allowed in certain jurisdictions and therefore advice has to be sought to determine whether the device is suitable. In addition, most licensing authorities have some latitude to allow some people to drive if their vision falls below the minimum driving standard, as long as adaptation can be demonstrated and the applicant passes a driving assessment by a qualified examiner [18].

15.1.4 Decreased Visual Acuity

Neurological causes of decreased binocular visual acuity range from diseases of the anterior visual pathways, typically bilateral optic neuropathies including Leber's hereditary optic neuropathy, toxic optic neuropathies, and severe bilateral optic neuritis, through to the posterior visual pathways that involve both optic radiations or visual cortices such as such as bilateral occipital infarction.

15.1.4.1 Decreased Visual Acuity and Reading

Typically, low-vision aids are provided to help people with visual impairment to read. These vision aids are typically hand-held or stand magnifiers, which can be provided with or without illumination. There have been two Cochrane reviews of the provision of these aids to adults [25] and to children and young people [26]. Neither of these reviews was able to provide firm conclusions regarding the benefit of the interventions due to the lack of appropriate evidence that met their criteria for inclusion. However, studies have suggested benefit from these interventions. In a study of 168 new referrals to a low-vision clinic with various causes of poor vision, although mainly age-related macular degeneration (ARMD), only 23% could read N8 or better and 40% were unable to even read large print (N14). After provision of suitable reading aids, 88% could read N8 ($p < 0.0001$) [27]. In a further study of 530 patients with ARMD, magnification aids improved the percentage of patients able to read N8 from 13% to 94% in patients with an improvement in reading speed from a mean 16 words/min to 72 words/min ($p < 0.0001$) [28]. Training needs to be provided in how to use the aids because the different types have different optimum working distances [29]. Optical aids become harder to use as magnification increases, since stronger optical lenses consist of an increasingly smaller aperture whilst also requiring a closer working distance to focus. Different magnifiers may therefore be needed for different reading tasks. The weakest needed to achieve the required visual acuity is usually recommended.

A randomized trial has occurred of low-vision intervention, including correction of refractive error, education on the eye disease diagnosis and prognosis, low-vision therapy, and prescribed low-vision devices. The intervention included five weekly sessions of approximately two hours each and one home visit. Compared with controls, who did not receive any intervention, participants reported an improvement in visual reading ability (difference 2.43, 95% p < 0.001) on the 48-item low-vision visual functioning questionnaire [1].

Patients who have central scotomas can learn to use eccentric fixation in an intact area of the visual field at the margin of the scotoma. The retinal area used now for reading does not have sufficient visual acuity to read normal newsprint, necessitating the use of magnifiers. Eccentric fixation usually occurs spontaneously, but training programmes exist for patients who still fixate centrally, although their benefit is not yet clear [29].

For people with very severe visual impairment, Braille script enables reading and writing and has been widely adapted to different languages [30]. There has, however, been a decline in recent years, with only about 10% of severely visually impaired people using it [31]. The reasons for this decline, particularly in the young, are complex and may involve the decline in people able to teach it and also the lack of compatibility with modern technology, although recent moves have been made to try and incorporate Braille into assistive technology devices [31, 32].

Assistive technology now has an increasing role in enabling people with visual impairment to access information. This can range from adjusting font size and screen brightness through to speech recognition, auditory feedback, haptic (touch-based) feedback, or multimodal interaction to reduce the need for vision. Technological devices are particularly popular in young people with visual impairment as they are viewed as non-stigmatizing [32]. In a recent study, although young people with visual impairment spent less time each day on the Internet compared with a control group (mean 2.64 hours per day versus mean 3.54 hours per day, p < 0.01), they visited discussion forums (p < 0.001), sent e-mails (p < 0.001), and used the Internet for learning purposes (p < 0.001) more frequently than students without visual impairment [33].

15.1.4.2 Decreased Visual Acuity and General Participation

For partially sighted individuals, optical aids in the form of small telescopes can allow street signs and bus numbers to be made out to assist with navigation. Cut-off filters and improved environmental illumination can also help by increasing contrast [29].

A Cochrane review has been performed regarding orientation and mobility training for adults with low vision [13]. This found a paucity of appropriate studies, but there were two small quasi-randomized trials with similar methods, where the intervention group received training in orientation (including sound localization, concepts, landmarks, turns, tactual discrimination, and systematic search patterns) and mobility (including motor balance, seating, stairs, trailing, diagonal cane, elevator, squaring off, and straight line, self-protection positions). The control group received programmed fitness exercises. Both studies did not find any clear benefits from orientation and mobility training, although there was a trend for the training, leading to improvements in the ability to travel indoors independently.

The low-vision intervention trial discussed earlier with respect to reading also looked at other visual ability domains. As well as improving reading, the intervention led to improvements of 0.84 logit (p = 0.001) for mobility, 1.38 logits (p = 0.001) for visual information processing, 1.51 logits (p = 0.001) for visual motor skills, and 1.63 logits (p = 0.001) for overall visual function [1].

In order to rehabilitate a visually impaired person to get them back into employment, a multidisciplinary process is required to assess level of current vision, to prescribe and dispense devices to assist with near, intermediate, and far distance, and then to undergo training to improve reading and writing skills. Lastly, a workplace assessment is needed to optimize the immediate workspace, to make the work environment easier to navigate, and to work with the employer to come up with a workable routine and pattern of work [34]. Many countries, as part of their disability discrimination legislation, require employers to make 'reasonable accommodation' to enable their employees to return to work following injury or illness [35].

In a study of 17 visually impaired participants in their use of assistive devices in daily living, optical and electronic vision-enhancement devices (41 currently used devices), mainstream aids of daily living (n = 22), adaptive computer technology (n = 15), audio players, recorders, note takers (n = 14), mobility devices (n = 7), and lighting and filters (n = 5) were in current usage. All but one respondent used some type of optical device and/or electronic vision-enhancement [36].

To assist with hazard avoidance, long canes are widely used. Two main techniques are employed in their use: the constant contact approach where the cane is swept from side to side with the tip in contact with the ground, and the two-point touch approach where the ground is touched with the cane tip on the opposite side of the forefoot. This is a cheap approach and does not require a long period of training [37]; however, some feel that their use is stigmatizing [36].

Guide dogs can have a substantial impact to improve the independence and mobility of visually impaired people. In a survey of guide dog users compared with visually impaired people who were not using a guide dog, the guide dog users tended to be younger and have more significant visual impairment than non-guide dog users [38]. A guide dog requires training, with significant costs both in the training period and in their subsequent upkeep. They also require care and attention from the visually impaired person partnered with them.

Both canes and guide dogs do not guarantee safe locomotion as the sensing range and information bandwidth are both limited [37]. Cane use can be supplemented with echolocation, in which the subject makes sonar emissions, such as mouth clicks, finger snaps, feet shuffles, hums, or can taps, and listens to the returning echoes to gain information about objects and obstacle nearby. This has been reported to be employed by up to 30% of severely visually impaired people and can particularly assist with mobility in unfamiliar surroundings [39].

Electronic ultrasonic echolocation can be incorporated into long canes to detect oncoming hazards by providing auditory or haptic alerts. In addition, assistive technology can assist with navigation. For indoor use, a combination of Wi-Fi and geographic information systems can be used. For outdoor use, a global positioning system can be used, which can be supplemented by environmentally embedded radio frequency identification (RFID) tags. An RFID reader within the long cane can detect and interpret such tags in the pavement to guide the visually impaired person. Mobile assistive technology can also assist on public transportation, including the RAMPE system that can connect a Wi-Fi enabled handheld device with fixed base stations installed at bus stops and a central system that sends real-time information about public transport to the base stations. Mobile devices can assist with shopping by helping with navigation about stores, but also by the use of barcode scanners with audio outputs to provide verbal information about products and their prices. A major advantage of using mobile devices, such as smartphones, for these purposes is that new functions can be easily programmed and customized without the need for a new device [32].

It has been found that 32.4% of canes and 26.5% of magnifiers owned by 1,056 frail elderly visually impaired people were actually currently in use. Although the reasons for non-use of canes was not explored in this study, the principal reasons for dissatisfaction with magnifiers were: magnification not strong enough (44%); device is too small (14%); vision has deteriorated too much so no longer helpful (14%); does not help (10%); and print appears blurry or distorted (5%) [40].

It is therefore necessary to understand the factors that affect the retention and use of devices by people with impaired vision [36]. Involvement of the users early on in the design process is vital, since 'lack of consideration of user opinion' is one of the most important factors leading to failure of update of devices [32].

One ultimate goal is to use technology to directly electrically stimulate the retina, optic nerve, lateral geniculate nucleus, or primary visual cortex in severely visually impaired people; however, there are still significant clinical, surgical, psychophysical, physiological, neuro-psychological, engineering, and surgical hurdles to overcome before these implants become available in practice [41].

15.1.4.3 Decreased Visual Acuity and Driving

Decreased visual acuity restricts the ability to read road signs, detect hazards, view highway markings, and perceive objects entering the road [24].

Approximately 3.3 million (2.76%) Americans aged 40 years and older are visually impaired (having a visual acuity of 20/40 or less) and are therefore not permitted to drive [42]. For those with reduced visual acuity, 34 states within the United States allow driving with a restricted licence with the use of bioptic telescopes, although they are not permitted in the European Union [43]. These are small telescopes mounted in the top half of a spectacle lens. They allow for reading road signs at greater viewing distances to allow more time to react, although their use requires training and adaptation to shift back and forth between the normal lens and the telescope lens. Their use is controversial. In a survey of 58 people with visual impairment who used bioptic telescopes, 74% rated the telescope as very helpful, and 90% would continue to use it for driving, even if it were not a licensing requirement. However, only 62% reported always wearing the bioptic telescope when driving, suggesting they are not always used according to the manufacturers' instructions. There is also a period of inattention blindness as the driver switches between the carrier lens and the bioptic [24]. Licensing a bioptic driver using such a device should occur after an driving assessment by a qualified examiner [18].

At present, the interventions possible to allow a visually impaired person to drive a motor vehicle are limited as they require the intervention used to improve vision to pass local licensing requirements. In the future, the vision requirements may change as more research is performed into other factors such as contrast sensitivity, colour vision, night vision, and useful field of vision, which are all important factors in the vision required for driving [24]. Assistive technology will certainly have a role to play. Currently available are devices such as verbal global position systems for easier navigation, adaptive cruise control, lane alert warnings, and self-parking cars [24]. Autonomous vehicles open up the possibility for more visually impaired people to be able to 'drive' [44], although the licensing requirements will complicated as well as deciding on whether the 'driver' or vehicle manufacturer is liable in the event of an accident [45].

15.2 Hemianopia

Hemianopia occurs due to damage to the post-chiasmal visual pathways. It occurs principally after stroke. In a population-based survey hemianopic visual field defects were found to affect 0.8% of people over 49 years of age [46]. The visual field defect can have a major effect on quality of life by restricting reading, general orientation, and driving [47].

15.2.1 Hemianopia and Reading

For left-to-right readers, the presence of a right hemianopic defect, if it splits the macular area, causes considerable difficulty in reading both by interrupting the viewing of each group of letters and by disrupting the saccadic eye movements to the right. This leads to prolonged fixations, reduced saccadic amplitude, and an increase in regressive saccades (i.e., saccades back to relook at an area). Reading speed and comprehension are therefore reduced [48]. The reading speed increases with the amount of macular sparing that occurs [49]. A left hemianopia in left-to-right readers leads to problems in finding the next line of text but also in accurately identifying the start of a word [6, 48].

Eccentric fixation may improve reading in some people with a macular splitting hemianopia. This will lead to a slight reduction in visual acuity, but causes a shift of the visual field defect towards the hemianopic side. In addition, people can develop unstable asymmetrical fixational eye movements with saccades towards the hemianopic side [5].

Simple measures, such as the use of a ruler or finger, may help reading by making it easier to follow words and in guiding people with left hemianopias to the start of the next line of text. Although these approaches seem intuitive, they have not been subject to any proper trials of their effectiveness [5]. Alternatively, the text could be re-orientated into different plains. A small study of this in 13 people with hemianopia did not show any clear benefits; however, there was a suggestion that 90° clockwise rotation may be useful in those with a right macular-splitting hemianopia [50].

In order to try and improve saccadic eye movements whilst reading to the right in people with right hemianopia, scrolled text training has been trialled as a way of inducing small-field optokinetic nystagmus. In a crossover design, 11 people with right hemianopia practised reading moving text that scrolled from right to left daily for two four-week blocks (group one), while the other eight (with three drop-outs) had sham therapy for the first block and then crossed over to moving text for the second (group two). Group one showed significant improvements in static text reading speed over both therapy blocks from a mean of 95 words per minute (wpm) to 112 wpm (p < 0.001), whereas group two only showed a non-significant improvement with sham therapy from 82 wpm to 86 wpm but an improvement to 101 wpm after moving text therapy (p = 0.007 compared with after sham therapy). The moving text therapy was associated with a direction-specific effect on saccadic amplitude for rightward- but not leftward-reading saccades [51].

A Cochrane review found that scanning training, such as outlined earlier, for people with visual field defects was more effective than control or placebo at improving reading ability, based on three studies with a total of 129 participants (standardized mean difference [SMD] 0.79, 95% confidence interval [CI] 0.29 to 1.29) [52].

This form of therapy for right hemianopia is available as a free-to-access web-placed application, called Read-Right (www.readright.ucl.ac.uk). An evaluation found that reading speed increased by 45.9% (p = 0.003) after 20 hours of practice [53].

15.2.2 Hemianopia and Participation

In order to improve mobility in the presence of hemianopia, some of the measures outlined earlier can be very useful, especially canes for obstacle avoidance in the blind hemifield. In addition, optical devices, such as prisms, can provide field-of-view relocation or expansion by transmitting the image from the hemianopic side to the functional side of the retina. The most successful are peripheral oblique prisms placed above and below the primary line of sight on the spectacle lens on the side of the field loss, providing visual field expansion. The prism images fall away from central vision, thereby preventing central diplopia [54]. A crossover study was performed, in which 61 people with hemianopia wore either real (57Δ) oblique prisms or sham (≤ 5Δ) horizontal prisms for four weeks before crossing over to the other prism. The study outcome was the answer to the question: 'If the study were to end today, would you want to continue with these prism glasses (i.e. the prism glasses worn in that period)?' The answer to this question being 'yes' was significantly higher when wearing real than sham prisms (64% versus 36%, p = 0.001). There was a significant improvement in the overall mobility score for both real and sham prism glasses; however, there was no significant difference in the amount of improvement between participants wearing real or sham prism glasses [55]. An earlier study found that 47% of hemianopic people still wore their 40Δ peripheral prism glasses more than eight hours per day after 12 months, finding subjective benefit in obstacle avoidance, with particular benefits when shopping and moving in crowded and unfamiliar areas [56]. Training is needed in prism use. The wearers should be advised to look through the central portion of their glasses and scan with their eyes as normal, without looking through the prisms, since this will cause diplopia. After detecting an object of interest in the periphery, they should turn their head to fixate on it [57].

People with hemianopias make more exploratory saccades into their blind hemifield; however, these saccades are usually not systematic and not accurate, resulting in much longer search times, but also adversely affecting the ability to avoid obstacles in the blind hemifield [57]. This spontaneous adaptation strategy can be supported by training [29]. A randomized controlled trial of explorative saccade training (EST) versus blind hemifield stimulation of flickering lights (FT) was performed in 28 hemianopic subjects for a period of six weeks. This found that EST led to reduced response times of 47% in a natural search task compared with pre-training, whereas the response time was unchanged in the FT group. Also, the number of fixations towards the blind hemifield increased by 238% after EST, whereas again it was unchanged after FT. The EST group also reported greater improvements in the World Health Organization questionnaire on the quality of life and social relationships domain (p 0.038) than the FT group [58].

A Cochrane review concluded that scanning training is more effective than control or placebo at improving visual scanning, based on three studies with 129 participants (SMD 1.14, 95% CI 0.29 to 2.00) [52]. This form of therapy is also available as a free-to-access web-placed application, called Eye-Search (www.eyesearch.ucl.ac.uk/index.php). A group of 78 suitable hemianopic people took part. After therapy of 800 trials over 11 days in 78 hemianopic subjects, participants, when tested on search times into their impaired hemifield, improved by a mean of 24% [59].

There is, however, no clear evidence to suggest that any form of what is termed 'visual restitution training' does lead to reductions in the size of the hemianopic visual field defect [52].

Hemispatial neglect is a very disabling condition where there is reduced awareness of stimuli on one side of space, even though there may be no sensory loss. It more often occurs after right cerebral hemisphere strokes, than left with contra-lesional neglect occurring. The difficult aspect in the rehabilitation of people with this phenomenon is that the nature of the deficit is that they are often unaware it is present [60]. There have been studies of visual scanning training and prism adaptation training for neglect; however, a Cochrane review concluded that the effectiveness of these interventions remains unproven [61].

15.2.3 Hemianopia and Driving

Hemianopia visual field defects have a major impact on the ability to detect and respond to hazards on the side of the field loss. In addition, they can impair visuo-motor control, causing problems with steering and lane position. The underlying brain injury may also cause other perceptual, attentional, cognitive, and motor impairments that could impair driving ability [62]. Most licensing authorities have stringent rules pertaining to visual field requirements, although many authorities will allow exceptions for people with stable defects to which they have fully adapted with no signs of neglect. They are, in addition, required to undergo a driving assessment.

A study compared masked evaluator driving performance using oblique prism glasses against sham oblique prism glasses in 12 people with hemianopia. The proportion of satisfactory responses to unexpected hazards on the hemianopia side was higher using oblique prisms than the sham prisms (80% versus 30%, p = 0.001), and there was no evidence of adverse effects on other aspects of driving, such as lane position or steering stability [54]. Recently, two people with hemianopia who had spectacles fitted with oblique peripheral prisms had been able to fulfil the licensing requirements of Minnesota in the United States and had been allowed to drive. Their angle of continuous, horizontal, binocular visual field improved from 95° to 115° and 82° to 112°, respectively. Both had subsequently driven without accidents for one and five years, respectively [63]. The use of prism devices is therefore promising but requires further study and assessment by more licensing authorities.

15.3 Diplopia

Neurological causes of diplopia arise from diseases affecting the innervation of the extra-ocular muscles. The disease may occur intra-axially by affecting the cranial nerve nuclei and their connections, or by affecting the cranial nerves themselves [2]. The double vision may be worse for far vision or for near. In the latter case, this is often caused by convergence insufficiency, a common condition affecting 2.25–8.3% of the population in which the eyes tend to drift outwards into exophoria when reading or working up close [64].

15.3.1 Diplopia and Reading

The simplest way of correcting diplopia to allow reading is to occlude either eye. The most efficient way is to use occluding tape over one spectacle lens, as this will still allow peripheral vision through that eye. For non-spectacle wearers, *plano* spectacles can be used with tape over one lens or an occlusive contact lens.

The use of prisms can restore single binocular vision. Fresnel prisms can be stuck onto the spectacle lens, alternatively when the defect is stable, prisms may be ground into the lens itself. In one study 68% of participants with strabismus obtained benefit from the use of prisms. In those that had their diplopia corrected, reading function, measured using the Adult Strabismus-20 questionnaire, improved from 57 (standard deviation [SD] 27) before the use of a prism to 69 (SD 27) with in-prism correction (p = 0.02) [65].

Sometimes different prisms are only required for near or distance, necessitating separate pairs of spectacles [2]. In cases of incommitent strabismus, it may not be possible to use a single prism to fuse the two images across the full range of eye movements; in these cases, occlusion is often the best option.

A Cochrane review of therapies for convergence insufficiency concluded that use of hospital-based orthoptist-guided vergence/accommodative therapy was more effective than home-based pencil push-up exercises or home-based computer therapy in children and young adults. It also concluded that using base-in prism reading glasses was not useful in children, but may be useful in presbyopic patients [64].

15.3.2 Diplopia and Participation

As well as assisting reading, the use of prisms to correct diplopia has been reported to lead to improvement in general function, as measured using the Adult Strabismus-20 scale, from 66 (SD 25) to 80 (SD 18) (p = 0.003). Self-perception and interaction scores, however, were not affected by their use (p > 0.02) [65]. In a study of 210 people who underwent strabismus surgery to correct diplopia, 52.38% had successful surgery, 38.09% had partially successful surgery, and 9.52% failed to gain any benefit from surgery. There were no differences between these groups on changes in functional quality of life from baseline to six months post surgery (p = 0.42); however, there were differences in changes in psychosocial quality of life (p = 0.02) [66].

15.3.3 Diplopia and Driving

If double vision can be corrected with a prism, then this is usually sufficient to satisfy driving licensing authorities. If occlusion of one eye is required, then this is also usually sufficient, as long as the eye being used satisfies the visual acuity and visual field requirements of the licensing authority. A number of authorities require a period off driving to allow functional adaptation to being monocular. It would be thought that the loss of stereoscopic vision would be a major handicap to driving; however, in the general population, the incidence of stereo blindness is 2–4%, with 10–15% having significant difficulties with random dot stereograms [67]. It is possible to perceive depth using monocular vision by using other cues, including motion parallax, the perceived size of an object, the perception of overlapping contours to decide which object is closer, and the need to converge and accommodate to view near objects. In one study, 88% of people who had an enucleation for a malignant melanoma were able to adapt so that they could drive safely again [68].

15.4 Nystagmus

The prevalence of nystagmus has been estimated at 24 per 10,000 population [69]. It can start in early childhood (infantile nystagmus) as pure infantile nystagmus or can occur in association with albinism, fusion maldevelopment nystagmus syndrome, spasmus nutans syndrome, and nystagmus associated with ocular disease. Acquired nystagmus is usually secondary to peripheral vestibular disease or disease affecting areas of the brain controlling eye movements, gaze stability, or afferent visual pathways, such as multiple sclerosis or stroke [69, 70]. Nystagmus leads to reduced visual acuity due to retinal slip preventing adequate foveation. In addition, in acquired nystagmus, oscillopsia can occur [71]. When assessed with the VF-14 visual impairment questionnaire, the impact of nystagmus on visual function was found to be similar to the effects of ARMD [72].

15.4.1 Nystagmus and Reading

As well as reducing visual acuity, nystagmus can reduce reading speed and performance by disrupting the sequence of fixations and saccades outlined earlier [73]. People with nystagmus often adopt a range of strategies to enable reading, including suppression of any corrective movements of the underlying involuntary drift, modulation of involuntary slow-phase movements by manipulating quick-phase, and correction of involuntary slow phases using quick phases [74]. Even with these strategies, reading performance in nystagmus is far more susceptible to limitations imposed by using small font sizes compared with controls. The effective reading visual acuity can be 6 logMAR lines worse than single-letter near-visual acuity in some individuals with nystagmus. Therefore, appropriate adjustments to font size are often needed for a person with nystagmus. When there is a limit to the font size available, then more time may be needed. This can be communicated to educational establishments or workplaces [73].

15.4.2 Nystagmus and Participation

In a qualitative study of 21 people with congenital nystagmus, difficulties with distance (n = 9) and near vision (n = 11) were commonly reported, leading to restriction of movement in the fields of education (n = 10), leisure (n = 16), and occupation (n = 17), amongst other things [75].

A trial of memantine and gabapentin versus placebo in congenital nystagmus found no significant differences between the three groups in terms of the change in Visual Function 14 (p = 0.50) and Social Function Questionnaire (p = 0.95) scores, even though drug treatment with both drugs led to significant improvement in visual acuity (p 0.004). At the end of the trial, 81% opted to continue taking the drug they were allocated [76].

Four-muscle tenotomy surgery (Anderson-Kestenbaum procedure) acts to centralize the nystagmus null position and so correct head (face) turns. In a study of nine participants who underwent this procedure, all had reductions in nystagmus amplitudes (14.6–37%) with associated increases in the duration of the foveation (11.2–200%), although the effects on overall visual quality of life and participation were not recorded [77].

15.4.3 Nystagmus and Driving

People with nystagmus often have reduced visual acuity such that they cannot pass the visual acuity requirement for licensing. On entry to a trial of drug therapy for nystagmus, the mean visual acuity of the different groups of patients ranged from 0.24 to 0.65 logMAR [76]. The cut-off for being able to drive in most countries is 6/12 (equivalent to 0.3 logMAR). In a survey of people with nystagmus, 10 out of 21 had a visual acuity better than 6/12, yet only four were currently driving [75]. The reasons for those not driving, yet apparently having sufficient visual acuity, were not explored in that article, although the article was based on a survey within the United Kingdom, which requires licensees to be able to read a standard number plate at 20 m as well as being able to read 6/12. Drug treatment with both gabapentin and memantine has been shown to improve visual acuity in both congenital and acquired nystagmus [71, 76], although the data are not available in the studies to determine who improved above the 6/12 threshold. In a patient with nystagmus and best corrected visual acuity close to the 6/12 threshold, with no other contraindications to driving, it may be worth a trial of either drug to see if vision can be improved so that the licensing requirement can be reached.

15.5 Conclusions

This chapter has discussed a range of rehabilitation strategies that can be employed for the major neurological causes of visual impairment. However, these disorders may not occur in isolation and coexisting deficits may be present, particularly when multi-focal brain disease has occurred. This can be the case, for example, in multiple sclerosis [71], stroke [78], cerebral palsy [79], and traumatic brain injury [80]. In such cases, there may be additional deficits of higher cortical function. A comprehensive multidisciplinary approach is usually therefore needed to be able to define what deficits are present and to individualize the approach to rehabilitation [29].

References

1. Stelmack JA, Tang XC, Reda DJ, et al. Outcomes of the Veterans Affairs Low Vision Intervention Trial (LOVIT). *Arch. Ophthalmol.* 2008; **126**: 608–17.

2. Singman EL, Matta NS, Silbert DI. Nonsurgical treatment of neurologic diplopia. *Am. Orthopt. J.* 2013; **63**: 63–8.

3. Royal National Institute of Blind People. Registering your sight loss. 2016. www.rnib.org.uk/eye-health/registering-your-sight-loss. (Accessed 8 November 2016).

4. Resnikoff S, Pascolini D, Etya'ale D, et al. Global data on visual impairment in the year 2002. *Bull. World Health Organ.* 2004; **82**: 844–51.

5. Trauzettel-Klosinski S. Rehabilitation for visual disorders. *J. Neuroophthalmol.* 2010; **30**: 73–84.

6. Grunda T, Marsalek P, Sykorova P. Homonymous hemianopia and related visual defects: Restoration of vision after a stroke. *Acta. Neurobiol. Exp. (Wars.)* 2013; **73**: 237–49.

7. Lamoureux EL, Hassell JB, Keeffe JE. The determinants of participation in activities of daily living in people with impaired vision. *Am. J. Ophthalmol.* 2004; **137**: 265–70.

8. Clements B, Douglas G, Pavey S. Which factors affect the chances of paid employment for individuals with visual impairment in Britain? *Work* 2011; **39**: 21–30.

9. Kaldenberg J. Vision. *Work* 2011; **39**: 1.

10. Ivers RQ, Cumming RG, Mitchell P, Attebo K. Visual impairment and falls in older adults: The Blue Mountains Eye Study. *J. Am. Geriatr. Soc.* 1998; **46**: 58–64.

11. Tsur A, Segal Z. Falls in stroke patients: Risk factors and risk management. *Isr. Med. Assoc. J.* 2010; **12**: 216–19.

12. Baig S, Diniz-Filho A, Wu Z, et al. Association of fast visual field loss with risk of falling in patients with glaucoma. *JAMA Ophthalmol.* 2016; **134**: 880–7.

13. Virgili G, Rubin G. Orientation and mobility training for adults with low vision. *Cochrane Database Syst. Rev.* 2010; **5**: CD003925.

14. de Haan GA, Heutink J, Melis-Dankers BJM, et al. Difficulties in daily life reported by patients with homonymous visual field defects. *J Neuroophthalmol.* 2015; **35**: 259–64.

15. O'Connor PM, Lamoureux EL, Keeffe JE. Predicting the need for low vision rehabilitation services. *Br. J. Ophthalmol.* 2008; **92**: 252–5.

16. Ragland DR, Satariano WA, MacLeod KE. Driving cessation and increased depressive symptoms. *J. Gerontol. A Biol. Sci. Med. Sci.* 2005; **60**: 399–403.

17. Carr DB, Schwartzberg JG, Manning L, Sempek J. *Physician's guide to assessing and counseling older drivers* (2nd edn.) Washington, DC:, National Highway Traffic Safety Association, 2010.

18. Colenbrander A, De Laey JJ. *Vision requirements for driving safety with emphasis on individual assessment.* Sao Paulo, Brazil: Report prepared for the International Council of Ophthalmology at the 30th World Ophthalmology Congress, 2006.

19. Austroads and the National Transport Commission (NTC). *Assessing fitness to drive for commercial and private vehicle drivers* (5th edn.). Sydney, Australia, Austroads Ltd, 2016.

20. Canadian Council of Motor Transport Administrators. *Determining driver fitness in Canada* (13th edn.). Ottawa, Canada, Canadian Council of Motor Transport Administrators, 2013.

21. Yazdan-Ashoori P, ten Hove M. Vision and driving: Canada. *J. Neuroophthalmol.* 2010; **30**: 177–85.

22. European Commission. Commission Directive 2009/113/EC of 25 August 2009 amending Directive 2006/126/EC of the European Parliament and of the Council on Driving Licences. *Official Journal of the European Union* 2009; **223**: 31–5.

23. Driver and Vehicle Licensing Agency. *Assessing fitness to drive: A guide for medical professionals.* Swansea, UK: Driver and Vehicle Licensing Agency, 2016.

24. Johnson CA, Wilkinson ME. Vision and driving: The United States. *J. Neuroophthalmol.* 2010; **30**: 170–6.

25. Virgili G, Acosta R, Grover LL, et al. Reading aids for adults with low vision. *Cochrane Database Syst. Rev.* 2013; **10**: CD003303.

26. Barker L, Thomas R, Rubin G, Dahlmann-Noor A. Optical reading aids for children and young people with low vision. *Cochrane Database Syst. Rev.* 2015; **3**: CD010987.

27. Margrain TH. Helping blind and partially sighted people to read: The effectiveness of low vision aids. *Br. J. Ophthalmol.* 2000; **84**: 919–21.

28. Nguyen NX, Weismann M, Trauzettel-Klosinski S. Improvement of reading speed after providing of low vision aids in patients with age-related macular degeneration. *Acta Ophthalmol.* 2009; **87**: 849–53.

29. Trauzettel-Klosinski S. Current methods of visual rehabilitation. *Dtsch. Arztebl. Int.* 2011; **108**: 871–8.

30. Roth GA, Fee E. The invention of Braille. *Am. J. Public Health* 2011; **101**: 454.

31. Wiazowski J. Can Braille be revived? A possible impact of high-end Braille and mainstream technology on the revival of tactile literacy medium. *Assistive Technology* 2014; **26**:227–30.

32. Hakobyan L, Lumsden J, O'Sullivan D, Bartlett H. Mobile assistive technologies for the visually impaired. *Surv. Ophthalmol.* 2013; **58**: 513–28.

33. Wrzesińska M, Tabała K, Stecz P. The online behavior of pupils with visual impairment: A preliminary report. *Disabil. Health J.* 2016; **9**: 724–9.

34. Markowitz M, Markowitz RE, Markowitz SN. The multi-disciplinary nature of low vision rehabilitation: A case report. *Work* 2011; **39**: 63–6.

35. Robertson D. Individualized functional work evaluation and vision: A case study in reasonable accommodation. *Work* 2011; **39**: 31–5.

36. Fok D, Polgar JM, Shaw L, Jutai JW. Low vision assistive technology device usage and importance in daily occupations. *Work* 2011; **39**: 37–48.

37. Kim Y, Moncada-Torres A, Furrer J, et al. Quantification of long cane usage characteristics with the constant contact technique. *Appl. Ergon.* 2016; **55**: 216–25.

38. Refson K, Jackson AJ, Dusoir AE, Archer DB. Ophthalmic and visual profile of guide dog owners in Scotland. *Br. J. Ophthalmol.* 1999; **83**: 470–7.

39. Thaler L. Echolocation may have real-life advantages for blind people: An analysis of survey data. *Front. Physiol.* 2013; **4**: 98.

40. Mann WC, Goodall S, Justiss MD, Tomita M. Dissatisfaction and nonuse of assistive devices among frail elders. *Assist. Technol.* 2002; **14**: 130–9.

41. Lewis PM, Ackland HM, Lowery AJ, Rosenfeld JV. Restoration of vision in blind individuals using bionic devices: A review with a focus on cortical visual prostheses. *Brain Res.* 2015; **1595**: 51–73.

42. Congdon N, O'Colmain B, Klaver CCW, et al. Causes and prevalence of visual impairment among adults in the United States. *Arch. Ophthalmol.* 2004; **122**: 477–85.

43. Bowers AR, Apfelbaum DH, Peli E. Bioptic telescopes meet the needs of drivers with moderate visual acuity loss. *Invest. Ophthalmol. Vis. Sci.* 2005; **46**: 66–9.

44. Leng T. Can driverless cars help people with vision loss? 2012. http://wp.me/p2kVu3-5v. (Accessed 9 November 2016).

45. Neumann PG. Risks of automation. *Commun. ACM* 2016; **59**: 26–30.

46. Gilhotra JS, Mitchell P, Healey PR, et al. Homonymous visual field defects and stroke in an older population. *Stroke* 2002; **33**: 2417–20.

47. Warren M. Pilot study on activities of daily living limitations in adults with hemianopsia. *Am. J. Occup. Ther.* 2009; **63**: 626–33.

48. Zihl J. Eye movement patterns in hemianopic dyslexia. *Brain* 1995; **118**: 891–912.

49. Papageorgiou E, Hardiess G, Schaeffel F. Assessment of vision-related quality of life in patients with homonymous visual field defects. *Graefes Arch. Clin. Exp. Ophthalmol.* 2007; **245**: 1749–58.

50. de Jong D, Kaufmann-Ezra S, Meichtry JR, et al. The influence of reading direction on hemianopic reading disorders. *J. Clin. Exp. Neuropsychol.* 2016 **38**: 1077–83.

51. Spitzyna GA, Wise RJS, McDonald SA, et al. Optokinetic therapy improves text reading in patients with hemianopic alexia: A controlled trial. *Neurology* 2007; **68**: 1922–30.

52. Pollock A, Hazelton C, Henderson CA, et al. Interventions for visual field defects in patients with stroke. *Cochrane Database Syst. Rev.* 2011; **10**: CD008388.

53. Ong Y-H, Brown MM, Robinson P, et al. Read-Right: A 'web app' that improves reading speeds in patients with hemianopia. *J. Neurol.* 2012; **259**: 2611–15.

54. Bowers AR, Tant M, Peli E. A pilot evaluation of on-road detection performance by drivers with hemianopia using oblique peripheral prisms. *Stroke Res. Treat.* 2012; **2012**: 176806.

55. Bowers AR, Keeney K, Peli E. Randomized crossover clinical trial of real and sham peripheral prism glasses for hemianopia. *JAMA Ophthalmol.* 2014; **132**: 214–19.

56. Bowers AR, Keeney K, Peli E. Community-based trial of a peripheral prism visual field expansion device for hemianopia. *Arch. Ophthalmol.* 2008; **126**: 657–64.

57. Goodwin D. Homonymous hemianopia: Challenges and solutions. *Clin. Ophthalmol.* 2014; **8**: 1919–27.

58. Roth T, Sokolov AN, Messias A, et al. Comparing explorative saccade and flicker training in hemianopia: A randomized controlled study. *Neurology* 2009; **72**: 324–31.

59. Ong Y-H, Jacquin-Courtois S, Gorgoraptis N, et al. Eye-Search: A web-based therapy that improves visual search in hemianopia. *Ann. Clin. Transl. Neurol.* 2014; **2**: 74–8.

60. Parton A, Malhotra P, Husain M. Hemispatial neglect. *J. Neurol. Neurosurg. Psychiatr.* 2004; **75**: 13–21.

61. Bowen A, Hazelton C, Pollock A, Lincoln NB. Cognitive rehabilitation for spatial neglect following stroke. *Cochrane Database Syst. Rev.* 2013; **7**: CD003586.

62. Bowers AR. Driving with homonymous visual field loss: A review of the literature. *Clin. Exp. Optom.* 2016; **99**: 402–18.

63. Moss AM, Harrison AR, Lee MS. Patients with homonymous hemianopia become visually qualified to drive using novel monocular sector prisms. *J. Neuroophthalmol.* 2014; **34**: 53–6.

64. Scheiman M, Gwiazda J, Li T. Non-surgical interventions for convergence insufficiency. *Cochrane Database Syst. Rev.* 2011; **3**: CD006768.

65. Hatt SR, Leske DA, Liebermann L, Holmes JM. Successful treatment of diplopia with prism improves health-related quality of life. *Am. J. Ophthalmol.* 2014; **157**: 1209–13.

66. McBain HB, MacKenzie KA, Hancox J, et al. Continuing medical education: Does strabismus surgery improve quality and mood, and what factors influence this? *Eye (Lond.)* 2016; **30**: 656–67.

67. Westlake W. Is a one eyed racing driver safe to compete? Formula one (eye) or two? *Br. J. Ophthalmol.* 2001; **85**: 619–24.

68. Edwards MG, Schachat AP. Impact of enucleation for choroidal melanoma on the performance of vision-dependent activities. *Arch. Ophthalmol.* 1991; **109**: 519–21.

69. Sarvananthan N, Surendran M, Roberts EO, et al. The prevalence of nystagmus: The Leicestershire nystagmus survey. *Invest. Ophthalmol. Vis. Sci.* 2009; **50**: 5201–6.

70. Thurtell MJ, Leigh RJ. Therapy for nystagmus. *J. Neuroophthalmol.* 2010; **30**: 361–71.

71. Hickman SJ, Raoof N, McLean RJ, Gottlob I. Vision and multiple sclerosis. *Multiple Sclerosis and Related Disorders* 2014; **3**: 3–16.

72. Pilling RF, Thompson JR, Gottlob I. Social and visual function in nystagmus. *Br. J. Ophthalmol.* 2005; **89**: 1278–81.

73. Barot N, McLean RJ, Gottlob I, Proudlock FA. Reading performance in infantile nystagmus. *Ophthalmology* 2013; **120**: 1232–8.

74. Thomas MG, Gottlob I, McLean RJ, et al. Reading strategies in infantile nystagmus syndrome. *Invest. Ophthalmol. Vis. Sci.* 2011; **52**: 8156–65.

75. McLean RJ, Windridge KC, Gottlob I. Living with nystagmus: A qualitative study. *Br. J. Ophthalmol.* 2012; **96**: 981–6.

76. McLean R, Proudlock F, Thomas S, et al. Congenital nystagmus: Randomized, controlled, double-masked trial of memantine/gabapentin. *Ann. Neurol.* 2007; **61**: 130–8.

77. Wang Z, Dell'Osso LF, Jacobs JB, et al. Effects of tenotomy on patients with infantile nystagmus syndrome: Foveation improvement over a broadened visual field. *J. AAPOS* 2006; **10**: 552–60.

78. Rowe F, Wright D, Brand D, et al. Reading difficulty after stroke: Ocular and non ocular causes. *Int. J. Stroke* 2011; **6**: 404–11.

79. Fazzi E, Signorini SG, La Piana R, et al. Neuro-ophthalmological disorders in cerebral palsy: Ophthalmological, oculomotor, and visual aspects. *Dev. Med. Child Neurol.* 2012; **54**: 730–6.

80. Brahm KD, Wilgenburg HM, Kirby J, et al. Visual impairment and dysfunction in combat-injured service members with traumatic brain injury. *Optom. Vis. Sci.* 2009; **86**: 817–25.

16

Management of Pressure Ulcers in Neurological Rehabilitation

Ramaswamy Hariharan and Anand Viswanathan

16.1 Introduction

A pressure ulcer is a focal injury to the skin and underlying tissues caused by unrelieved pressure or shear, or both [1]. This usually occurs over bony prominences. Pressure ulcers are also known as pressure sores, bedsores, or decubitus ulcers, and most commonly affect people with reduced mobility following long-term neurological conditions. They occur due to and are one of the most frequent causes of unplanned hospitalization among people with spinal cord injury. They can present as persistently hyperaemic, blistered, broken, or necrotic skin that can extend to underlying structures including muscle and bone and sometimes even joint spaces. They can affect up to one-third of people in hospitals or community care and one-fifth of nursing home residents.

Pressure ulcers pose a huge burden not just on those living with them but also on their families, care providers, and the healthcare system as a whole. The prevention of pressure ulcers is therefore a high priority [2]. At a time when resources are constrained, it is imperative to calculate the cost of preventing and treating pressure ulcers to assess the impact it has on the healthcare system and society.

The prevalence of pressure ulcers of grade 2 and above ranges between 4.4% and 26% in European and North American settings [3]. These proportions could increase significantly if grade 1 pressure ulcers were included in these data.

16.1.1 Aetiology

Pressure ulcers generally arise because of sustained pressure on the soft tissue layers over bony prominences. Tissues can withstand large pressures for brief periods, but continuous pressures above the arterial capillary pressure can impair the flow of nutrients and oxygen to the tissues. Similarly, continuous pressure greater than the venous capillary closing pressure over

a long period of time can impede the return of blood flow and can lead to accumulation of toxic metabolites, lymphatic stasis, and tissue damage. This leads to reactive capillary dilatation, increased vascular permeability, oedema, blistering, and thrombosis. Tissue ischaemia ensues, leading to necrosis and ulceration. The tissues are capable of sustaining pressure on the arterial side of around 30–32 mm Hg for only a small duration of time. But when pressure increases even slightly above this capillary filling pressure, it causes microcirculatory occlusion and this in turn initiates a downward spiral towards ischaemia, tissue death, and ulceration [4, 5].

Tissue distortion also obstructs lymphatic flow, resulting in accumulation of metabolic waste products in the affected tissue, which further influences tissue damage [6].

The thickness of tissue cover and the characteristics of the blood vessels over bony prominences are key factors in pressure ulcer development. Vasculature in the soles of the feet are able to withstand significant pressures for long durations, in contrast to those on the sacrum and ischial tuberosity, areas not adept at weight-bearing and hence at higher risk of ulcer formation.

16.1.2 Causes

The causes for developing a pressure ulcer can be broadly divided into intrinsic and extrinsic. Intrinsic factors include loss of sensations, paralysis, age, vascular disease, and diabetes. Extrinsic factors are pressure, shear, friction, and maceration.

Pressure, when unrelieved, can cause tissue ischaemia. Necrosis and ulceration could occur if such unrelieved pressure persists for as briefly as two hours [7].

Shearing happens when patients are positioned at inappropriate inclines. This could cause distortion of vessels in tissues and thereby ischemia, though to a smaller extent than due to pressure [8]. Ischial tuberosities, heels, shoulder blades, and elbows are believed to be particularly susceptible.

Friction could lead to shear in deeper tissues, increasing the risk of ulceration. Direct skin breakdown due to friction is not categorized as pressure ulcer [9].

Maceration refers to the superficial skin changes following prolonged exposure to moisture, usually due to urinary or faecal incontinence. This reduces the threshold for skin breakdown due to pressure. Maceration also predisposes to skin infections and dermatitis [10].

16.2 Risk Factors

A risk factor is an identifiable intrinsic or extrinsic characteristic that increases a patient's susceptibility to forces that causes tissue damage. These include:

1. Age-related physiological alterations like increase in the fragility of blood vessels and connective tissue, loss of subcutaneous fat, and thinning of muscles can lead to a reduced capacity to dissipate pressure, lowering the threshold for pressure-induced injury in elderly patients.
2. Co-morbid conditions that are associated with prolonged, impaired wound healing such as diabetes mellitus.
3. Other medical conditions like heart failure, atrial fibrillation, myocardial infarction, and chronic obstructive pulmonary disease that are associated with a low tissue–oxygen tension [11].
4. Peripheral vascular disease
5. Contractures and spasticity can contribute by repeatedly exposing tissues to pressure through abnormal positions.
6. Immobility and sensory loss renders the skin more susceptible to the pressure, shear, and friction.
7. Malnutrition, hypoproteinaemia, and anaemia can cause significant delays in wound healing and hasten the formation of pressure ulcers [12].
8. Mental health conditions such as severe schizophrenia or depression could increase risk of pressure ulcers, by affecting diet and the ability to self-care adequately.

16.3 Prevention

Clinical guidelines recommend many strategies for prevention of pressure ulcers. They include patient and family/caregiver education, use of appropriate support surfaces, frequent skin inspection, and repositioning to relieve pressure. A high level of knowledge about skin care is necessary to successfully prevent pressure ulcers, which makes indispensable educating all healthcare personnel, patients, and their carers about the principles of pressure ulcer prevention. The efficacy of preventive interventions should be carefully assessed, avoiding those that have measured outcomes that are merely proxies for ulceration such as interface pressure and skin blood flow. Timely and tailored information should be offered to people who have been assessed as being at high risk of developing a pressure ulcer, and their family or carers [2]. The information should be delivered by a trained or experienced healthcare professional and include the causes of a pressure ulcer, the early signs of a pressure ulcer, ways to prevent a pressure ulcer, and the implications of having a pressure ulcer (for example, for general health and treatment options and the risk of developing pressure ulcers in the future). The team should also demonstrate techniques and equipment used.

16.4 Classification of Pressure Ulcers

Pressure ulcers are classified based on their severity, and help to plan management options and also assess response to treatment. The European Pressure Ulcer Advisory Panel (EPUAP) and the American National Pressure Ulcer Advisory Panel (NPUAP) have developed a Quick Reference Guide, an evidence-based guidance on pressure ulcer prevention and treatment [1].

16.4.1 International EPUAP–NPUAP Classification

Pressure ulcers are graded as one of the four categories, depending on the depth of the tissue involved. Commonly, deep tissue injuries as well as unclassified/unstageable ulcers are graded as 'IV'. If osteomyelitis is suspected, it needs to be confirmed by X-rays or histopathological examination of the bone, and does not alter the classification.

16.4.1.1 Category/Stage I

In Category/Stage I, non-blanchable erythema appears in intact skin of a localized area, usually over a bony prominence. Discoloration of the skin, warmth, oedema, hardness, or pain may also be present. Darkly pigmented skin may not have visible blanching; its colour may differ from the surrounding area. The area may be painful, firm or soft, and warmer or cooler as compared with adjacent tissue. Category I may be difficult to detect in individuals with dark skin tones and may indicate 'at-risk' persons.

16.4.1.2 Category/Stage II

In Category/Stage II, partial thickness loss of dermis presents as a shallow open ulcer with a reddish pink wound bed, without slough. A Stage II ulcer may also present as an intact or open/ruptured serum-filled or serosanguinous fluid-filled blister. It can present as a shiny or dry shallow ulcer without slough or bruising (deep tissue injury). This category should not be used to describe skin tears, tape burns, incontinence-associated dermatitis, maceration, or excoriation.

16.4.1.3 Category/Stage III

Full thickness tissue loss occurs in Category/Stage III. Subcutaneous fat may be visible, but bone, tendon, or muscles are not exposed. Slough may be present but does not obscure the depth of the tissue loss. The ulcer may include undermining and tunnelling. The depth of a Category/Stage III ulcer varies by anatomical location. The bridge of the nose, ear, occiput, and malleoli do not have (adipose) subcutaneous tissue and can have shallow Category/Stage III ulcers. In contrast, areas of significant adiposity can develop extremely deep Category/Stage III ulcers. Bone/tendon is not visible or directly palpable.

16.4.1.4 Category/Stage IV

Full thickness tissue loss with exposed bone, tendon, or muscle can appear in Category/Stage IV. Slough or eschar may be present. Ulcers can often demonstrate undermining and tunnelling. The depth of a Category/Stage IV pressure ulcer varies by anatomical location. The bridge of the nose, ear, occiput, and malleoli do not have (adipose) subcutaneous tissue and ulcers in these locations can be shallow. Category/Stage IV ulcers can extend into muscle and/or supporting structures (e.g., fascia, tendon, or joint capsule), increasing the likelihood of osteomyelitis or osteitis. Exposed bone/muscle is visible or directly palpable.

16.5 Risk Assessments

Determining the 'risk' of a person developing a pressure ulcer is an essential element of pressure ulcer prevention. Assessment of a pressure ulcer is necessary not only to plan treatment options but also to assess response to the treatment. Numerous pressure ulcer risk calculators have been developed since the 1960s. Common among them are the Norton Pressure Ulcer Risk Assessment Score (Table 16.1), Waterlow Scale (Table 16.2), and Braden tools [13–15]. There is a lack of conclusive evidence on whether such assessments lead to reduced incidence of pressure ulcers [16]. Also, there is only inconclusive evidence to suggest one tool is better than any other. A structured risk assessment as per the consensus of the treating team is therefore recommended [1]. This needs to be always supplemented by a clinical assessment, preferably by a person knowledgeable in pressure ulcer evaluation and management.

The Norton Scale was one of the first pressure ulcer risk scoring systems. This assessment is based on physical and mental conditions, incontinence, activity, and mobility, each of which is scored 1–4 in the descending order of risk. The Braden Scale is based on a concept that the critical determinants for development of pressure ulcers are the intensity and duration of pressure on the one hand, and the tolerance of the skin and supporting structures for pressure on the other. The scale is composed of six subscales: mobility, activity, sensory perception, moisture, nutritional status, and friction and shear. The maximum total score is 23, with a lower score predicting a higher risk. The Waterlow Scale consists of seven items: build/weight, height, visual assessment of the skin, sex/age, continence, mobility, and appetite, and special risk factors, divided into tissue malnutrition, neurological deficit, major surgery/trauma, and medication. The tool identifies three 'at risk' categories, with a higher score indicating a higher risk.

16.6 Ulcer Healing

Regular clinical assessment is recommended to look for signs of ulcer healing such as the amount of exudate, size of the ulcer, and the ulcer bed. Serial photographs help with documentation of progress. The Pressure Ulcer Scale for Healing (PUSH) tool is used to measure the status of pressure ulcer healing

Table 16.1 The Norton Pressure Ulcer Risk Assessment Score

Physical condition		Mental Condition		Incontinence	
Good	4	Alert	4	Not	4
Fair	3	Apathetic	3	Occasional	3
Poor	2	Confused	2	Usually urine	2
Very bad	1	Stuporous	1	Doubly incontinent	1
Activity		**Mobility**			
Ambulant	4	Full	4		
Walks with help	3	Limited	3		
Chair-bound	2	Very limited	2		
In bed	1	Immobile	1		

over time [17]. It recommends that the tool be used on a regular basis, at least weekly or whenever the patient or wound status changes. The PUSH tool measures three parameters that are considered most indicative of healing: wound size, exudate amount, and tissue type. Instructions for its use are given in Appendix 16.1.

16.7 Complications of Pressure Ulcers

Pressure ulcers could lead to increase in therapy time and prolong the hospital stay. Infection from pressure ulcers can result in septicaemia and death [18, 19]. Ulcers extending to the bone could cause periostitis, osteomyelitis, and heterotopic bone formation. They can also necessitate amputation. In persons with mid thoracic and higher spinal cord injury, pressure ulcers distally may result in autonomic dysreflexia. Drainage from pressure ulcers could lead to ongoing loss of protein.

16.8 Management

16.8.1 Conservative

Conservative treatment methods share three common objectives: pressure relief, wound debridement, and infection control.

16.8.1.1 Pressure Relief

Pressure is the primary cause for pressure ulcers; complete relief of pressure is therefore essential for healing. When there are multiple pressure points, which is not uncommon in people with long-term neurological conditions, complete relief of pressure at regular intervals must be provided to all affected areas. This can be accomplished physically by frequent turning of the patient, or mechanically by means of a surface that provides alternating pressure support. The frequency and interval between turning are very critical. Previously, use of special support surfaces and turning all vulnerable patients every two hours was recommended [20]. European best practice guidelines suggest individualizing the need for and the frequency of repositioning [1, 21]. Wheelchair users with ischial pressure ulcers are traditionally advised bed rest until wound healing [22].

16.8.1.2 Support Surfaces

Pressure-relieving equipment plays a key role in the prevention and treatment of pressure ulcers. Special beds, mattresses, overlays, seat cushions, foam pads, or pillows that support the body in a bed or chair have been used to reduce interface pressure between the skin and the support surface.

High-specification foam mattresses and medical-grade sheepskin overlays are likely to be better than standard hospital mattresses in helping with pressure ulcer healing [23]. Other low-technology surfaces that are used in ulcer treatment include mattresses filled with air, beads, fibre, gel, or water.

Alternating-pressure air mattresses, air-fluidized beds, and low-air-loss beds are high-technology, constant low-pressure devices that afford maximal pressure redistribution [24]. Air-fluidized beds consist of

Table 16.2 The Waterlow Scale

Build/Weight for height		Appetite	
Average	0	Average	0
Above average	1	Poor	1
Obese	2	NG tube/fluids only	2
Below	3	NBM/anorexic	3
Continence		**Tissue malnutrition**	
Completely catheterized	0	Terminal cachexia	8
Occasionally incontinent	1	Cardiac failure	5
Catheterized/incontinent of faeces	2	Peripheral vascular disease	5
Double incontinent	3	Anaemia	2
		Smoking	1
Skin type: Visual risk area		**Neurological deficit**	
Healthy	0	Diabetes, MS, CVA	4–6
Tissue paper	1	motor/sensory	
Dry	1	Paraplegia	
Oedematous	1		
Clammy (temp increase)	1		
Discoloured	2		
Broken/spot	3		
Mobility		**Major surgery/trauma**	
Fully	0	Orthopaedic – below waist, spinal	5
Restless/fidgety	1	On table for more than two hours	5
Apathetic	2		
Restricted	3		
Inert/traction	4		
Chair-bound	5		
Sex/Age		**Medication**	
Male	1	Cytotoxics	4
Female	2	High doses of steroids	
14–49	1	anti-inflammatory	
50–64	2		
65–74	3		
75–80	4		
81+	5		

a container sheet filled with tiny ceramic beads resembling fine sand through which air is continuously forced by a blower, causing the beads to assume a fluid-like character. Interface pressures when positioned on these are among the lowest. Low-air-loss beds consists of a series of 18 to 20 air-filled sacks, each of which can be individually pressurized so that weight can be shifted from one body part to another.

16.8.1.3 Wound Debridement

With tissue necrosis being the inevitable outcome of ischaemia caused due to pressure, cleaning of the ulcer by removal of the dead tissue is important. The purpose of wound debridement is to remove necrotic tissue/eschar that promotes infection, delays granulation, and impedes healing. Accurate ulcer staging cannot be made until necrotic tissue is removed. Removing the slough from the pressure ulcer using sharp instruments is the traditional method of debridement. This could be done as a bedside procedure or under controlled conditions in an operating theatre.

In mechanical debridement, the necrotic tissue is loosened and removed by forceful irrigation, whirlpool treatments, or use of special dressing materials.

16.8.1.4 Wound Dressings

Pressure ulcer dressings are done to maintain a moist wound environment that is ideal for healing, to prevent leakage of exudate, and to minimize wound infection. Traditionally dressings were done using saline-soaked gauze. A variety of materials are now available for dressing pressure ulcers, including hydrogel, hydrocolloid, alginate, permeable films, and foam. Though best practice guidelines recommend that gauze should not be used as a primary dressing material [1], there is insufficient evidence to suggest any other dressing is better than saline-moistened gauze [3].

16.8.1.5 Wound Healing

Topical pharmacological agents and a few physical modalities have been explored for a role in expediting wound healing. Negative pressure wound therapy is helpful for deeper wounds after adequate debridement [1, 25]. Direct contact capacitive electrical stimulation, pulsed electromagnetic field treatment, and pulsed radiofrequency energy application could also be considered in recalcitrant ulcers. Other modalities such as topical phenytoin, glyceryl trinitrate, therapeutic ultrasound, and LASER are also used as per the preferences of treating teams.

16.8.1.6 Infection Control

Topical antiseptics that are tissue appropriate and non-cytotoxic could be used for a limited period along with debridement to control surface bacterial load. Commonly used antiseptics include iodine compounds, silver compounds, chlorhexidine, medical-grade honey, and acetic acid. Caution should be exercised with hydrogen peroxide and sodium hypochlorite, which are toxic to tissues and should be avoided in cavity wounds [26, 27].

Topical antibiotics are not recommended for routine use in pressure ulcers. An open wound that is draining well does not usually warrant treatment with systemic antibiotics. If there are definitive signs of local or systemic sepsis, oral or parenteral antibiotics should be considered. In such instances, debridement should also be performed as necessary to ensure adequate unhindered drainage from the wound.

16.8.1.7 Surgical Intervention

When conservative measures have failed or are unlikely to ensure adequate healing of pressure ulcers, surgical interventions are resorted to [28]. Surgery is usually performed as a single- or multi-stage intervention for closure of Stage III and IV pressure ulcers once other factors such as general condition, functional status, and nutrition have been addressed. Principles underpinning surgical interventions are (1) removal of infected nonviable tissue, including bursa and osteomyelitic bone, to facilitate growth of healthy granulation tissue; and (2) covering the ulcer defect with adequate tissue and skin cover to prevent recurrence. Ulcer closure is achieved by skin grafts for superficial ulcers, direct tissue approximation, and flaps. Multipronged post-operative care is essential to ensure adequate healing and prevention of recurrence. These include bed rest with pressure relief for three to four weeks, appropriate antibiotics for a limited duration, graded resumption of mobilization to facilitate scar maturation, assessment and provision of appropriate seating surfaces, continued pressure-relieving manoeuvres at regular intervals, lifestyle modifications as necessary, and patient education about all these aspects.

References

1. *National Pressure Ulcer Advisory Panel, European Pressure Ulcer Advisory Panel, Pan Pacific Pressure Injury Alliance: Prevention and treatment of pressure ulcers: Quick reference guide.* Perth, Australia, Cambridge Media, 2014.

2. National Institute for Health and Care Excellence. *Pressure ulcers: Prevention and management. NICE guideline (CG179).* 2014.

3. Westby MJ, Dumville JC, Soares MO, Stubbs N, Norman G. Dressings and topical agents for treating

pressure ulcers. *Cochrane Database Syst. Rev.* 2017. doi:10.1002/14651858.CD011947.pub2

4. Gefen A. Reswick and Rogers pressure-time curve for pressure ulcer risk. Part 1. *Nurs. Stand. R. Coll. Nurs. G. B.* 2009; **23**: 64, 66, 68 passim.

5. Gefen A. Reswick and Rogers pressure-time curve for pressure ulcer risk. Part 2. *Nurs. Stand. R. Coll. Nurs. G. B.* 2009; **23**: 40–4.

6. Bhattacharya S, Mishra RK.Pressure ulcers: Current understanding and newer modalities of treatment. *Indian J. Plast. Surg. Off. Publ. Assoc. Plast. Surg. India* 2015; **48**: 4–16.

7. Kuffler DP Techniques for wound healing with a focus on pressure ulcers elimination. *Open Circ. Vasc. J.* 2010; **3**: 72–84.

8. Hoogendoorn I, Reenalda J, Koopman BFJM, Rietman JS. The effect of pressure and shear on tissue viability of human skin in relation to the development of pressure ulcers: A systematic review. *J. Tissue Viability* 2017; **26**: 157–71.

9. Brienza D, Antokal S, Herbe L, Logan S, Maguire J, Van Ranst J, et al. Friction-induced skin injuries – are they pressure ulcers? An updated NPUAP white paper. *J. Wound Ostomy Cont. Nurs. Off. Publ. Wound Ostomy Cont. Nurses Soc.* 2015; **42**: 62–4.

10. Beeckman D. A decade of research on incontinence-associated dermatitis (IAD): Evidence, knowledge gaps and next steps. *J. Tissue Viability* 2017; **26**: 47–56.

11. Li C, DiPiro ND, Cao Y, Szlachcic Y, Krause J. The association between metabolic syndrome and pressure ulcers among individuals living with spinal cord injury. *Spinal Cord* 2016; **54**: 967–72.

12. Langemo D, Anderson J, Hanson D, Hunter S, Thompson P, Posthauer ME. Nutritional considerations in wound care. *Adv. Skin Wound Care* 2006; **19**: 297–8, 300, 303.

13. Norton D, Exton-Smith AN, McLaren R. *An investigation of geriatric nursing problems in hospital.* Edinburgh; New York, NY: Churchill Livingstone, 1975 [cited August 28, 2017]. Available from http://trove.nla.gov.au/version/26132113.

14. Waterlow J. Pressure sores: A risk assessment card. *Nurs. Times* 1985; **81**: 49–55.

15. Bergstrom N, Braden BJ, Laguzza A, Holman V. The Braden Scale for predicting pressure sore risk. *Nurs. Res.* 1987; **36**: 205–10.

16. Moore ZE, Cowman S. Risk assessment tools for the prevention of pressure ulcers. *Cochrane Database Syst.*

Rev. 2014; **5**(2): CD006471. doi:10.1002/14651858. CD006471.pub3

17. Thomas DR, Rodeheaver GT, Bartolucci AA, Franz RA, Sussman C, Ferrell BA, et al. Pressure ulcer scale for healing: Derivation and validation of the PUSH tool. The PUSH Task Force. *Adv. Wound Care J. Prev. Heal.* 1997; **10**: 96–101.

18. Guttmann SL. *Spinal cord injuries: Comprehensive management and research* (2nd edn.). Oxford, UK: Blackwell Science Ltd., 1976.

19. Redelings MD, Lee NE, Sorvillo F Pressure ulcers: More lethal than we thought? *Adv. Skin Wound Care* 2005; **18**: 367–72.

20. Reswick JB, Rogers JE. Experience at Rancho Los Amigos Hospital with devices and techniques to prevent pressure Sores. In Kenedi RM, Cowden JM eds. *Bed sore biomechanics.* London, UK: MacMillan Education, 1976; 301–10.

21. Moore ZE, Cowman S Repositioning for treating pressure ulcers. *Cochrane Database Syst. Rev.* 2015. doi:10.1002/14651858.CD006898.pub4

22. Moore ZE, Van Etten MT, Dumville JC. Bed rest for pressure ulcer healing in wheelchair users. *Cochrane Database Syst. Rev.* 2016. doi:10.1002/14651858. CD011999.pub2

23. McInnes E, Jammali-Blasi A, Bell-Syer SE, Dumville JC, Middleton V, Cullum N. Support surfaces for pressure ulcer prevention. *Cochrane Database Syst. Rev.* 2015. doi:10.1002/14651858. CD001735.pub5

24. Vanderwee K, Grypdonck M, Defloor T. Alternating pressure air mattresses as prevention for pressure ulcers: A literature review. *Int. J. Nurs. Stud.* 2008; **45**: 784–801.

25. Dumville JC, Webster J, Evans D, Land L. Negative pressure wound therapy for treating pressure ulcers. *Cochrane Database Syst. Rev.* 2015. doi:10.1002/ 14651858.CD011334.pub2

26. Norman G, Dumville JC, Moore ZE, Tanner J, Christie J, Goto S. Antibiotics and antiseptics for pressure ulcers. *Cochrane Database Syst. Rev.* 2016. doi:10.1002/14651858.CD011586.pub2

27. Jull AB, Cullum N, Dumville JC, Westby MJ, Deshpande S, Walker N. Honey as a topical treatment for wounds. *Cochrane Database Syst. Rev.* 2015. doi:10.1002/14651858.CD005083.pub4

28. Wong JK, Amin K, Dumville JC. Reconstructive surgery for treating pressure ulcers. *Cochrane Database Syst. Rev.* 2016. doi:10.1002/14651858. CD012032.pub2

Appendix 16.1

Instructions for Using the PUSH Tool

To use the PUSH Tool, the pressure ulcer is assessed and scored on the three elements in the tool:

Length x Width —> scored from 0 to 10

Exudate Amount —> scored from 0 (none) to 3 (heavy)

Tissue Type —> scored from 0 (closed) to 4 (necrotic tissue)

Step 1: Using the definition for length x width, a centimetre ruler measurement is made of the greatest head-to-toe diameter. A second measurement is made of the greatest width (left to right). Multiply these two measurements to get square centimetres and then select the corresponding category for size on the scale and record the score.

Step 2: Estimate the amount of exudate after removal of the dressing and before applying any topical agents. Select the corresponding category for that amount and record the score.

Step 3: Identify the type of tissue. Note: If there is ANY necrotic tissue, it is scored a 4. Or, if there is ANY slough, it is scored a 3, even though most of the wound is covered with granulation tissue.

Step 4: Sum the scores on the three elements of the tool to derive a total PUSH Score.

Step 5: Transfer the total score to the Pressure Ulcer Healing Graph. Changes in the score over time provide an indication of the changing status of the ulcer. If the score goes down, the wound is healing. If it gets larger, the wound is deteriorating.

Management of Disorders of Blood Pressure Control in Neurorehabilitation

Ellen Merete Hagen

17.1 Introduction

Management of blood pressure is important to secure circulation to the brain, the spinal cord, and other vital organs in neurorehabilitation. Cardiovascular autonomic dysfunction is common in many neurological disorders and may be the most disabling part of the disorder.

Blood pressure is mainly controlled by autonomically mediated circulatory reflexes that secure the needs of the individual tissues, especially the brain and the spinal cord (Figures 17.1, 17.2).

The afferent pathway transfers information from arterial baroreceptors in the carotid artery and the aortic arch. This information reaches the vasomotor centre in the medulla oblongata. The efferent pathway regulates two basic cardiovascular responses: heart rate and vascular tone. The hypothalamus can then activate vasopressin release as additional regulatory mechanisms. Higher brain functions can modulate autonomic cardiovascular responses [1].

17.1.1 Baroreflex

The baroreflex or baroreceptor reflex is a homeostatic mechanism that enables us to maintain blood pressure at nearly constant levels when changing from supine or seated to standing (Figure 17.2). It provides a rapid feedback loop between blood pressure and heart rate; increased blood pressure activates the baroreceptor reflex, causing reduced heart rate and reduced blood pressure through negative feedback, and vice versa. The baroreflex responds to changes in fractions of a second and is vital for preventing postural hypotension and syncope. Dysfunction may lead to cardiac dysrhythmias and abnormal blood pressure responses to normal activities of daily living [2].

Many disorders can cause impaired autonomic function. The most severe cases are primary neurodegenerative diseases affecting the autonomic nervous system, resulting in pathologic lesions at different levels of the baroreflex pathways [3].

17.2 Clinical Challenges

Disorder of the autonomic nervous system can occur either alone or as the result of another disease: multiple system atrophy (MSA), Parkinson's disease, or diabetes. It can be generalized, or localized such as in spinal cord injury (SCI) and multiple sclerosis (MS) [4]. Many commonly used drugs affect the autonomic nervous system. Diminished function of the autonomic nervous system often leads to hypotension and bradycardia, while increased function leads to hypertension and tachycardia. Intermittent autonomic dysfunction is common in many neurological conditions and after prolonged bedrest, while chronic failure of the autonomic nervous system is less frequent. Identification and treatment of both intermittent and chronic conditions will facilitate neurorehabilitation.

Intermittent dysfunction is commonly seen in patients with:

- Orthostatic hypotension/intolerance
- Syncope
- Postural tachycardia syndrome (PoTS).

Chronic failure is seen in patients with:

- Pure autonomic failure
- Multiple system atrophy
- Parkinson's disease with orthostatic hypotension
- Traumatic brain injury
- Spinal cord injury
- Familial dysautonomia

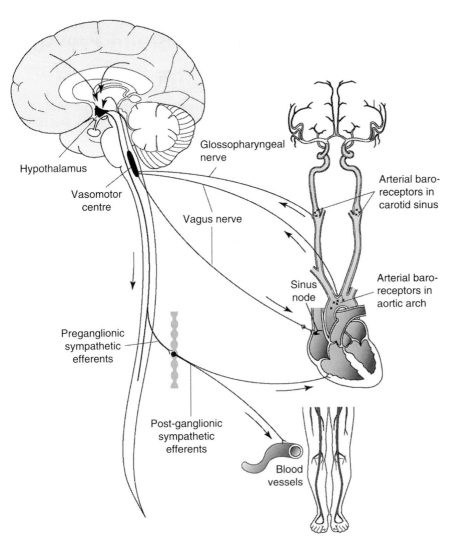

Figure 17.1 Baroreceptor reflex. *Printed with permission Ricci F, De CR, Fedorowski A. J Am Coll Cardiol 2015* [1]]

17.2.1 Hypotension

17.2.1.1 Orthostatic (Postural) Hypotension (OH)

Autonomic Response to Orthostatic Change

Orthostatic hypotension (OH) is a fall in blood pressure upon standing, compromising the perfusion to the brain. This is normally prevented by compensatory mechanisms involving the baroreceptor reflex [5]. When we change position, the baroreceptor-mediated reflex response keeps the blood pressure stable with a slow heart rate rise. The systolic blood pressure (SBP) may decrease 5–10 mmHg, the diastolic blood pressure (DBP) increases 5–10 mmHg, and the heart rate (HR) increases 10–20 bpm, due to initial

venous pooling, followed by plasma loss to the interstitial fluid [6].

OH is an independent predictor of mortality and a cause of significant morbidity associated with falls. OH is a common problem in frail older people. It is age dependent, ranging from 5% in patients < 50 years to 30% in patients > 70 years [1]. Common causes are drugs (e.g., α-adrenergic blocker tamsulosin used for benign prostate hypertrophy), diseases causing neuropathy (e.g., diabetes mellitus), and Parkinson's disease.

17.2.1.2 Definition of OH

Orthostatic hypotension is by definition a sustained reduction of SBP of ≥ 20 mmHg or DBP ≥ 10 mmHg

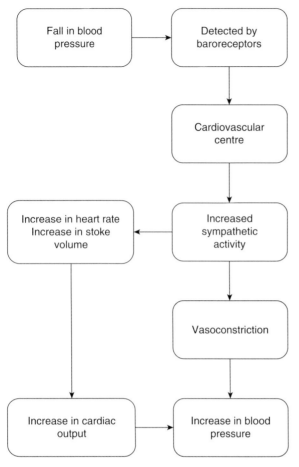

Figure 17.2 Blood pressure regulation

within three minutes of standing or head-up tilt to at least 60° on a tilt table (Figure 17.3) [7, 8].

Orthostatic hypotension can further be divided according to time of blood pressure fall [7, 8]:

1. **Initial:** Transient blood pressure fall (within 15 seconds): SBP ≥ 40 mmHg and/or DPS ≥ 20 mmHg
2. **Common:** Blood pressure reduction within three minutes of standing: SBP ≥ 20 mmHg and/or DBP ≥ 10 mmHg
3. **Delayed:** Blood pressure reduction after three minutes of standing: SBP ≥ 20 mmHg and/or DBP ≥ 10 mmHg

17.2.1.3   Typical Symptoms of OH

- Cerebral hypoperfusion causing dizziness/light-headedness, pre-syncope, syncope, visual disturbance, impaired cognition

- Muscle hypoperfusion causing aches across the neck and shoulders that are relieved by lying down ('coat hanger pain')
- Hypoperfusion of organs: cardiac leading to angina, renal leading to oliguria
- Non-specific symptoms: weakness, fatigue, lethargy, nausea, headache, dyspnoea, and falls [9, 10].

17.2.1.4   Triggers of OH

Common physical triggers are sitting up, standing up, standing still, bending down/forward, or raising arms above the head, dehydration, eating, warm ambient temperature, including showers or baths, and infections. Common psychological triggers are pain, fear, and anxiety.

17.2.1.5   Twenty-Four-Hour Ambulatory Blood Pressure Measurements

Ambulatory blood pressure monitoring (ABPM) measures blood pressure at regular intervals. A 24-hour ABPM allows the detection of OH, and assesses cardiovascular autonomic dysfunction in relation to various daily stimuli, such as food, alcohol, exercise, and drugs [12]. Information about the circadian rhythm of blood pressure and heart rate can be obtained and establish whether or not a patient has a fall of blood pressure at night (i.e., 'dipper' versus non-'dipper'). The information about nocturnal blood pressure may also allow the investigation or detection of disorders such as sleep dysfunction, nocturnal movement disorders, and obstructive sleep apnoea. Additionally, a 24-hour ABPM should be conducted to examine the effectiveness of OH therapy [12].

17.2.1.6   Treatment of OH

Treatment is dependent on the severity of OH (Figure 17.4). Non-pharmacological measures should always be part of treatment. Non-pharmacological measures include measures to avoid, measures to introduce, and measures to use [13]. This includes prevention strategies like physical counter manoeuvres [14]. Non-pharmacological strategies should always be implemented and continued together with pharmacological strategies when needed. The use of pharmacological treatment is dependent on the clinical findings.

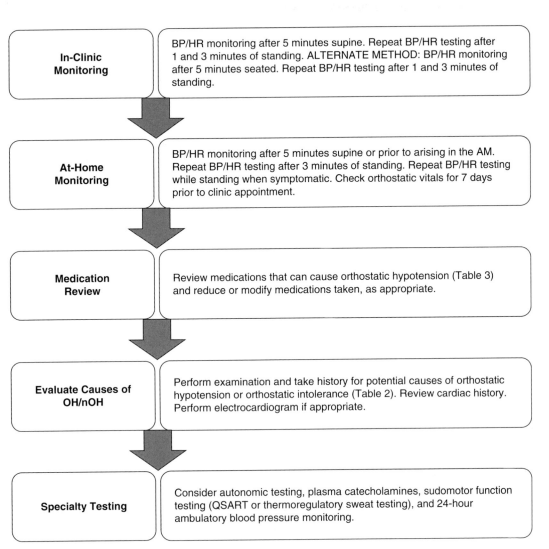

In-Clinic Monitoring	BP/HR monitoring after 5 minutes supine. Repeat BP/HR testing after 1 and 3 minutes of standing. ALTERNATE METHOD: BP/HR monitoring after 5 minutes seated. Repeat BP/HR testing after 1 and 3 minutes of standing.
At-Home Monitoring	BP/HR monitoring after 5 minutes supine or prior to arising in the AM. Repeat BP/HR testing after 3 minutes of standing. Repeat BP/HR testing while standing when symptomatic. Check orthostatic vitals for 7 days prior to clinic appointment.
Medication Review	Review medications that can cause orthostatic hypotension (Table 3) and reduce or modify medications taken, as appropriate.
Evaluate Causes of OH/nOH	Perform examination and take history for potential causes of orthostatic hypotension or orthostatic intolerance (Table 2). Review cardiac history. Perform electrocardiogram if appropriate.
Specialty Testing	Consider autonomic testing, plasma catecholamines, sudomotor function testing (QSART or thermoregulatory sweat testing), and 24-hour ambulatory blood pressure monitoring.

Figure 17.3 Stepwise approach to diagnosis of OH
Printed with permission: Gibbons CH, Schmidt P, Biaggioni I, Frazier-Mills C, Freeman R, Isaacson S, et al. J. Neurol. 2017 [11]

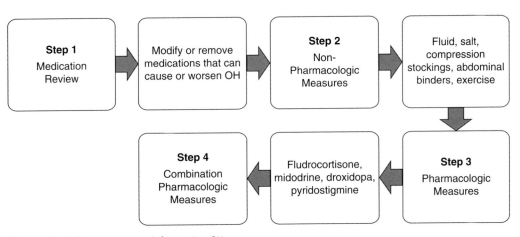

Figure 17.4 A four-step approach for treating OH
Printed with permission: Gibbons CH, Schmidt P, Biaggioni I, Frazier-Mills C, Freeman R, Isaacson S, et al. J. Neurol. 2017 [11]

17.2.1.7 Non-Pharmacological Measures of OH

Key factors in prevention and management of OH include avoiding activities and medication that promote OH, introduce activities that prevent OH, and adhere to activities that counteract OH [13].

Activities to Avoid

- Sudden head-up postural change (especially on waking – start the day slowly)
- Prolonged recumbency
- High environmental temperatures
- Large meals (especially of refined carbohydrates)
- Alcohol
- Excessive exertion
- Medications that may cause OH or exacerbate the symptoms of OH (Table 17.1).

Other drugs with vasodepressor and/or vasodilator properties that may cause or aggravate OH and syncope are antipsychotics, hypnotics, anaesthetics, barbiturates, phenothiazines, and monoamine oxidase (MAO) inhibitors.

Activities to Be Introduced

- High salt intake (only in non-hypertensive patients) [13]
- Water repletion
- Small, frequent meals

Table 17.1 Medications that may cause OH or exacerbate the symptoms of OH

Class of medications	Common examples
Dopaminergic agents	Levodopa, dopamine agonists
Antidepressants	Especially tricyclic agents: amitriptyline, nortriptyline
Anticholinergics	Atropine, glycopyrrolate, hyoscyamine
Antihypertensive agents	
Preload reducers	
• Diuretics[a]	Furosemide, torsemide, acetazolamide, hydrochlorothiazide, spironolactone
• Nitrates[a]	Nitroprusside, isosorbide dinitrate, nitroglycerin
• Phosphodiesterase E5 inhibitors	Sildenafil, vardenafil, tadalafil
Vasodilator	
• α1-adrenergic agonists[a]	Alfuzosin, doxazosin, prazosin, terazosin, tamsulosin (when used primarily)
• Dihydropyridine calcium channel block	Amlodipine, nifedipine, nicardipine
• Other direct vasodilators	Hydralazine, minoxidil
Negative inotropic/chronotropic agents	
β-adrenergic blockers	Propranolol, metoprolol, atenolol, bisoprolol, nebivolol (also vasodilator), carvediol (also α1-antagonist), labetalol (also α1-antagonist)
• Non-dihydropyridine calcium channel blockers	Verapamil, diltiazem
Central sympatholytic agents	
• Centrally acting α2-agonists	Clonidine
• False neurotransmitters	α-methyldopa
Renin-angiotensin system (RAS) antagonists	
• Angiotensin-converting enzyme (ACE) inhibitors	Captopril, enalapril, perindopril
• Angiotensin receptor type II blockers (ARB)	Losartan, telmisartan, candesartan

[a] Agents that may cause more significant worsening of OH

Printed with permission: Gibbons CH, Schmidt P, Biaggioni I, Frazier-Mills C, Freeman R, Isaacson S, et al. J. Neurol. 2017 [11]

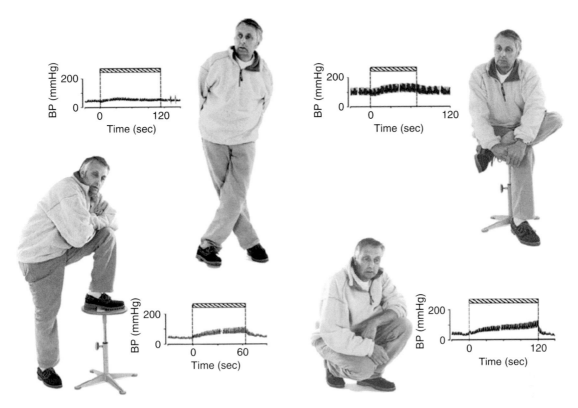

Figure 17.5 Physical counter manoeuvres to boost blood pressure Physical counter manoeuvres using isometric contractions of the lower limbs and abdominal compression. The effects of leg crossing in standing and sitting position, placing a foot on a chair and squatting, on finger arterial blood pressure (FINAP) in a 54-year-old male patient with pure autonomic failure and incapacitating orthostatic hypotension. The patient was standing (sitting) quietly prior to the manoeuvres. Bars indicate the duration of the manoeuvres. Note the increase in blood pressure and pulse pressure during the manoeuvres (Harms and Wieling, unpublished, with written permission of the patient). *Reprinted with permission from Wieling W, Colman N, Krediet CT, Freeman R. Clin. Auton. Res. 2004* [14]

- Head-up tilt at night
- Physical counter manoeuvres (Figure 17.5)
- Sensible regular exercise; regular endurance training is shown to improve symptoms in patients with orthostatic intolerance [15]
- Liquorice

Activities to Be Used

- Elastic stockings [13]
- Abdominal binders [16]
- Physical countermeasures to increase orthostatic tolerance [14].

If possible, non-pharmacological measurements should be used for three months before adding medication.

17.2.1.8 Pharmacological Treatment of OH

If non-pharmacological measurements are not sufficient, or the OH is severe, pharmacological measurements may be necessary [3].

- Starter – volume expansion
  - Fludrocortisone (increases the blood pressure both day and night)
  - Erythropoietin to treat anaemia
- Sympathomimetics – replacing noradrenergic stimulation
  - Midodrine, ephedrine, droxidopa (short-acting pressor)
- Harnessing the residual sympathetic tone
  - Pyridostigmine

- Yohimbine
- Atomoxetine
- Targeting specific problems
  - Post-prandial hypotension: octreotide [17]
  - Nocturnal polyuria: desmopressin [18]
  - Overactive bladder: oxybutynin, solifenacin, tolterodine (antimuscarinics) [19], mirabegron (β3-adrenoceptor agonist) [20]

17.2.1.9 Prevention: Patient Teaching and Education

It is important that the patients are aware of triggers and try to avoid these as much as possible by using the recommendation of what to avoid, what to introduce, and what to use.

After long recumbency, a graded activity plan for reconditioning may be beneficial.

Suggested graded activity plan after prolonged bedrest:

Stage 1: Sitting upright in bed

Stage 2: Sitting with legs over the side of bed

Stage 3: Sitting in reclining chair, standing transfers

Stage 4: Walking with two people

Stage 5: Walking short distances unaided.

Before starting any activity, it is important that the patient has developed a routine of preparing the circulation for activity, which will prevent symptoms. Immediately before moving, the patient should:

- Have a drink of water
- Pump calf muscles for a few seconds to stimulate circulation
- Move or start the activity on a breath out, keeping the shoulders and chest relaxed.

It is important that the patient is able to adhere to each stage for a longer period before moving to the next stage.

17.2.2 Postprandial Hypotension (PPH)

Postprandial hypotension is a common condition in neurorehabilitation. Postprandial hypotension (PPH) is defined as a decrease in SBP of ≥ 20 mmHg, or a decrease below 90 mmHg if pre-prandial SBP was ≥ 100 mmHg, within two hours after a meal [21].

PPH is more common in older than younger people. Prevalence rates vary between 36% among patients in care homes and 67% among hospitalized patients [22]. PPH can cause dizziness, falls,

confusion, visual disturbances, nausea, tiredness, syncope, and poor quality of life [22], and is present in half of those with 'unexplained' syncope [17]. There is an increased risk of PPH in patents with pure autonomic failure, Parkinson's disease, diabetes mellitus, and SCI [21].

PPH is also associated with acute vascular events such as stroke and angina pectoris, and with increased risk of mortality [23].

The postprandial reduction in blood pressure is independent of systemic hypertension [22] and also independent of antihypertensive medication [24]. The reduction in blood pressure after food mirrors the failure of the normal homeostatic mechanisms to maintain blood pressure levels in the face of a reduction of the systemic vascular resistance due to splanchnic and peripheral vasodilation which has not been compensated for by an increase in cardiac output [21, 25].

Risk factors for PPH are medications, especially polypharmacy (more than three medications) and diuretics, and carbohydrate-rich meals, breakfast, hot meals, and alcohol [21]. Non-pharmacological measures to counteract PPH consist of [21]:

- Water before meals
- Frequent, smaller meals
- Assume a recumbent or sitting position after a meal
- Avoid alcohol before and after a meal
- Dietary modification, reduce intake of refined carbohydrates
- Water with the meal
- Abdominal binders.

17.2.2.1 Pharmacological Treatment of PPH

- Caffeine 250 mg (two cups) either 30 minutes before a meal or by the end of the meal [26]
- Midodrine 10 mg with a meal [26]
- Octreotide 25–50 µg subcutaneous 30 minutes before a meal [26]
- α-glucosidase inhibitor
  - Acarbose 25–100 mg tds [22]
  - Voglibose 0.2–0.5 mg tds [27]
- Guar gum 9 g [22]

17.2.3 Exercise-Related Hypotension

Exercise-related hypotension is not well known, but it is still important. It is a common condition in neurorehabilitation. It was first reported in a group of patients with autonomic failure who were cycling in supine position [28]. Aerobic exercises can induce a post-exercise hypotension due to the vasodilatation of the exercised muscle during the exercise recovery period. A centrally mediated decrease in sympathetic nerve activity, combined with reduced signal transduction from sympathetic nerve activation resulting in vasoconstriction, and local vasodilator mechanisms, leads to a fall in arterial blood pressure after exercise [29].

17.2.3.1 Definition of Exercise-Related Hypotension

Exercise-induced hypotension (EIH) is defined as a fall in SBP during exercise of $\geq$ 10 mmHg [30]. EIH is due to a fall in total peripheral resistance caused by impairment of sympathetic vasoconstriction. It can be a significant symptom in patients with pure autonomic failure, MSA, and SCI. The severity is higher during dynamic compared to static exercise [30, 31].

Post-exercise hypotension (PEH) is a sustained reduction in systolic and/or diastolic arterial blood pressure below control levels after a single bout of exercise which can last for up to three hours after the exercise [32]. Studies have demonstrated PEH in patients with hypertension [33], diabetes mellitus [34], and SCI [35].

This response may be similar to the Bezold-Jarisch reflex, triggering the vasovagal reaction in exercise-induced neurally mediated syncope [36]. The Bezold-Jarisch reflex is a trio of responses (apnoea, bradycardia, and hypotension). It is dependent on intact vagal nerves and is mediated through the cranial part of the medullary centres controlling respiration, heart rate, and vasomotor tone [37].

17.2.3.2 Non-Pharmacological Measures

- Adequate hydration prior to exercise [36]
- Avoiding food intake for several hours before exercise to prevent postprandial hypotension [36]
- Increased daily salt intake [38]
- Prevention of dehydration after exercise by oral water intake during exercise [36]
- Muscle tensing [38]
- Use of abdominal compression/binders and lower limb elastic stockings [38]
- Mild physical exercise [38]

- Reducing risk factors by exercise training in the supine position (swimming, rowing) [30, 39].

17.2.3.3 Guidelines for Fluid Replacement [36]

1. Consume a balanced diet and drink adequate fluids during the 24 hours preceding exercise.
2. Drink 500 mL (two 8-oz. glasses) of fluid two hours before exercising.
3. During exercise, drink fluids early and at regular intervals. The goal is to replace fluid at a rate equal to what is lost in sweating (up to what can be tolerated).
4. Fluids should be cooler than ambient temperature (15–22°C), flavoured for palatability, and readily available.
5. If exercise will last longer than one hour, proper amounts of carbohydrates and/or electrolytes should be included in the fluids.

   A. The addition of carbohydrates should allow for 30–60 g/hour. This can be achieved by consuming 600–1,200 mL/hour of a 4–8% carbohydrate solution.

   B. The addition of sodium at 0.5–0.7 g/L increases palatability, promotes fluid retention, and avoids hyponatremia.

17.2.3.4 Pharmacological Treatment

Unfortunately, studies have not found octreotide and midodrine to be effective on exercise-induced hypotension [38]. Still, an increase in the overall blood pressure may be beneficial for reducing fatigue [40].

17.3 Syncope

Syncope is defined as transient loss of consciousness associated with the inability to maintain postural tone, followed by spontaneous recovery [41]. Syncope is synonymous with fainting, blackouts, and loss of consciousness. It is potentially disabling and relatively common. The Framingham Study found that 3% of men and 3.5% of women had experienced syncope. It accounts for 1% of all hospital admissions, and 3% of A&E visits. Although it is commonly not serious, the medical costs are high [42, 43]. The age distribution is bimodal, with a preponderance among young females aged 15–20 years and older people of both genders from age 80 years and upwards [44].

Causes of syncope [45]

- Neurally mediated (vasovagal/reflex) syncope
  a. Vasodepressor
  b. Cardioinhibitory
  c. Mixed
- Situational syncope (vasovagal in nature)
- Carotid sinus syncope
- Orthostatic/postural syncope
- Non-neurogenic causes
  - Cardiac arrhythmias
  - Structural cardiac or cardiopulmonary disease
  - Cerebrovascular
  - Non-cardiovascular/non-syncopal causes of transient loss of consciousness

17.3.1 Pathophysiology

Neurally mediated syncope results when the circulatory reflexes fail to secure the cerebral perfusion, causing vasodilatation and/or bradycardia and a fall in blood pressure. Stretch-activated baroreceptors located in the carotid sinus and aortic arch transmit afferent signals through the glossopharyngeal and vagal nerves, respectively, to the nucleus tractus solitaries in the brainstem.

Neurally mediated syncope is classified according to physiological mechanism:

- Vasodepressor type: characterized by loss of upright vasoconstrictor tone
- Cardioinhibitory type: characterized by bradycardia
- Mixed type: characterized by occurrence of both.

17.3.2 Triggers of Syncope

Triggers of syncope are similar to OH. Frequent triggers are standing still, heat, dehydration, eating, alcohol, and exertion [46]. Psychological triggers are emotional (pain, fear, and anxiety) or situational (having blood tests taken). Syncope is often divided into neurally mediated (vasovagal/reflex) syncope, situational syncope (vasovagal in nature), and carotid sinus super sensitivity [46].

17.3.3 Situational Syncope

Situational syncope (vasovagal in nature) is linked to activities: defecation, micturition, coughs, sneezes, laughter, post exercise, vomiting, swallowing, weightlifting, and during orgasm [44].

Prevention of defecation syncope includes softening of the stools to avoid straining and seating position

during opening of the bowels. In some patients, the use of abdominal binder may be effective to prevent a fall in blood pressure during opening of the bowels.

Micturition syncope is more frequent in middle-aged men, during the evening hours, especially in men taking vasodilators or after drinking alcohol [44]. Prevention of micturition syncope, if it's recurrent, is to sit on the toilet while opening the bladder.

17.3.4 Carotid Sinus Stimulation/ Hypersensitivity

This syndrome is defined as situational syncope with carotid sinus massage resulting in either asystole of more than three seconds or a fall in SBP of > 50 mmHg, or both, and inducing a spontaneous syncope. The incidence is 35–40 patients/year/million, with a male:female ratio of 4:1. It is more frequent in the elderly, especially in diabetic patients with atherosclerosis. Precipitating factors are often sudden movements of the head and neck, cervical compressions, and use of a tight neck tie [41].

Management is avoiding provoking activities, volume expansion if the main component is vasodepressor, and, rarely, a pacemaker if there is a strong cardioinhibitory component [41].

17.3.5 Treatment of Syncope

The most effective forms of treatment are education of patients, avoidance of triggers, physical counter manoeuvres (Figure 17.5), and hydration or intravascular volume expansion. Pharmacologic interventions may be appropriate for some patients but, in general, they have limited evidence of efficacy in preventing syncope [44].

17.3.5.1 Non-Pharmacological Measurements

Treatment strategies include information and education of patients with special emphasis on potential predisposing factors and recognition of prodromal symptoms. Education about possible pre-syncopal symptoms can help avert a syncopal episode by assuming a seated or supine position when possible. Increased fluid and salt intake may also help avoiding the development of syncope and should always be tried first. Other non-pharmacological measurements include lower limb exercise, counter manoeuvres (Figure 17.5), use of stockings, avoidance of triggers like heat, and standing still for a long period, as well as exercise and tilt training.

Water and increasing salt intake increase plasma volume. The increase in blood pressure is evident within five minutes after drinking water, reaches a maximum after approximately 20–30 minutes, and is sustained for more than 60 minutes [47]. The recommended daily intake of water is 1.5–2 L/day, and 6–10 g of sodium chloride is either incorporated into meals or taken as supplement tablets [48].

Carefully controlled and individualized exercise training such as swimming, aerobics, cycling, and walking if possible can improve OH and counteract syncope.

17.3.5.2 Pharmacological Treatment

In patients with the cardioinhibitory form of syncope, a dual-chamber pacemaker may be of value; however, the pacemaker will not improve the vasodepressor component of the syncope.

Pharmacotherapy includes beta-blockers, which inhibit the activation of mechanoreceptors; fludrocortisone, which expands central fluid volume via retention of sodium; and vasoconstrictors and selective serotonin reuptake inhibitors, which may have a role in regulating sympathetic nervous system activity. In patients with mixed syncope, the aim is to treat the dominating source.

17.4 Postural Tachycardia Syndrome (PoTS)

Postural tachycardia syndrome (PoTS) is characterized by tachycardia and orthostatic symptoms, with postural changes in the absence of significant hypotension. The symptoms include palpitations, dizziness, and, in some patients, syncope, usually upon standing, and may be exacerbated by modest exertion, food ingestion, and heat [49].

PoTS affects predominantly young females with a 5:1 ratio over males, and most patients are between 20 and 40 years of age [49]. There is a strong link to joint hypermobility syndrome, also known as Ehlers-Danlos syndrome (EDS) type III or hypermobility. Symptoms may be brought on by infection, trauma, surgery, or stress. Possible pathophysiological mechanisms include alterations in neural control, humoral factors, vascular properties, and intravascular volume, as well as physical deconditioning [49].

17.4.1 Non-Pharmacological Measurements

Measurements preventing hypotension and counteracting tachycardia are increased fluid and salt intake, lower limb exercise, counter manoeuvres, and use of stockings. Gentle and gradually increasing core-strengthening exercises like Pilates and swimming may be useful, especially for those with a diagnosis of EDS.

17.4.2 Pharmacological Treatment

Pharmacological treatment for PoTS is similar to that used for orthostatic hypotension [49] by boosting the blood pressure by using fludrocortisone, ephedrine, and midodrine. To lower the heart rate, a low-dose beta-blocker or ivabradine may be beneficial. Associated disorders, such as joint hypermobility syndrome and pain, need to be addressed. With time many patients get less symptomatic.

17.5 Supine Hypertension

Supine hypertension is defined as an SBP ≥ 150 mmHg or DBP ≥ 90 mmHg [7]. It is common in autonomic failure patients, but, unfortunately, it is frequently overlooked; more than half of patients with autonomic failure have this problem [50]. Due to their absent baroreflex function, patients are unable to compensate, not only for the drop in blood pressure upon standing, but also for the mechanisms that drive hypertension with aging. The cause may be an unmasked essential hypertension or the development of unique pathophysiological mechanisms of hypertension.

The supine hypertension of autonomic failure can be severe: blood pressure as high as 230/140 mmHg has been described and is associated with end-organ damage, including left ventricular hypertrophy and impaired renal function [50].

17.5.1 Non-Pharmacological Measurements

Non-pharmacological measurements should always be applied. Ways to counteract supine hypertension are:

- Avoid supine position during daytime
- Avoid pressor medications after 6 PM
- Elevate the bed head (20–30 cm)
- Have a snack just before going to bed (inducing postprandial hypotension)
- Fludrocortisone may worsen the supine hypertension – change to a short-acting pressor agent
- Avoid medications that increase blood pressure: nasal decongestants, eye drops containing sympathomimetics, and NSAIDs

17.5.2 Pharmacological Treatments

A single dose given at bedtime is recommended [11, 51]:

- Losartan (angiotensin II receptor antagonist) 50 mg
- Transdermal nitroglycerin (vasodilator) 0.05–0.2 mg/h only during night
- Hydralazine (peripheral smooth muscle relaxant) 10–50 mg
- Short-acting nifedipine (calcium channel blocker) 30 mg
- Clonidine (central α2-agonist) 0.1–0.2 mg early in the evening/with evening meal – clonidine has a long half-life, which may exacerbate morning OH
- Sildenafil (phosphodiesterase 5 inhibitor) 25 mg
- Minoxidil (vasodilator) 2.5 mg
- Captopril (ACE inhibitor) 25 mg.

17.6 Hypertensive Emergencies

17.6.1 Paroxysmal Sympathetic Storm/Hyperactivity/Traumatic Brain Injury

Paroxysmal sympathetic storm is a rare syndrome seen in severe traumatic brain injury. It is characterized by:

- Episodic hypertension: SBP > 160 mmHg or pulse pressure > 80 mmHg
- Hyperhidrosis/excessive diaphoresis
- Hyperthermia: body temperature > 38.3°C
- Tachycardia: heart rate > 120 bpm (or > 100 bpm if the patient is treated with a beta-blocker)
- Tachypnea: respiratory rate > 30 breaths per minute
- Posturing or severe dystonia, change in posturing, or spontaneous posturing
- Rigidity or spasticity.

Paroxysmal sympathetic hyperactivity is associated with prolonged length of hospital stay, poorer outcome, and death. It is described in patients with lesions of the central nervous system and is attributed to damage at the diencephalic level [52]. It has been reported in other conditions than traumatic brain injury, including hypoxic injury, brain tumours, hydrocephalus, and subarachnoid haemorrhage [53].

17.6.1.1 Treatment of Other Causes

It is important to increase hydration, treat possible triggers like infection, pulmonary embolism, hydrocephalus, and epilepsy, and give effective analgesia [54].

17.6.1.2 Pharmacological Treatment

The pharmacological approach is to inhibit the central sympathetic outflow, inhibit the afferent sensory process, and block end-response organs of the sympathetic nervous system [54].

Medications Used for the Treatment of PSH

- Non-selective beta-blockers (propranolol) is effective on hypertension, tachycardia, and fever – 20–60 mg every four to six hours enteric.
- Morphine is effective on tachycardia, peripheral vasodilation, and end-organ response – 2–8 mg IV.
- Clonidine is effective on hypertension – 0.1–0.3 mg tds enteric.
- Bromocriptine is effective on dystonia, fever, posturing – 1.25 mg by bd enteric.
- Oral baclofen is effective on pain, clonus, rigidity – 5 mg tds.
- Intrathecal baclofen is effective on pain, clonus, rigidity.
- Benzodiazepines are effective on agitation, hypertension, tachycardia, posturing.
  - Midazolam: 1–2 mg IV
  - Lorazepam: 2–4 mg IV
  - Diazepam: 5–10 mg IV
- Gabapentin is effective on spasticity and end-organ response – 300–900 mg/d.

17.6.2 Autonomic Dysreflexia (AD): SCI

An SCI at the T6 segment or above interrupts the supraspinal control of the sympathetic nervous system, causing an imbalance between the sympathetic and the parasympathetic nervous systems. Autonomic dysreflexia (AD) is characterized by a sudden, uncontrolled sympathetic response, resulting in a dramatic rise in arterial blood pressure – usually triggered by a noxious or irritant stimulus – and by episodic hypertension and bradycardia [55].

Patients with SCI above T6 have a lower blood pressure and lower noradrenaline levels compared with able-bodied subjects, normally SBP of

90–110 mmHg. Decreased sympathetic nervous activity appears to be responsible for the low SBP together with a lower basal heart rate compared to paraplegics [56].

A pressure rise of 20–40 mmHg above the usual of 90–110 mmHg is a sign of AD. SBP above 250–300 mmHg and DBP above 200–220 mmHg have been reported [56]. The lifetime prevalence of AD ranges from 19% to 70%. AD occurs more frequently in patients with cervical lesions and with complete injury and it is more frequent the first two to four months after injury [55].

17.6.2.1 Typical Signs and Symptoms of AD

- Pounding headache
- Nasal stuffiness
- Facial flush
- Blotchy rash and flushing above the level of lesion
- Increased spasticity
- Elevated blood pressure
- Profuse sweating
- Bradycardia
- Goosebumps
- Chills without fever
- Blurred vision
- Nausea
- Anxiety [55].

Many patients use slight symptoms of AD as a tool to monitor their bladder, bowel, and skin.

17.6.2.2 Common Causes of AD

The most common causes of AD are irritation of bladder, bowel (constipation, ulcer), and skin (ingrown toenail).

Other causes can be infection, sexual intercourse, labour and childbirth, fractures, acute abdominal disease, investigations, e.g., cystoscopy, or any stimulus that would cause pain and discomfort in a person without SCI [55].

17.6.2.3 Complications of AD

Untreated AD can lead to retinal haemorrhage, subarachnoid haemorrhage, intracerebral haemorrhage, myocardial infarct, seizures, and death.

17.6.2.4 Twenty-Four-Hour Ambulatory Blood Pressure Measurements

Ambulatory blood pressure measurements (ABPMs) indicate loss of circadian blood pressure rhythm (sympathetic control) with preserved heart rate rhythm (parasympathetic regulation) in patients with complete tetraplegia. In 70% of patients with symptoms of autonomic dysreflexia, the AMBP recordings were pathological. By using ABPM recordings, the occurrence of episodes of autonomic dysreflexia over 24 hours and the effectiveness of therapeutically treatment can be assessed [57]. The acute treatment of AD consists of: [55]

- Elevate the patient – prevents further increase in blood pressure
- Rapid survey of triggering factors
- Monitor blood pressure every two to five minutes
- If pressure hasn't improved after one minute, consider pharmacological treatment.

If the **blood pressure is > 150 mmHg** systolic, consider pharmacological therapy.

If the **blood pressure is > 170 mmHg** systolic, drug therapy needs to be commenced to reduce the risk of a cerebral incident and to give more time to identify and treat the cause.

17.6.2.5 Pharmacological Treatment

- Nitroglycerine sublingual or topical paste (one-half inch)
- Nifedipine 10 mg orally – instruct the patient to bite the capsule, then swallow it
- Prazosin 1–3 mg po
- Clonidine 0.1–0.2 mg po
- Hydralazine 10–20 mg im/IV

17.6.2.6 Prevention

General measures are wearing loose clothing, careful control of bladder or bowel, frequent relief of pressure in the chair/bed, and careful control of status of skin and toenails. It is important that patients, patients' families, friends, and caregivers learn to recognize the symptoms and triggers of AD, and how to help them through an episode.

17.6.2.7 Procedures Causing AD

Some procedures may cause AD more frequently, and hence precautions are warranted [58].

- **Bladder procedures**: studies have found botulinum toxin, anticholinergics, sacral denervation, and bladder and urethral sphincter surgery all to be beneficial to avoid eliciting AD.
- **Anorectal procedures**: 1% lidocaine is recommended to avoid eliciting AD.

- *Pregnancy and labour*: epidural anaesthesia is recommended to avoid eliciting AD.
- *Surgery*: general anaesthesia and spinal anaesthesia prevent AD during procedures.

17.6.2.8 'Boosting'

- The intentional induction of autonomic dysreflexia to try and enhance athletic performance
- A type of doping that is unique to the Paralympics
- Boosting is the act of deliberating triggering autonomic dysreflexia, and is characterized by a rise in blood pressure.
- How is it achieved? Athletes block their catheters so that their bladders overfill and distend.
- A 'boost' is estimated to improve performance by as much as 15%, but the practice is extremely dangerous.

  ABC of Autonomic Dysreflexia: http://wp-dev .jibc.ca/abcofad/

17.6.3 Autonomic Crisis: Familial Dysautonomia

Familial dysautonomia (FD) is due to a genetic deficiency of a protein (IKAP), which affects the development of peripheral neurons. Patients with FD display complex abnormalities of the baroreflex of unknown cause. FD affects the development and survival of sensory, sympathetic, and parasympathetic neurons. It is a progressive neuronal degeneration. Elevated plasma levels of catecholamines and dopamine are observed during autonomic crises. FD has a high mortality rate and is associated with a high incidence of sudden death [59].

Due to the absence of normal baroreflex buffering which prevents blood pressure from rising and falling excessively, the patients have extreme labile blood pressure with hypertension and hypotension, which lead to organ damage.

17.6.3.1 Typical Cardiovascular Autonomic Symptoms

- Hypertension
- Transient hypertensive surges
- Hypertensive vomiting attacks
- Dysautonomic crises
- Sustained hypertension
- Tachycardia
- Orthostatic hypotension
- Occasional faint (vasovagal syncope)

17.6.3.2 Transient Hypertensive Surges

Hypertension can be triggered by cognitive/emotional and physical stressors. The hypertensive peaks are frequently associated with nausea and retching. Transient hypertensive surges occur with everyday activities. They are common when awakening from sleep, while eating, or when a patient is anxious, excited, or frustrated. Hypertensive surges are present from infancy and are accompanied by reddish blotching of the skin and excessive sweating.

Treatment of transient hypertensive surges includes relaxation and/or distraction, standing or walking, and medications.

17.6.3.3 Hypertensive Vomiting Attacks

Hypertensive vomiting attacks are a characteristic feature of FD. They are due to an increase in the secretion of epinephrine, norepinephrine, and plasma dopamine. The increase in plasma dopamine is believed to activate D2 and D3 receptors in the chemoreceptor trigger zone of the area postrema outside of the blood–brain barrier and cause vomiting.

17.6.3.4 Dysautonomic Crises

These episodes can last for several days. Common triggers include emotions, infection/illness or surgery, constipation, and bladder distension. Attacks are sometimes unpredictable and without obvious cause, but one should always suspect infection.

The episodes may be associated with excessive secretion of vasopressin, anti-diuresis, water retention, and hyponatremia. Hyponatremic seizures should be corrected. Carbidopa, a reversible dopa-decarboxylase inhibitor, can reduce the frequency and severity of hypertensive vomiting attacks.

17.6.3.5 Pharmacological Treatment of Hypertensive, Retching and Vomiting Crises

- Carbidopa oral/ GT: 200 mg three times/day (600 mg/day)
- Clonidine oral/ GT: 0.10–0.5 (or 0.005 mg/kg) every three to four hours
- Transdermal patch: constant dose over 24 hours (0.1 mg/day). Each patch lasts for seven days.
- Diazepam oral/ GT: 5–7.5 mg (or 0.1 mg/kg) every four to six hours. Rectal: 0.1 mg/kg every three to four hours.
- Metoclopramide oral, GT or IV: 5 mg every eight hours (0.1 mg/kg every eight hours in children < 10 years)

- Domperidone oral or GT: 10 mg every six to eight hours
- Ondansetron oral, GT or IV: 8 mg every six to eight hours
- Pregabalin oral: 25–50 mg twice daily or maximum of 6 mg/kg per day
- Tocotrienols oral: 25–400 mg

Sustained supine hypertension is usually present in FD patients with advanced chronic kidney disease. The pharmacological treatment of tachycardia consists of: [59]

- Propranolol oral/GT: 20 mg three times a day (60 mg/day); can be increased up to 120 mg/day.
- Labetalol IV: 20 mg bolus over two minutes. Additional doses of 40 mg, then 80 mg may be administered every 10 minutes as needed. Total maximum dose of 300 mg/day.

17.7 Summary

- Identification of intermittent dysfunction and chronic failure of the cardiovascular system is important for neurorehabilitation.
- Treatment should always start with non-pharmacological measurements and, if needed, add on pharmacological measurements.
- Education is crucial to understand, recognize, and prevent dysfunction of blood pressure.

References

1. Ricci F, De CR, Fedorowski A. Orthostatic hypotension: Epidemiology, prognosis, and treatment. *J. Am. Coll. Cardiol.* 2015; **66**(7): 848–60. Printed with permission.

2. Gall A, Craggs M. *Autonomic nervous system dysfunction.* In Craggs AGAM. ed. Oxford, UK: Oxford Textbook of Neurorehabilitation, 2015; 89–111.

3. Biaggioni I. The pharmacology of autonomic failure: From hypotension to hypertension. *Pharmacol. Rev.* 2017; **69**(1): 53–62.

4. Mathias CJ. Autonomic dysfunction and hypotension. In Willerson J, Wellens H, Cohn J, Holmes D, eds. *Cardiovascular medicine.* London, UK: Springer, 2007; 1883–1910.

5. Gupta D, Nair MD. Neurogenic orthostatic hypotension: Chasing 'the fall'. *Postgrad. Med. J.* 2008; **84**(987): 6–14.

6. Smit AA, Halliwill JR, Low PA, Wieling W. Pathophysiological basis of orthostatic hypotension in autonomic failure. *J. Physiol.* 1999; **519** Pt. 1: 1–10.

7. Freeman R, Wieling W, Axelrod FB, Benditt DG, Benarroch E, Biaggioni I, et al. Consensus statement on the definition of orthostatic hypotension, neurally mediated syncope and the postural tachycardia syndrome. *Auton. Neurosci.* 2011; **161**(1–2): 46–8.

8. Wieling W, Krediet CT, Van DN, Linzer M, Tschakovsky ME. Initial orthostatic hypotension: Review of a forgotten condition. *Clin. Sci. (Lond.)* 2007; **112**(3): 157–65.

9. Cariga P, Ahmed S, Mathias CJ, Gardner BP. The prevalence and association of neck (coat-hanger) pain and orthostatic (postural) hypotension in human spinal cord injury. *Spinal Cord* 2002; **40**(2): 77–82.

10. Oldenburg O, Kribben A, Baumgart D, Philipp T, Erbel R, Cohen MV. Treatment of orthostatic hypotension. *Curr. Opin. Pharmacol.* 2002; **2**(6): 740–7.

11. Gibbons CH, Schmidt P, Biaggioni I, Frazier-Mills C, Freeman R, Isaacson S, et al. The recommendations of a consensus panel for the screening, diagnosis, and treatment of neurogenic orthostatic hypotension and associated supine hypertension. *J. Neurol.* 2017: 1–16.

12. Stuebner E, Vichayanrat E, Low DA, Mathias CJ, Isenmann S, Haensch CA. Twenty-four hour non-invasive ambulatory blood pressure and heart rate monitoring in Parkinson's disease. *Front. Neurol.* 2013; **4**: 49.

13. Lahrmann H, Cortelli P, Hilz M, Mathias CJ, Struhal W, Tassinari M. EFNS guidelines on the diagnosis and management of orthostatic hypotension. *Eur. J. Neurol.* 2006; **13**(9): 930–6.

14. Wieling W, Colman N, Krediet CT, Freeman R. Nonpharmacological treatment of reflex syncope. *Clin. Auton. Res.* 2004; **14**, Suppl. 1: 62–70.

15. Winker R, Barth A, Bidmon D, Ponocny I, Weber M, Mayr O, et al. Endurance exercise training in orthostatic intolerance: A randomized, controlled trial. *Hypertension* 2005; **45**(3): 391–8.

16. Fanciulli A, Goebel G, Metzler B, Sprenger F, Poewe W, Wenning GK, et al. Elastic abdominal binders attenuate orthostatic hypotension in Parkinson's disease. *Mov. Disord. Clin. Pract.* 2016; **3**(2): 156–60.

17. Armstrong E, Mathias CJ. The effects of the somatostatin analogue, octreotide, on postural hypotension, before and after food ingestion, in primary autonomic failure. *Clin. Auton. Res* 1991 1991; 135–40.

18. Freeman R. Treatment of orthostatic hypotension. *Semin. Neurol.* 2003; **23**(4): 435–42.

19. Madersbacher HG. Neurogenic bladder dysfunction. *Curr. Opin. Urol.* 1999; **9**(3): 303–7.

20. Rosa GM, Ferrero S, Nitti VW, Wagg A, Saleem T, Chapple CR. Cardiovascular safety of

beta3-adrenoceptor agonists for the treatment of patients with overactive bladder syndrome. *Eur. Urol.* 2016; **69**(2): 311–23.

21. Jansen RW, Lipsitz LA. Postprandial hypotension: Epidemiology, pathophysiology, and clinical management. *Ann. Intern. Med.* 1995; **122**(4): 286–95.

22. Ong ACL, Myint PK, Potter JF. Pharmacological treatment of postprandial reductions in blood pressure: A systematic review. *J. Am. Geriatr. Soc.* 2014; **62**(4): 649–61.

23. Vaitkevicius PV, Esserwein DM, Maynard AK, O'Connor FC, Fleg JL. Frequency and importance of postprandial blood pressure reduction in elderly nursing-home patients. *Ann. Intern. Med.* 1991; **115** (11): 865–70.

24. Lipsitz LA, Nyquist RP, Jr, Wei JY, Rowe JW. Postprandial reduction in blood pressure in the elderly. *N. Engl. J. Med.* 1983; **309**(2): 81–3.

25. Heseltine D, Dakkak M, Woodhouse K, Macdonald IA, Potter JF. The effect of caffeine on postprandial hypotension in the elderly. *J. Am. Geriatr. Soc.* 1991; **39** (2): 160–4.

26. Freeman R, Kaufmann H. Disorders of orthostatic tolerance–orthostatic hypotension, postural tachycardia syndrome, and syncope. *Continuum: Lifelong Learning in Neurology* 2007; **13**(6, Autonomic Disorders).

27. Maruta T, Komai K, Takamori M, Yamada M. Voglibose inhibits postprandial hypotension in neurologic disorders and elderly people. *Neurology* 2006; **66**(9): 1432–4.

28. Marshall RJ, Schirger A, Shepherd JT. Blood pressure during supine exercise in idiopathic orthostatic hypotension. *Circulation* 1961; **24**: 76–81.

29. Halliwill JR, Buck TM, Lacewell AN, Romero SA. Postexercise hypotension and sustained postexercise vasodilatation: What happens after we exercise? *Exp. Physiol.* 2013; **98**(1): 7–18.

30. Low DA, da Nóbrega ACL, Mathias CJ. Exercise-induced hypotension in autonomic disorders. *Auton. Neurosci.* 2012; **171**(1–2): 66–78.

31. da Nóbrega ACL, Low DA, Mathias CJ. Exercise-induced hypotension in autonomic disorders. In Mathias CJ, Bannister R. eds. *Autonomic failure: A textbook of clinical disorders of the autonomic nervous system.* 5th edn. Oxford, UK: Oxford University Press, 2013; 381–94.

32. Hayes PM, Lucas JC, Shi X. Importance of post-exercise hypotension in plasma volume restoration. *Acta Physiol. Scand.* 2000; **169**(2): 115–24.

33. MacDonald JR. Potential causes, mechanisms, and implications of post exercise hypotension. *J. Hum. Hypertens.* 2002; **16**(4): 225–36.

34. Lima LCJ, Assis GV, Hiyane W, Almeida WS, Arsa G, Baldissera V, et al. Hypotensive effects of exercise performed around anaerobic threshold in type 2 diabetic patients. *Diabetes Res. Clin. Pract.* 2008; **81**(2): 216–22.

35. Rimaud D, Calmels P, Pichot V, Bethoux F, Roche F. Effects of compression stockings on sympathetic activity and heart rate variability in individuals with spinal cord injury. *J. Spinal Cord Med.* 2012; **35**(2): 81–8.

36. Krediet CT, Wilde AA, Wieling W, Halliwill JR. Exercise related syncope, when it's not the heart. *Clin. Auton. Res.* 2004; **14** Suppl. 1: 25–36.

37. Aviado DM, Guevara Aviado D. The Bezold-Jarisch reflex: A historical perspective of cardiopulmonary reflexes. *Ann. N. Y. Acad. Sci.* 2001; **940**: 48–58.

38. Figueroa JJ, Basford JR, Low PA. Preventing and treating orthostatic hypotension: As easy as A, B, C. *Cleve. Clin. J. Med.* 2010; **77**(5): 298–306.

39. Maule S, Papotti G, Naso D, Magnino C, Testa E, Veglio F. Orthostatic hypotension: Evaluation and treatment. *Cardiovasc. Hematol. Disord. Drug Targets* 2007; **7**(1): 63–70.

40. Butler JE, Ribot-Ciscar E, Zijdewind I, Thomas CK. Increased blood pressure can reduce fatigue of thenar muscles paralyzed after spinal cord injury. *Muscle Nerve* 2004; **29**(4): 575–84.

41. Costantino G, Casazza G, Reed M, Bossi I, Sun B, Del Rosso A, et al. Syncope risk stratification tools vs clinical judgment: An individual patient data meta-analysis. *Am. J. Med.* 2014; **127**(11): 1126.e.13-1126.e.25.

42. Ruwald MH, Hansen ML, Lamberts M, Hansen CM, Hojgaard MV, Kober L, et al. The relation between age, sex, comorbidity, and pharmacotherapy and the risk of syncope: A Danish nationwide study. *Europace* 2012; **14**(10): 1506–14.

43. Chen L, Chen MH, Larson MG, Evans J, Benjamin EJ, Levy D. Risk factors for syncope in a community-based sample (the Framingham Heart Study). *Am. J. Cardiol.* 2000; **85**(10): 1189–93.

44. Cheshire WP, Jr. Syncope. *Continuum* (Minneap. Minn.). 2017; **23**(2, Selected Topics in Outpatient Neurology): 335–58.

45. Bassetti CL. Transient loss of consciousness and syncope. *Handb. Clin. Neurol.* 2014; **119**: 169–91.

46. da Silva RM. Syncope: Epidemiology, etiology, and prognosis. *Front. Physiol.* 2014; **5**: 471.

47. Jordan J. Acute effect of water on blood pressure. What do we know? *Clin. Auton. Res.* 2002; **12**(4): 250–5.

48. Wieling W, Ganzeboom KS, Saul JP. Reflex syncope in children and adolescents. *Heart* 2004; **90**(9): 1094–1100.

49. Mathias CJ, Low DA, Iodice V, Owens AP, Kirbis M, Grahame R. Postural tachycardia syndrome: Current experience and concepts. *Nat. Rev. Neurol.* 2012; **8**(1): 22–34.

50. Biaggioni I. The pharmacology of autonomic failure: From hypotension to hypertension. *Pharmacological Reviews* 2017; **69**(1): 53–62.

51. Low PA, Tomalia VA. Orthostatic hypotension: Mechanisms, causes, management. *J. Clin. Neurol.* 2015; **11**(3): 220–6.

52. Rey M, Borrallo JM, Vogel CM, Pereira MA, Varela MA, Diz JC. Paroxysmal sympathetic storms after type a dissection of the aorta. *J. Cardiothorac. Vasc. Anesth.* 2005; **19**(5): 654–5.

53. Perkes IE, Menon DK, Nott MT, Baguley IJ. Paroxysmal sympathetic hyperactivity after acquired brain injury: A review of diagnostic criteria. *Brain Inj.* 2011; **25**(10): 925–32.

54. Feng Y, Zheng X, Fang Z. Treatment progress of paroxysmal sympathetic hyperactivity after acquired brain injury. *Pediatr. Neurosurg.* 2015; **50**(6): 301–9.

55. Hagen EM, Faerestrand S, Hoff JM, Rekand T, Gronning M. Cardiovascular and urological dysfunction in spinal cord injury. *Acta Neurol. Scand. Suppl.* 2011; **124**(191): 71–8.

56. Weaver LC, Fleming JC, Mathias CJ, Krassioukov AV. Chapter 13 – Disordered cardiovascular control after spinal cord injury. In John JVA. ed. *Handbook of clinical neurology: Spinal cord injury*. Volume **109**. Elsevier, 2012; 213–33.

57. Curt A, Nitsche B, Rodic B, Schurch B, Dietz V. Assessment of autonomic dysreflexia in patients with spinal cord injury. *J. Neurol. Neurosurg. Psychiatry* 1997; **62**(5): 473–7.

58. Krassioukov A, Warburton DE, Teasell R, Eng JJ. A systematic review of the management of autonomic dysreflexia after spinal cord injury. *Arch. Phys. Med. Rehabil.* 2009; **90**(4): 682–95.

59. Palma J-A, Norcliffe-Kaufmann L, Fuente-Mora C, Percival L, Mendoza-Santiesteban C, Kaufmann H. Current treatments in familial dysautonomia. *Expert Opin. Pharmacother.* 2014; **15**(18): 2653–71.

18

Management of Neurogenic Lower Urinary Tract Dysfunction

Mahreen Pakzad and Pierre Denys

18.1 Introduction

The management of patients with neurogenic lower urinary tract (LUT) dysfunction is an everyday challenge for specialists in neurorehabilitation. In fact, bladder-sphincter physiology is under a strong and complex neurological control, which explains the very high prevalence of bladder-sphincter disorders in all types of neurological diseases such as dementia, stroke, Parkinson's disease, multiple sclerosis (MS), spinal cord injury (SCI), peripheral nerve lesions, disc prolapse, or polyneuropathies. However, the terms 'neurogenic LUT dysfunction' or 'neurogenic bladder' are an oversimplification and encompass diverse conditions which are influenced by the level of neurological lesion and the type of disease, as well as the disease burden.

One method of describing the different aetiologies of neurogenic LUT dysfunction is to separate them according to the level of the neurological lesion, i.e. suprapontine, infrapontine suprasacral lesions, conus medullaris, and infrasacral lesions (Table 18.1). This classification is helpful as it reflects different types of pathophysiologies and clinical presentations (Table 18.2).

Bladder-sphincter integrative physiology [1] controls two main functions, continence and micturition. Basically, continence involves the storage of urine at low pressure. This low-pressure storage is a result of a combination of the inhibition of detrusor contractions and the viscoelastic properties of the bladder wall. At the same time, the urethral sphincter adapts its resistance to filling and to various stress conditions. The opposite occurs during the micturition cycle, when the detrusor contracts and synergistically the sphincters are open. Micturition should be voluntary, complete, and of short duration.

Over time, knowledge about the physiological role of the different components of the nervous system has increased significantly. Simply and comprehensively, the brain controls socially adapted behaviour. Usually, brain lesions result in incontinence due to detrusor overactivity, but the synergy between the detrusor and the sphincter is preserved. The pontine micturition centre (PMC) is responsible for the coordination of the various spinal effectors to coordinate detrusor contraction and internal sphincter relaxation during micturition. This explains why in cases of infrapontine and suprasacral lesions, there is a lack of coordination between the different effectors. The spinal cord is the place where sympathetic, sacral parasympathetic, and somatic centres are located. The peripheral nervous system conveys both bladder and urethral sensation and is responsible for the efferent control on the bladder and the sphincters.

18.2 The Aims of Treatment

The two primary goals when treating patients with neurogenic LUT dysfunction are to preserve kidney

Table 18.1 Major aetiologies of lower urinary tract dysfunction depending on the level of injury

	Medical	Surgical	Degenerative	Congenital
Suprapontine	Stroke Multiple sclerosis	Tumours Trauma	Parkinson's disease	Cerebral palsy
Infrapontine suprasacral	Multiple sclerosis Infection	Trauma		
Conus medullaris				myelomeningocele
Peripheral lesion		Disc prolapse		myelomeningocele

Table 18.2 Pathophysiology of lower urinary tract dysfunction according to level of neurological lesion

	Bladder	Sphincter	Symptoms	Risk of complications
Suprapontine	Detrusor overactivity	Preserved synergia	Overactive bladder	
Infrapontine suprasacral	Detrusor overactivity	Detrusor sphincter dyssynergia	Incontinence and voiding difficulties	High risk for renal impairment
Conus medullaris	Detrusor overactivity or areflexic bladder or low compliance	Detrusor sphincter dyssynergia or non-relaxing sphincter		High risk for renal impairment
Peripheral lesion	Areflexic bladder	Sphincter deficiency		

function and to improve quality of life/urinary continence. This is particularly the case in patients with spinal cord lesions, where despite major advances in therapies during recent decades, LUT dysfunction is still the second most common cause for morbidity, and the most common cause for rehospitalization in the long term. In fact the association of neurogenic detrusor overactivity and detrusor sphincter dyssynergia may result in a high-risk situation due to the association of chronic urinary retention and high intravesical pressures. The potential effects this might have on the renal functions are real challenge for all physicians involved in the field, reinforced by the fact that injury usually occurs during the third decade. This means that bladder management must be considered in the long term, as well as the short term, for the patient. The clinician must recognize that the bladder needs of the patient may change during their lifetime.

The other goal of treatment is to improve quality of life, by restoring continence when feasible. The impact of incontinence is not isolated. Not only does it pertain directly to the use of continence aids or potential medical or surgical treatments, but it can also affect other major functions, such as sexual function. Incontinence is the number one limiting factor for sexual satisfaction after SCI, in both genders.

18.3 Holistic Evaluation of the Patient

Holistic evaluation is a prerequisite before planning therapy. A failure to do so may result in catastrophic consequences for an already compromised patient. For example, the clinician must record the patient's cognitive state as many antimuscarinic drugs prescribed for the management of overactive bladder (OAB) can have a negative effect on cognition. Several questions should be addressed: Is the patient manually dexterous? Will they be able to handle the demands of intermittent self-catheterization? How mobile is the patient? Will they be able to transfer to the toilet or commode independently? Do they suffer from adductor spasticity, making it difficult for them to access their urethral meatus? To improve perineal access in tetraplegic patients, has intrathecal baclofen or tendon transfer surgery been considered?

Answers to questions such as these play an integral part in the management of these patients. Therapeutic intervention for non-bladder functional problems is sometimes required to improve neurogenic bladder management, per se.

Some complications, such as the development of pressure ulcers and concomitant urinary incontinence, often require a coordinated input from the different medical or surgical specialties involved in the patient's treatment.

Global evaluation of the patient's medications and an awareness of polypharmacy is mandatory. For example, medications taken for spasticity control or neuropathic pain may have side effects on other bodily functions (baclofen and ejaculation; tricyclics for neuropathic pain may have an anticholinergic effect on the bladder or on the colon).

A multidisciplinary approach team (MDT) is therefore vital in the management of patients with neurogenic LUT dysfunction. This is qualified in the National Institute of Care Excellence (NICE) guidance document published in 2012 on the management of LUT in neurological disease [2]. NICE encourages holistic care and the involvement of family and primary carers with the patient's permission. Another strength of the document is that it was written by a multidisciplinary team, including urological surgeons, rehabilitation physicians, and specialist neurological nurses.

The MDT needs to take into account the patient's age at injury. For example, the effects of placing a urethral catheter in a younger patient could be interpreted as predominantly negative, where an elderly patient may be delighted with this form of urinary incontinence management.

Gender also influences management of neurogenic LUT dysfunction. Containment devices such as penile urinary sheaths (convene) are useful in men but of course not for female patients, who may require pads or pants. However, wet pads and constant contact of urine with the skin increase the risk for pressure ulcers and skin complications, such as ammoniacal dermatitis.

Ultimately, disease aetiology and natural history, as well as life expectancy of the patient, will have a strong influence on the choice of treatment for management of the neuropathic bladder.

18.4 Urinary Tract Infections

Neurological patients are at particular risk of a urinary tract infection (UTI) because of a myriad of factors. The most obvious factor is the inefficiency of the neurogenic LUT, culminating in poor bladder emptying, high post-void residuals (PVRs), or urinary retention. The resulting bladder soup is a potential breeding ground for bacteria, which can multiply and pathologically invade the urothelium.

Secondly, the patients may be immunosuppressed. For example, there is evidence to suggest that stroke causing brain injury results in both local and systemic inflammation as evidenced by raised levels of brain and plasma inflammatory cytokines immediately after stroke. A second phase of the immune response, however, appears to involve systemic immunosuppression, occurring in a delayed fashion, possibly related to splenic apoptosis and loss or redistribution of immune calls, again, resulting in an increased risk of infection.

Furthermore, these patients may already be affected by a chronic disease, such as diabetes mellitus, which increases the risk of UTI. Other factors increasing risk include immobility and having a catheter of some sort, which is dealt with later in the chapter.

An important issue pertaining to UTI treatment is the potential for antibiotic resistance developing in this group of patients. Although antibiotics have undoubtedly revolutionized the treatment of UTIs, the international vogue is to take a step back from these agents, and think twice about prescribing. This view has been triggered by the reported global increase in antibiotic resistance.

18.4.1 UTI Treatment

The incidence and prevalence of UTIs in patients with neurogenic bladder is very high [3, 4]. This is particularly well described in the SCI population of patients where UTIs are one of the major causes of morbidity in the long term and the first cause of rehospitalization [5]. On the other hand, the percentage of patients who are carrying a multi-drug resistant (MDR) microorganism increases with time and due to antibiotic over-usage. In fact patients and physicians should be aware of the phenomenon of multidrug resistance and should endeavour to reduce MDR in the long term [6], with a clear strategy for diagnosis, prevention, and treatment of UTIs.

In terms of diagnosis, there is a consensus that due to the very high percentage of chronic bacteriuria, only symptomatic UTI must be treated. Moreover, treatment of chronic asymptomatic bacteriuria did not demonstrate any clinically relevant improvement for the patient. This is particularly the case for patients using indwelling catheters or intermittent catheterization. Symptoms, for example, in the SCI population, are not specific, and may include general weakness, cloudy urine, incontinence, spasticity, or autonomic dysreflexia. Urine culture is mandatory to assess antibiotic sensitivity before introduction of an antibiotic course. According to European Association of Urology (EAU) guidance, a five-day course is probably sufficient and a good compromise between efficacy and the risk of resistance [7].

Risk factors for recurrent UTI must be identified. They may be due to suboptimal management of neurological symptoms. The patient should undergo checks of residual volume, detrusor pressure, reflux, and urinary tract stone formation and should complete a bladder diary to control risk factors before discussing more complex strategy.

If despite a good control of risk factors patients still suffer from recurrent symptomatic UTIs, an individualized management plan should be constructed. The chronic administration of low doses of antibiotics was not proven to be efficacious in term of symptoms, and rather is associated with increasing the risk for MDR organisms. Weekly oral cyclic antibiotics may be used, but still need confirmation of efficacy in double-blind controlled studies [8]. Bladder inoculation of a non-pathogenic strain of E. coli seems efficient to prevent symptomatic UTI [9]. The role of D-Mannose in UTI reduction has been recently published in a small pilot study indicating promising results in the MS population. The number of monthly proven UTIs decreased in both catheter users and non-users (p < 0.01) with no adverse effects reported [10].

18.5 Investigations

Fluid intake and urine output measurements are best recorded by means of a bladder diary, ideally for seven days. On this chart, the patient records fluid intake, time and volume of voids, incontinence episodes, and catheterization episodes. If completed fully, it can provide information about functional bladder capacity.

Many central nervous system diseases are associated with sleep disorders; this is particularly the case in stroke or Parkinson's disease. Both may modify the regulation of nocturnal diuresis. Nocturnal polyuria can be identified from the analysis of a well-kept bladder diary, as can nocturia and nocturnal enuresis. All these symptoms, once correctly identified, can be treated, albeit by different modalities.

Non-invasive urodynamics is centred upon measuring the flow rate of the urine voided, i.e. the amount of urine passed within a period of time, expressed in millilitres per second (mL/s). It also identifies the total volume actually voided by the patient. After the void, the patient undergoes a bedside ultrasound scan of their bladder, in order to document the PVR (mL). There is much debate within urological circles as to exactly which volume left in the bladder constitutes a significant volume; however, it is widely accepted that a PVR of more than 300 mL corresponds to chronic urinary retention [11]. However, amongst neurological patients, a lower PVR is considered significant, and this is because of a reduced

bladder capacity and greater risk for upper urinary tract damage; values greater than 100–150 mL are often considered significant [2, 12].

Those patients who are symptomatic for recurrent UTI may undergo bedside urinalysis using urine dipstick testing kits, which have more than 90% positive predictive value for identifying a UTI, if leucocytes+/- nitrites are positive, in men. However, a negative dipstick cannot exclude a UTI. In women, the positive predictive value is far lower at 76%; hence urine should always be sent on for culture [13]. If urine positivity correlates with clinical symptomatology, then empirical antibiotics (according to local laboratory advice) should be given. This prescription may need to be altered, once the definitive urine culture result returns; however, currently there is no consensus on the correct duration of antibiotic treatment and discussion with the microbiologist is advisable. As many of the patients may have an indwelling urinary catheter, even at this stage of initial evaluation, it is recommended that the urine sample is taken wherever possible from the catheter port or a freshly inserted intermittent sterile catheter. A sample taken directly from the bag will always be contaminated. It is debated whether it is necessary to treat the patient with asymptomatic bacteriuria with antibiotics. Nicolle et al. [14] have shown no benefit in treating this group of patients despite their dysfunctional LUTs, and in the catheterized patient.

More invasive investigations such as flexible cystoscopy may be required, especially where the patient describes visible haematuria, there is a history of recurrent UTIs, or for patients who have had an indwelling urethral catheter for several years.

Invasive urodynamics (cystometry) is a valuable investigation which can delineate the LUT functions during both the storage and voiding phases of the micturition cycle. Video urodynamics using contrast agents to fill the bladder instead of saline (as per conventional urodynamics) is of added benefit as it involves an additional fluoroscopy phase. This live radiographic screening during the study enables the urodynamicist to document any anatomical abnormalities, such as urethral stricture, bladder outflow obstruction, or stress urinary incontinence.

Upper urinary tract imaging is useful in excluding any pre-existing renal dysfunction, such as hydronephrosis or renal tract calculi. Regular renal imaging is desirable, particularly in those patients with SCI, who are at real risk of renal deterioration, if left unchecked, due to potentially high bladder pressures.

18.6 Treatment

Once the holistic neurological evaluation has been completed, treatment can be tailored to the patient, with the expectation that specific needs will require addressing. The family and primary carers should be involved in this treatment pathway.

Urodynamics studies allow a precise delineation of the type of LUT dysfunction. The urodynamic diagnosis of detrusor overactivity (DO) can lead to urinary incontinence with or without urgency. DO can also be associated with detrusor sphincter dyssynergia, resulting in difficulty in voiding, and may lead to chronic urinary retention. Sphincter deficiency is the consequence of peripheral sacral lesions, and is a cause for severe stress neurogenic incontinence. The detrusor can be acontractile in case of peripheral lesions as well, leading to overflow incontinence and dysuria.

The general principles of treatment are that one should be as conservative as possible and efficient in preventing complications and UTIs. Several options of treatment are usually possible for one patient at one time and need to be discussed extensively with the patient, family, and caregivers. Figure 18.1 indicates a treatment algorithm for a typical SCI patient, to support discussion about alternatives of treatment.

18.7 Conservative Treatment: Non-Pharmacological

18.7.1 Pelvic Floor Muscle Training (PFMT)

PFMT is a well-established treatment for stress, mixed, or urge incontinence in the general population, recommended as a first-line therapy by NICE and the EAU. Very few studies specifically address the efficacy of PFMT in the neurogenic population [15]. Some efficacy was reported in the MS population on incontinence, frequency, and quality of life after PFMT. The level of evidence is, however, poor. In practice, PFMT is only really feasible for those with incomplete neurological lesions, or patients with a low level of disability.

18.7.2 Triggered Voiding

After the spinal shock phase of SCI, reflex detrusor contraction reappears. If the sacral reflex is preserved, it is possible to induce detrusor contractions by

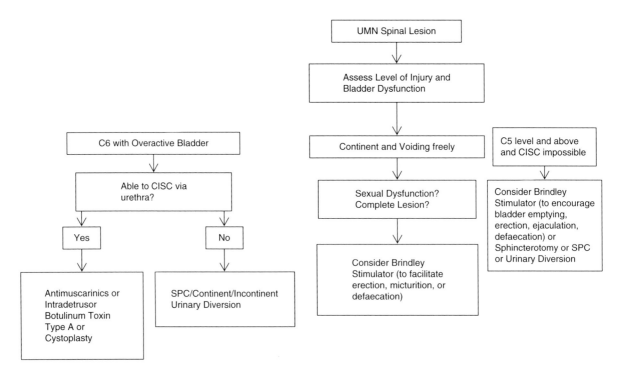

Figure 18.1 Algorithm for treatment of patients with SCI and neurogenic lower urinary tract dysfunction

stimulation of the pelvic region. Techniques include tapping of the suprapubic region, scratching of the perineal skin, or anal/rectal stimulation. This method was the gold standard treatment of spinal neurogenic bladder before the introduction of intermittent catheterization. In fact this method is efficient to induce reflex detrusor contraction, but then of course it may result in incontinence due to neurogenic detrusor overactivity and difficulty in voiding due to detrusor-sphincter dyssynergia (DSD). The former demands that the patient wear a containment device and the latter demands some method of bladder drainage.

The ultimate goal is to obtain 'balanced voiding', with low storage pressures and complete bladder emptying. Patients who manage their bladder by a 'triggered voiding' regime are considered at high risk of renal complications [16, 17]. Patients should have a regular follow-up with urodynamic checks of bladder function. The typical target population is a male high tetraplegic unable to perform catheterization. Although it is quite clear from the literature that this method increases the risk for renal dysfunction compared with intermittent catheterization, there are very few studies reporting the outcomes of triggered voiding and sphincterotomy and little about the long-term tolerance of penile sheaths.

18.7.3 Toileting and Behavioural Therapy

Toileting or behavioural therapy involves assistance by caregivers to help the patient to void at regular intervals of time. This is usually done for patients with dementia [18] or after stroke, to reduce incontinence episodes. This therapy is only useful if the physiology of micturition is preserved, i.e. those with suprapontine lesions.

18.7.4 Crede Manoeuvre

The Crede manoeuvre is a method of bladder emptying that relies on the patient increasing abdominal pressure, by applying even pressure from the umbilicus down to the pubis. It is a non-physiological micturition, hence the urethral sphincter does not open during this manoeuvre. This method was used in patients with peripheral lesions with areflexic or acontractile bladders before the introduction of intermittent catheterization. Pelvic organ prolapse and vesicoureteric reflux are potential long-term complications and thus the Crede manoeuvre has fallen out of favour [19].

18.7.5 Catheterization

Catheterization may be intermittent or permanent (indwelling), and if permanent may be either urethral or suprapubic. Intermittent catheterization (IC) is a well-established and reliable method of voiding for patients with neurogenic LUT dysfunction and chronic urinary retention. Intermittent catheterization was described by Lapides [20], and the first patient treated was a female patient with MS suffering recurrent UTIs due to chronic urinary retention. The benefit was a significant decrease of UTI episodes and an improvement in continence. Since this publication, numerous studies have reinforced the benefits of IC, and this option is uniformly recommended as the first-line management for urinary retention across different guidelines.

For patients with myelomeningocele, it has been established that early use of IC by caregivers or the patient is the best technique for the prevention of upper urinary tract damage.

In the SCI population, large cohort studies demonstrated the benefits for the upper urinary tract of less reflux, better renal function, and less upper urinary tract lithiasis than alternative modes of bladder emptying such as reflex voiding or indwelling catheterization [16, 21].

In MS patients, IC has been shown to be a good method of bladder emptying in case of chronic urinary retention, or if botulinum toxin injections are needed to control OAB by recent phase 3 onabotulinumtoxin A studies using 200 units [22].

Techniques of IC may be sterile or clean. In practice, most patients can achieve the clean technique, whereas hospital care aims to provide sterile IC, with the use of sterile gloves, forceps, and a no-touch technique. The type of catheter is also a matter of much debate – reusable silicone or PVC catheters versus non-reusable coated catheters. A recent Cochrane meta-analysis concluded that there was no scientific evidence to support the sterile over the clean technique in terms of UTIs, and no evidence of benefits using a non-reusable catheter over a reusable PVC or silicone catheter. The Cochrane review [21], however, highlighted the poor quality of studies, which were usually under powered and short term, and used different definitions of UTIs. In terms of clinical relevance, sterile IC is not practical in day-to-day life for the majority of patients. Regarding the second part of the conclusion, a good-quality study comparing reusable versus non-reusable with an appropriate definition of UTI as the primary end-point and a long-term follow-up is still waiting to conclude. The cost of non-reusable catheters should be a consideration when advising IC. Regarding the frequency of catheterization, Lapides in his first paper had remarkable intuition, stating that frequency is more important than sterility. He recommended catheterization more than five times per day with an appropriate diuresis. The usual recommendation in SCI patients is between four and six catheterizations per day [12].

There appears to be a very low risk of long-term urethral complications with IC [23, 24]. The major concern is UTIs, which may still be a problem despite appropriate technique. Some authors have described the benefit of using intra-detrusor botulinum injections to reduce the risk of symptomatic UTI [24]. This is not currently worldwide practice and not advocated by most guidelines.

18.7.6 Indwelling Catheters

Before the description of IC, indwelling catheters were the method adopted for patients who were unable to void properly. Large cohort studies demonstrated that chronic indwelling catheters exposed the patient to a long list of complications: urethral trauma, hypospadias, urethral cleavage, fistulae, bladder stones, UTI, and bladder carcinoma. There is also a higher risk for complications of the upper urinary tract such as lithiasis, reflux dilatation, or renal function. This is the reason why in most countries IC is preferred over indwelling catheters.

Long-term suprapubic catheters (SPC) have several advantages over indwelling urethral catheters, such as the prevention of urethral complications, ease of catheter change, improved perineal hygiene, and permitting of sexual activity [25]. In case of indwelling urethral catheters and silicone catheters, closed drainage systems are recommended to reduce complications [12]. For the management of UTIs, both irrigation and chronic antibiotic therapy failed to demonstrate any benefit.

The merits of screening cystoscopy in patients with long-term indwelling catheters are debated, with no clear guidance on how frequently it should be conducted. NICE guidance encourages discussion with the patient and/or family members and carers that there may be an increased risk of bladder cancer in people with neurogenic LUT dysfunction, in

particular those with a long history of dysfunction and with complicating factors, such as recurrent UTIs. Patients and carers should be educated about warning signs such as haematuria or recurrent UTIs, both of which warrant urgent urological review [26].

Some centres recommend that paraplegic patients with long-term indwelling catheters [27] undergo annual cystoscopy and urine cytology with random bladder biopsies every one to two years. Others advocate annual cystoscopic review for 10 years following SCI, and in patients with recurrent or chronic UTI [28]. There is no clear consensus and indeed this school of thought is challenged. Hamid et al. [29] summarized that screening cystoscopy in patients with neurogenic LUT dysfunction and chronic indwelling SPCs could not be validated.

18.7.7 Diet and Fluid Intake Control

Fluid intake control is a major and relevant issue for the majority of patients with neurogenic bladder. There is clear evidence that in case of intermittent catheterization, the frequency and timing of catheterization depends on the fluid intake. This is also relevant in cases of behavioural therapy, such as prompted or timed voiding. For patients who lose bladder filling sensation because of the disease, fluid intake and frequency become major factors in the attempt to control continence. This reinforces the role of education and the bladder diary. Another point is the risk of high nocturnal diuresis in this population due to the interplay of several different mechanisms, including sleep disorders and modification of circadian regulation of creatinine clearance as well as water diuresis [30].

18.8 Conservative Treatment: Pharmacological

Pharmacological modulation of the LUT was originally developed for non-neurogenic patients; however, several patients have been evaluated in the neurogenic population. Pharmacology can be used alone for a subgroup of moderate severity in the neurogenic population, for example Parkinson's disease, stroke, or MS patients suffering from detrusor overactivity without detrusor sphincter dyssynergia. For more severely symptomatic patients, pharmacotherapy can be used in combination with IC, e.g., the MS or SCI patient suffering with urinary incontinence due to

DO could be offered onabotulinum toxin A 200U in association with IC.

Pharmacotherapy often has two main goals: to improve micturition (by treating detrusor sphincter dyssynergia), or to improve continence, detrusor pressure, and bladder capacity.

18.8.1 To Improve Micturition

18.8.1.1 Alpha-Blockers

Only tamlusosin was evaluated in the neurogenic population. Alpha adrenergic receptors are present mainly in the bladder base and in the posterior urethra. The rationale was to improve voiding difficulties due to detrusor sphincter dyssynergia by acting on the smooth muscle component of sphincters. One double-blind, placebo-controlled, international multi-centric study assessed the efficacy of 0.4 mg and 0.8 mg in MS and SCI patients. The study failed to demonstrate efficacy on the primary endpoint (MUP) [31], but showed some improvement in the storage and voiding urodynamic parameters, and symptoms assessed by the International Prostate Symptom Score in the long-term extension. The two dosages show the same type of moderate benefits.

18.8.1.2 Botulinum Toxin

For the same purpose (DSD treatment), injection of the urethral sphincter with botulinum toxin type A was found to improve micturition and to reduce detrusor pressure and residual volume. This was the first urological indication of botulinum toxin in the early 1990s. Several independent studies were performed to assess efficacy. One double-blind placebo-controlled study was conducted to assess the efficacy of transperineal injection of 100 U onabotulinumtoxin A compared to placebo in a population of MS [32] with chronic urinary retention. This study failed to demonstrate a significant decrease of residual volume at one month. Some improvement in maximal detrusor pressure and bladder capacity was observed. Based on this well-designed study, it is difficult to recommend this treatment in the MS population. Moreover, there is no good level of evidence for use in the SCI population.

18.9 Pharmacological Agents to Improve Storage

18.9.1 Parasympatholytic Drugs (Antimuscarinics, Anticholinergics)

Parasympatholytic drugs are used to increase bladder capacity, to decrease detrusor pressure, and to decrease urinary incontinence due to neurogenic detrusor overactivity (NDO). In fact there are two ways to use parasympatholytics. On the one hand, for patients suffering from neurogenic OAB without retention due to DSD, titration is an appropriate way to be in the best balance between efficacy and side effects and to preserve complete micturition. This is typically the case for Parkinson's disease, stroke, or moderately disabled MS patients. Close, careful follow-up is necessary to assess efficacy with a micturition diary and to review cognitive side effects and effects on the bowels, such as constipation, as well as measurement of the PVR volume. This monitoring enables adaptation of both the dose and the drug.

The majority of parasympatholytic agents listed in what follows were developed for the treatment of idiopathic OAB. Few of them were assessed in the neurogenic population, usually on urodynamic parameters only, and very few on symptoms [33].

18.9.1.1 Oxybutynin

Gajewski reported in a prospective randomized trial that oxybutynin was more effective that probantheline in MS patients [34]. Stohrer demonstrated in a randomized study that there was a decrease in incontinence episodes and an improvement in maximal cystometric capacity [35]. In this study, which compared oxybutynin to propiverine, 67% of patients reported a dry mouth in the oxybutynin group.

A recent study assessed different formulations of oxybutynin for the treatment of NDO in children with a significant improvement of all formulations on clinical parameters as well as in urodynamic parameters [36].

18.9.1.2 Propiverine hydrochloride

Propiverine hydrochloride is one of the most-studied drugs in the field of NDO with Stohrer publishing numerous studies [35, 37]. Double-blind studies show a significant benefit in terms of urinary incontinence as well as with cystometric parameters on NDO. There were fewer reports of dry mouth, compared with oxybutynin.

18.9.1.3 Trospium

Trospium as well as propiverine was specifically assessed in the neurogenic population and results in significant benefit in urinary incontinence and cystometric parameters also [38].

The cognitive effects of an antimuscarinic drug depend on the ability of the drug to cross the blood–brain barrier, which in turn depends on the polarity and the size of the molecule; trospium is relatively impermeable to the blood–brain barrier. This side effect should be a major consideration when prescribing antimuscarinics to patients with diseases of the brain.

18.9.1.4 Tolterodine

Tolterodine was studied by Ethans [39] in the neurogenic population in a prospective randomized double-blind crossover study versus oxybutynin and placebo. Tolterodine when used at self-selected doses was comparable in outcome to oxybutynin but with fewer side effects. It seems that doses larger than 2 mg twice daily are mandatory to achieve satisfactory efficiency.

For children, different formulations were tested (oral solution and extended release) in the neurogenic population [40]. The number of incontinence and catheterization episodes was reduced in all groups.

18.9.1.5 Solifenacin

The SONIC study was a double-blind, randomized, active, and placebo-controlled study which demonstrated the efficacy of solifenacin 10 mg once a day on urodynamic parameters at one month [41]. Solifenacin significantly improved quality of life versus placebo in this population. Darifenacin and fesoterodine are approved for the treatment of OAB, but have not been studied in the neurogenic population. Moreover, some authors reported the benefit of association of two anticholinergics mostly in the case of SCI patients [42].

18.9.2 Mirabegron

Mirabegron belongs to a new class of medications, beta-3-receptor agonists, used for the treatment of OAB. Very few data are available for the treatment of neurogenic detrusor overactivity. Pannek published in 2016 preliminary experience with 15 patients [43]. A significant improvement on incontinence episodes and a decrease of urodynamic severity parameters was reported. Side effects include palpitations and are mainly limited to elevation of blood pressure. Placebo-controlled studies and studies comparing mirabegron with anticholinergics are required, however, to clearly determine outcomes.

18.9.3 Treatment of Nocturnal Polyuria

The pathophysiology of nocturnal polyuria in the neurogenic population may have different origins. It may be due to sleep apnoea or modification of blood pressure regulation, and therefore treatment should be tailored, based on a strict diagnostic evaluation [30]. A seven-day bladder diary charting fluid input and bladder output is a vital tool to evaluate this when suspected.

18.9.4 Botulinum Toxins to Improve Storage

Since the first description by Brigitte Schurch [44] of the efficacy of intra-detrusor onabotulinumtoxin A for the treatment of refractory NDO, large, multi-centric, controlled studies have confirmed the results with the best level of evidence [45, 46]. Onabotulinumtoxin A is now registered in several countries across the world for the treatment of urinary incontinence in adult neurological patients with inadequate response to anticholinergic drugs. EAU, International Continence Society (ICS), and International Consultation on Incontinence (ICI) guidelines recommend onabotulinumtoxin A as a second-line treatment for refractory NDO.

Abobotulinumtoxin A was also studied at 500, 750 U with a significant efficacy on incontinence reduction and improvement on urodynamic parameters and quality of life [47]. Phase 3 studies are running to support approval. Dosage, therapeutic window, and pharmacokinetics of the two botulinum toxin A are not interchangeable, and no direct head-to-head comparative studies are available.

In terms of efficacy, clinical studies confirm a dramatic clinical improvement at two weeks post injection with 200 U of onabotulinumtoxin A, with reduction of incontinence episodes, associated with an improvement of relevant urodynamic parameters such as maximal cystometric capacity, reflex volume, detrusor pressure at first contraction, and quality of life. Median duration of treatment with 200 U is around 42 weeks for MS patients and 36 weeks for SCI patients. The percentage of patients fully continent at six weeks is 37%.

The populations studied are mostly SCI and MS patients. Some differences in epidemiological characteristics and mode of micturition may explain variations in efficacy. The percentage of patients fully continent at six weeks is higher in MS (60% versus 32%) and the duration of effect is longer. More MS patients had to use clean IC after botulinum toxin injections, but fewer MS patients used IC at inclusion in the phase 3 studies. A recent placebo-controlled study assessing lower dosage of 100 U of onabotulinumtoxin A in MS patients not using clean IC and with low residual urine showed efficacy, with a lower risk of urinary retention requiring clean IC after injection.

Few studies assessed specifically the efficacy of intra-detrusor botulinum toxin in other aetiologies. Limited open studies report favourable outcomes in Parkinson's disease [48] and stroke populations. This effect must be confirmed by larger studies in these populations where the use of IC is questionable due to poor comprehension or cognitive disorders.

A post hoc analysis showed no benefit in terms of efficacy of concomitant anticholinergic drugs. However, the studies were not designed to show such a difference and need to be further specifically examined. A plateau effect can explain no difference at six weeks, but some authors reported in clinical practice a prolonged effect when using anticholinergic drugs when the efficacy of onabotulinum toxin A decreases.

Botulinum toxin injections are performed under cystoscopic guidance, using either a flexible cystoscope under local anaesthesia or a rigid cystoscope under general anaesthesia. The use of an intra-urethral anaesthetic gel is always recommended in patients with SCI even if the patient has no bladder sensation, in order to reduce the risk of autonomic dysreflexia. For onabotulinumtoxin A, the recommended technique is to perform 30 sites of 1 mL injections in the detrusor sparing the trigone.

In terms of safety, the most frequent side effect is directly related to the mode of action of the drug and is the risk of increasing residual volume, UTI, and the need to perform clean IC after injection. One interesting point is the risk of UTIs; some studies shows in patients using clean IC a reduction of symptomatic UTIs after injections. No risk of exacerbation of MS was noted after injections.

18.10 Tibial Nerve Stimulation

Electrical stimulation can be used to treat neurogenic OAB by stimulating the tibial nerve and modulating the micturition reflex. Electrical stimulation can be delivered either by a needle (percutaneous tibial nerve stimulation) (PTNS) or a transcutaneous (transcutaneous tibial nerve stimulation) electrode. Different studies show a moderate but real effect on symptoms of OAB in the neurogenic population [49], especially in the MS population. The main advantages are that this is a non-invasive or minimally invasive technique, and the treatment does not impair voiding functions.

18.11 Surgery

18.11.1 Surgery for Bladder Storage Dysfunction

18.11.1.1 Sacral Neuromodulation (SNM)

Although the exact mechanism of SNM is unknown, it is thought that the application of an electrical current to the sacral afferents may inhibit sacral efferent activity, in patients with NDO. SNM is not thought to have a direct motor influence on the detrusor muscle. The two-stage surgical procedure can be performed under sedation, which gives it a great advantage over other operations for bladder storage dysfunction. SNM is nevertheless a costly intervention, and long-term outcomes in the NDO group are uncertain.

Studies have been limited by the rather heterogeneous group of neurological patients selected. One such study by Wallace et al. reported outcomes of 33 patients with diagnoses ranging from MS to Parkinson's disease [50]. The number of incontinence episodes and voids in a 24-hour period dropped by 68% and 43%, respectively.

A more recent evaluation by Engeler et al. prospectively reviewed the efficacy and safety of SNM in 17 patients with MS [51]. Sixteen had a positive test phase and at three years, the median voided volume, PVR, and micturition frequency reduced significantly, as did the number of incontinence episodes. The median subjective degree of satisfaction was high, at 80%.

18.11.1.2 Augmentation Cystoplasty

Augmentation cystoplasty is reserved for those patients refractory to medical therapy and minimally invasive surgical procedures. The typical patient will have a poorly compliant, small-capacity bladder, with NDO that may trigger urinary incontinence, such as those with myelomeningocele, or indeed an SCI. Absolute contraindications include inflammatory bowel disease, short bowel syndrome, and radiation or haemorrhagic colitis.

Any bowel/stomach segment may be used, although ileum is preferred, and the most surgically accessible segment, in order to increase bladder capacity and suppress detrusor contractions. The long-term outcomes remain excellent with continence rates of more than 90% during both the day and night [52]. Overall patient satisfaction with the procedure is high, with a reported improvement in quality of life scores also at more than 90% [53]. There is a high likelihood that neurogenic patients will have to self-catheterize in order to empty the augmented bladder, and therefore they should be taught and consented for this preoperatively. For those unable to reach the urethra, a Mitrofanoff continent catheterizable stoma is also an option. A channel is surgically fashioned which connects the umbilicus to the augmented bladder. The appendix is the appendage of choice for the Mitrofanoff channel. It is also possible to use the Fallopian tube or indeed a short section of ileum. The main complications that bother patients in the long term are problems with stenosis of the channel and skin fistulation [54].

Recent advances point to the possibility in the future of replacing a patient's neurogenic bladder with a laboratory-grown artificial urinary bladder, using the patient's own urothelial cells [55]. The technique is not yet approved by the Food and Drug Administration as further clinical trials are required; however, initial results are extremely promising.

18.11.1.3   Urinary Diversion

For severely incontinent patients, urinary diversion is a valid alternative. This surgical diversion may be continent (using the Mitrofanoff channel, described earlier) or incontinent, in the form of an ileal conduit. For those unable to catheterize, or those with deteriorating renal function or severe disability, the ileal conduit is a reliable operation. The external stoma appliances may be changed by the patient or a carer. The surgical revision rate is lower compared with the Mitrofanoff channel; however, the overall complication rate appears to be high, and up to 50%, in patients with MS [56].

18.11.2   Surgery for Bladder Outlet Dysfunction

Bladder outlet dysfunction may result in either difficulty in voiding or urinary incontinence. The outlet maybe functionally obstructed, most commonly in neurogenic patients, due to DSD. The lack of coordination between the bladder and the external urethral sphincter muscle (EUS) in DSD can result in poor bladder emptying and high bladder pressures, which may lead to progressive renal damage. Historically, patients were given medical therapy in the form of alpha-1 sympathetic blockade, with medications such as tamsulosin and alfuzosin. There is no convincing evidence that alpha-blockers reduce functional obstruction [57]; however, they may be useful in treating those who continue to suffer voiding dysfunction despite surgery.

Various surgical techniques have been employed to reduce this functional obstruction. These include: balloon dilatation of the EUS (risks stricture formation, which may require surgical intervention), intra-sphincteric botulinum toxin injections (a therapy which needs to be repeated for continued efficacy), surgical sphincterotomy, and placement of a sphincteric stent. Stents placed across the surgical sphincter are associated with the possible complications of stent migration, encrustation, and urethral stone formation, which would require surgical removal of the stent [58].

18.11.2.1   Surgical External Sphincterotomy

Surgical external sphincterotomy performed endoscopically is undoubtedly an effective treatment for DSD; however, high intra-renal pressure may not resolve, which increases the risk of long-term renal dysfunction [59]. Resection of the sphincter is usually performed with a Collins knife, at 12 o'clock position to minimize haemorrhage. Post-operatively, the male patient will need to wear an external urinary containment device, such as a penile sheath. In a study reported by Pan et al., 68% of the 84 patients experienced recurrent UTIs and upper tract dilatation on imaging, but there were no reports of progressive renal failure [60].

18.11.2.2   The Artificial Urinary Sphincter (AUS)

This is a treatment for neuropathic external urethral sphincter weakness. It should only be offered once any detrusor overactivity has been tackled as in some patients, reducing the bladder pressure by means of anticholinergics, intra-detrusor botulinum toxin, or augmentation cystoplasty may be sufficient to achieve continence. The AMS800^{TM} is a three-part device which consists of an inflatable cuff, which can be placed around the bladder neck in men and women or around the bulbar urethral sphincter in men. Fluid-filled tubing from the cuff connects to a pressure-regulating balloon in the extra-peritoneal space and to a labial/scrotal pump, which is used to activate or deactivate the system. The cuff supplies continuous compression to the urethra. When the patient wishes to void, the pump is squeezed and fluid exits the cuff and moves to the balloon. It takes three minutes for the cuff to fill again and voiding should be completed during this time.

Urinary continence is achieved in 73% (61–96), with complication rates of 12% (3–33) for mechanical failure of the device [61]. There are recent reports of success rates in female adult neurological patients of 57.7% with median follow-up of 7.5 years [62]. Most erosions occur in the first year after implantation, and primary implant infection rates are 1–5% [63].

Although the AUS has stood the test of time, there are alternatives such as intra-sphincteric injection of bulking agents. However, these lose efficacy and need to be repeated regularly.

18.11.2.3 Minimally Invasive Surgical Treatments

Recently, minimally invasive approaches are gaining popularity for the treatment of male SUI. Slings are cheaper than the AUS, are an easier operation to perform, and avoid the need to operate a mechanical device to void. The transobturator AdVanceXP® male sling supports the urethra, and is thought to improve urinary continence in a non-compressive manner, by relocating the proximal urethra more proximally [64]. After a mean follow-up of almost three years, 46% of the patients could be classified as cured and 29% as improved on the basis of pad use and a 24-hour pad test. A significant decrease in mean pad use per day was reported, along with improvement of scores on the International Consultation on Incontinence Questionnaire and Incontinence Quality of Life Questionnaire [65]. Despite its attributes, the male sling still risks urethral erosion, osteitis pubis, urinary retention, and chronic perineal pain.

The ProACT^{TM} device consists of two silicone balloons placed at either side of the bladder neck. Each balloon is attached to a titanium port placed in the scrotum, aiming to achieve continence through static extrinsic compression and support of the urethra. Potential advantages over both the AUS and male sling include the lack of circumferential compression (therefore reducing the risk of urethral atrophy), and balloon volumes may be adjusted postoperatively in the outpatient department in order to achieve maximum continence; minimal chances of mechanical failure, except balloon deflation; and, lastly, the operative procedure is far easier than placement of an AUS device [64].

In terms of outcome, the AUS had the highest percentage of success, followed by the urethral sling procedures, compared to the urethral bulking agents, which reported the highest rate of failure. However with the AUS, there was a higher reoperation rate per patient as compared with the sling procedure (66).

18.11.3 Surgery to Improve Both Continence and Micturition in Spinal Cord Injured Patients: The Brindley Stimulator

The Brindley stimulator is a surgical solution consisting of an implantable sacral anterior nerve stimulator to stimulate on demand detrusor contraction and a posterior sacral root deafferentation from S2 to S5. Basically the goal is to achieve complete continence by sacral deafferentation of the micturition reflex and micturition by anterior sacral root stimulation without catheterization. The prototypical patient who may benefit is a stable, complete paraplegic patient. Although the stimulator is very well tolerated and has a very long life expectancy, many patients decline the Brindley stimulator as a treatment option for their bladder (continence achieved in up to 85%), because of the impact on erectile function and also on defecation, although specific programmes can be used to restore those functions. This procedure requires the backing of a highly specialized team, in order to carefully select the patient, to perform the procedure, and to follow up with the patients in the long term [67].

18.12 Long-Term Follow-Up

The authors recommend annual review, at the very least, of patients with neurogenic LUT dysfunction. The aim is to prevent urological complications developing, such as lithiasis, recurrent UTIs, and upper urinary tract deterioration, as well as to improve quality of life.

Neurology and urology are not exclusive subspecialties. For example, a patient with Parkinson's disease could be suffering with neurogenic LUT dysfunction, but equally could have benign prostatic hyperplasia, causing bladder outflow obstruction, or both. The paraplegic patient with cauda equina syndrome could have intrinsic urethral sphincter deficiency due to neurological disease, but could equally suffer from concomitant pelvic organ prolapse, independent from the neurogenic dysfunction. Coordinated multidisciplinary input is vital for successful management of neurological patients with bladder dysfunction.

References

1. de Groat WC, Griffiths D, Yoshimura N. Neural control of the lower urinary tract. *Comprehensive Physiology* 2015; **5**(1): 327–96.

2. National Institute for Health and Care Excellence. *Urinary incontinence in neurological disease: Management of lower urinary tract dysfunction in neurological disease.* London, UK: National Institute for Health and Care Excellence: Guidance, 2012.

3. Esclarin de Ruz A, Garcia Leoni E, Herruzo Cabrera R. Epidemiology and risk factors for urinary tract infection in patients with spinal cord injury. *Journal of Urology* 2000; **164**(4): 1285–9.

4. Garcia Leoni ME, Esclarin De Ruz A. Management of urinary tract infection in patients with spinal cord injuries. *Clinical Microbiology and Infection: The Official Publication of the European Society of Clinical Microbiology and Infectious Diseases* 2003; **9**(8): 780–5.

5. Cardenas DD, Hoffman JM, Kirshblum S, McKinley W. Etiology and incidence of rehospitalization after traumatic spinal cord injury: A multicenter analysis. *Archives of Physical Medicine and Rehabilitation* 2004; **85**(11): 1757–63.

6. Murphy DP, Lampert V. Current implications of drug resistance in spinal cord injury. *American Journal of Physical Medicine & Rehabilitation.* 2003; **82**(1): 72–5.

7. Darouiche RO, Al Mohajer M, Siddiq DM, Minard CG. Short versus long course of antibiotics for catheter-associated urinary tract infections in patients with spinal cord injury: A randomized controlled noninferiority trial. *Archives of Physical Medicine and Rehabilitation* 2014; **95**(2): 290–6.

8. Poirier C, Dinh A, Salomon J, Grall N, Andremont A, Bernard L. Prevention of urinary tract infections by antibiotic cycling in spinal cord injury patients and low emergence of multidrug resistant bacteria. *Medecine et maladies infectieuses* 2016; **46**(6): 294–9.

9. Darouiche RO, Green BG, Donovan WH, Chen D, Schwartz M, Merritt J, et al. Multicenter randomized controlled trial of bacterial interference for prevention of urinary tract infection in patients with neurogenic bladder. *Urology* 2011; **78**(2): 341–6.

10. Phé V, Pakzad M, Curtis C, Porter B, Haslam C, Chataway J, Panicker JN. Urinary tract infections in multiple sclerosis. *Mult. Scler.* 2016; **22**(7): 855–61. doi:10.1177/1352458516633903

11. Abrams PH, Dunn M, George N. Urodynamic findings in chronic retention of urine and their relevance to results of surgery. *British Medical Journal* 1978; **2**(6147): 1258–60.

12. Drake MJ, Apostolidis A, Cocci A, Emmanuel A, Gajewski JB, Harrison SC, et al. Neurogenic lower urinary tract dysfunction: Clinical management recommendations of the Neurologic Incontinence committee of the fifth International Consultation on Incontinence 2013. *Neurourology and Urodynamics* 2016; **35**(6): 657–65.

13. Deville WL, Yzermans JC, Van Duijn NP, Bezemer PD, Van der Windt DA, Bouter LM. The urine dipstick test useful to rule out infections: A meta-analysis of the accuracy. *BMC Urology* 2004; **4**: 4.

14. Nicolle LE. Urinary tract infections in patients with spinal injuries. *Current Infectious Disease Reports* 2014; **16**(1): 390.

15. De Ridder D, Vermeulen C, Ketelaer P, Van Poppel H, Baert L. Pelvic floor rehabilitation in multiple sclerosis. *Acta neurologica Belgica.* 1999; **99**(1): 61–4.

16. Weld KJ, Dmochowski RR. Effect of bladder management on urological complications in spinal cord injured patients. *Journal of Urology* 2000; **163**(3): 768–72.

17. Killorin W, Gray M, Bennett JK, Green BG. The value of urodynamics and bladder management in predicting upper urinary tract complications in male spinal cord injury patients. *Paraplegia* 1992; **30**(6): 437–41.

18. Averbeck MA, Altaweel W, Manu-Marin A, Madersbacher H. Management of LUTS in patients with dementia and associated disorders. *Neurourology and Urodynamics* 2017; **36**(2): 245–52.

19. Abrams P, Agarwal M, Drake M, El-Masri W, Fulford S, Reid S, et al. A proposed guideline for the urological management of patients with spinal cord injury. *BJU Int.* 2008;**101**(8):989–94.

20. Lapides J, Diokno AC, Silber SJ, Lowe BS. Clean, intermittent self-catheterization in the treatment of urinary tract disease. *Journal of Urology* 1972; **107**(3): 458–61.

21. Moore KN, Fader M, Getliffe K. Long-term bladder management by intermittent catheterisation in adults and children. *Cochrane Database of Systematic Reviews* 2007; **4**: CD006008.

22. Herschorn S, Gajewski J, Ethans K, Corcos J, Carlson K, Bailly G, et al. Efficacy of botulinum toxin A injection for neurogenic detrusor overactivity and urinary incontinence: A randomized, double-blind trial. *Journal of Urology* 2011; **185**(6): 2229–35.

23. Lindehall B, Abrahamsson K, Jodal U, Olsson I, Sillen U. Complications of clean intermittent catheterization in young females with myelomeningocele: 10 to 19 years of followup. *Journal of Urology* 2007; **178**(3 Pt. 1): 1053–5.

24. Game X, Castel-Lacanal E, Bentaleb Y, Thiry-Escudie I, De Boissezon X, Malavaud B, et al. Botulinum toxin A detrusor injections in patients with neurogenic detrusor overactivity significantly decrease the incidence of symptomatic urinary tract infections. *European Urology* 2008; **53**(3): 613–18.

25. Feifer A, Corcos J. Contemporary role of suprapubic cystostomy in treatment of neuropathic bladder dysfunction in spinal cord injured patients. *Neurourology and Urodynamics* 2008; **27**(6): 475–9.

26. National Institute for Health and Care Excellence. *Urinary incontinence in neurological disease (CG148)*. London, UK: National Institute for Health and Care Excellence, 2012.

27. Broecker BH, Klein FA, Hackler RH. Cancer of the bladder in spinal cord injury patients. *Journal of Urology* 1981; **125**(2): 196–7.

28. Navon JD, Soliman H, Khonsari F, Ahlering T. Screening cystoscopy and survival of spinal cord injured patients with squamous cell cancer of the bladder. *Journal of Urology* 1997; **157**(6): 2109–11.

29. Hamid R, Bycroft J, Arya M, Shah PJ. Screening cystoscopy and biopsy in patients with neuropathic bladder and chronic suprapubic indwelling catheters: Is it valid? *Journal of Urology* 2003; **170**(2 Pt. 1): 425–7.

30. Denys MA, Viaene A, Goessaert AS, Van Haverbeke F, Hoebeke P, Raes A, et al. Circadian rhythms in water and solute handling in adults with a spinal cord injury. *Journal of Urology* 2017; **197**(2): 445–51.

31. Abrams P, Amarenco G, Bakke A, Buczynski A, Castro-Diaz D, Harrison S, et al. Tamsulosin: Efficacy and safety in patients with neurogenic lower urinary tract dysfunction due to suprasacral spinal cord injury. *Journal of Urology* 2003; **170**(4 Pt. 1): 1242–51.

32. Gallien P, Reymann JM, Amarenco G, Nicolas B, de Seze M, Bellissant E. Placebo controlled, randomised, double blind study of the effects of botulinum A toxin on detrusor sphincter dyssynergia in multiple sclerosis patients. *Journal of Neurology, Neurosurgery, and Psychiatry* 2005; **76**(12): 1670–6.

33. Madhuvrata P, Singh M, Hasafa Z, Abdel-Fattah M. Anticholinergic drugs for adult neurogenic detrusor overactivity: A systematic review and meta-analysis. *European Urology* 2012; **62**(5): 816–30.

34. Gajewski JB, Awad SA. Oxybutynin versus propantheline in patients with multiple sclerosis and detrusor hyperreflexia. *Journal of Urology* 1986; **135**(5): 966–8.

35. Stohrer M, Murtz G, Kramer G, Schnabel F, Arnold EP, Wyndaele JJ, et al. Propiverine compared to oxybutynin in neurogenic detrusor overactivity: Results of a randomized, double-blind, multicenter clinical study. *European Urology* 2007; **51**(1): 235–42.

36. Franco I, Horowitz M, Grady R, Adams RC, de Jong TP, Lindert K, et al. Efficacy and safety of oxybutynin in children with detrusor hyperreflexia secondary to neurogenic bladder dysfunction. *Journal of Urology* 2005; **173**(1): 221–5.

37. Stohrer M, Madersbacher H, Richter R, Wehnert J, Dreikorn K. Efficacy and safety of propiverine in SCI-patients suffering from detrusor hyperreflexia: A double-blind, placebo-controlled clinical trial. *Spinal Cord* 1999; **37**(3): 196–200.

38. Stohrer M, Bauer P, Giannetti BM, Richter R, Burgdorfer H, Murtz G. Effect of trospium chloride on urodynamic parameters in patients with detrusor hyperreflexia due to spinal cord injuries: A multicentre placebo-controlled double-blind trial. *Urologia internationalis* 1991; **47**(3): 138–43.

39. Ethans KD, Nance PW, Bard RJ, Casey AR, Schryvers OI. Efficacy and safety of tolterodine in people with neurogenic detrusor overactivity. *Journal of Spinal Cord Medicine* 2004; **27**(3): 214–18.

40. Reddy PP, Borgstein NG, Nijman RJ, Ellsworth PI. Long-term efficacy and safety of tolterodine in children with neurogenic detrusor overactivity. *Journal of Pediatric Urology* 2008; **4**(6): 428–33.

41. Amarenco G, Sutory M, Zachoval R, Agarwal M, Del Popolo G, Tretter R, et al. Solifenacin is effective and well tolerated in patients with neurogenic detrusor overactivity: Results from the double-blind, randomized, active- and placebo-controlled SONIC urodynamic study. *Neurourology and Urodynamics* 2017; **36**(2): 414–21.

42. Amend B, Hennenlotter J, Schafer T, Horstmann M, Stenzl A, Sievert KD. Effective treatment of neurogenic detrusor dysfunction by combined high-dosed antimuscarinics without increased side-effects. *European Urology* 2008; **53**(5): 1021–8.

43. Wollner J, Pannek J. Initial experience with the treatment of neurogenic detrusor overactivity with a new beta-3 agonist (mirabegron) in patients with spinal cord injury. *Spinal Cord* 2016; **54**(1): 78–82.

44. Schurch B, Stohrer M, Kramer G, Schmid DM, Gaul G, Hauri D. Botulinum-A toxin for treating detrusor hyperreflexia in spinal cord injured patients: A new alternative to anticholinergic drugs? Preliminary results. *Journal of Urology*. 2000; **164**(3 Pt. 1): 692–7.

45. Schurch B, de Seze M, Denys P, Chartier-Kastler E, Haab F, Everaert K, et al. Botulinum toxin type a is a safe and effective treatment for neurogenic urinary incontinence: Results of a single treatment, randomized, placebo controlled 6-month study. *Journal of Urology* 2005; **174**(1): 196–200.

46. Cruz F, Herschorn S, Aliotta P, Brin M, Thompson C, Lam W, et al. Efficacy and safety of onabotulinumtoxinA in patients with urinary incontinence due to neurogenic detrusor overactivity: A randomised, double-blind, placebo-controlled trial. *European Urology* 2011; **60**(4): 742–50.

47. Denys P, Del Popolo G, Amarenco G, Karsenty G, Le Berre P, Padrazzi B, et al. Efficacy and safety of two administration modes of an intra-detrusor injection of 750 units dysport(R) (abobotulinumtoxinA) in patients suffering from refractory neurogenic detrusor overactivity (NDO): A randomised placebo-controlled phase IIa study. *Neurourology and Urodynamics* 2017; **36**(2): 457–62.

48. Giannantoni A, Conte A, Proietti S, Giovannozzi S, Rossi A, Fabbrini G, et al. Botulinum toxin type A in patients with Parkinson's disease and refractory overactive bladder. *Journal of Urology* 2011; **186**(3): 960–4.

49. de Seze M, Raibaut P, Gallien P, Even-Schneider A, Denys P, Bonniaud V, et al. Transcutaneous posterior tibial nerve stimulation for treatment of the overactive bladder syndrome in multiple sclerosis: Results of a multicenter prospective study. *Neurourology and Urodynamics* 2011; **30**(3): 306–11.

50. Wallace PA, Lane FL, Noblett KL. Sacral nerve neuromodulation in patients with underlying neurologic disease. *Am. J. Obstet. Gynecol.* 2007; **197**(1): 96 e1-5.

51. Engeler DS, Meyer D, Abt D, Muller S, Schmid HP. Sacral neuromodulation for the treatment of neurogenic lower urinary tract dysfunction caused by multiple sclerosis: A single-centre prospective series. *BMC Urology* 2015; **15**: 105.

52. Mundy AR, Stephenson TP. 'Clam' ileocystoplasty for the treatment of refractory urge incontinence. *British Journal of Urology* 1985; **57**(6): 641–6.

53. Khastgir J, Hamid R, Arya M, Shah N, Shah PJ. Surgical and patient reported outcomes of 'clam' augmentation ileocystoplasty in spinal cord injured patients. *European Urology* 2003; **43**(3): 263–9.

54. Perrouin-Verbe MA, Chartier-Kastler E, Even A, Denys P, Roupret M, Phe V. Long-term complications of continent cutaneous urinary diversion in adult spinal cord injured patients. *Neurourology and Urodynamics* 2016; **35**(8): 1046–50.

55. Atala A. Tissue engineering of artificial organs. *J. Endourol.* 2000; **14**(1): 49–57.

56. Legrand G, Roupret M, Comperat E, Even-Schneider A, Denys P, Chartier-Kastler E. Functional outcomes after management of end-stage neurological bladder dysfunction with ileal conduit in a multiple sclerosis population: A monocentric experience. *Urology* 2011; **78**(4): 937–41.

57. Chancellor MB, Erhard MJ, Rivas DA. Clinical effect of alpha-1 antagonism by terazosin on external and internal urinary sphincter function. *J. Am. Paraplegia Soc.* 1993; **16**(4): 207–14.

58. Hussain M, Greenwell TJ, Shah J, Mundy A. Long-term results of a self-expanding wallstent in the treatment of urethral stricture. *BJU Int.* 2004; **94**(7): 1037–9.

59. Reynard JM, Vass J, Sullivan ME, Mamas M. Sphincterotomy and the treatment of detrusor-sphincter dyssynergia: Current status, future prospects. *Spinal Cord* 2003; **41**(1): 1–11.

60. Pan D, Troy A, Rogerson J, Bolton D, Brown D, Lawrentschuk N. Long-term outcomes of external sphincterotomy in a spinal injured population. *Journal Urology* 2009; **181**(2): 705–9.

61. Hussain M, Greenwell TJ, Venn SN, Mundy AR. The current role of the artificial urinary sphincter for the treatment of urinary incontinence. *Journal Urology* 2005; **174**(2): 418–24.

62. Phe V, Leon P, Granger B, Denys P, Bitker MO, Mozer P, et al. Stress urinary incontinence in female neurological patients: Long-term functional outcomes after artificial urinary sphincter (AMS 800TM) implantation. *Neurourology and Urodynamics* 2017; **36**(3): 764–9.

63. Lai HH, Hsu EI, Teh BS, Butler EB, Boone TB. 13 years of experience with artificial urinary sphincter implantation at Baylor College of Medicine. *Journal of Urology* 2007; **177**(3): 1021–5.

64. Gilling PJ, Bell DF, Wilson LC, Westenberg AM, Reuther R, Fraundorfer MR. An adjustable continence therapy device for treating incontinence after prostatectomy: A minimum 2-year follow-up. *BJU Int.* 2008; **102**(10): 1426–30; discussion 30–1.

65. Bauer RM, Grabbert MT, Klehr B, Gebhartl P, Gozzi C, Homberg R, et al. 36-month data for the AdVance XP(R) male sling: Results of a prospective multicentre study. *BJU Int.* 2017; **119**(4): 626–30.

66. Farag F, Koens M, Sievert KD, De Ridder D, Feitz W, Heesakkers J. Surgical treatment of neurogenic stress urinary incontinence: A systematic review of quality assessment and surgical outcomes. *Neurourology and Urodynamics* 2016; **35**(1): 21–5.

67. Ren J, Chew DJ, Biers S, Thiruchelvam N. Electrical nerve stimulation to promote micturition in spinal cord injury patients: A review of current attempts. *Neurourology and Urodynamics* 2016; **35**(3): 365–70.

Chapter 19

Management of Neurogenic Bowel Dysfunction

Anton Emmanuel

19.1 Introduction

Bowel control (entailing voluntary control of colonic voiding and ability to defer when socially inappropriate) is a complex function, dependent on the integrity of the bidirectional brain-gut axis [1]. It is therefore predictable that central nervous system (CNS) diseases influence these functions, resulting in constipation and faecal incontinence. These neurological diseases have a major impact on patients' lives, and bowel dysfunction carries with it considerable anxiety and restriction of quality of life [2, 3].

For patients with spinal cord injury (SCI), whether supraconal or cauda equina, the prevalence of bowel dysfunction is between 42% and 95% of individuals [1, 4–6]. Constipation is the most common manifestation, but as many as 75% experience faecal incontinence [5]. Bowel dysfunction is ranked as the second most restricting consequence of spinal injury [2], ahead of pain and sexual dysfunction. The severity and likelihood of bowel dysfunction increase with the completeness of [5] and time since [7] injury. Amongst children with spina bifida 79% have symptoms of bowel dysfunction [8] with little diminution of symptom burden with age [9]. In multiple sclerosis (MS), up to two-thirds of patients experience bowel symptoms during the course of their illness, and these are associated with significant reduction in quality of life [10, 11]. Constipation occurs in more than 50% of patients with established Parkinson's disease, and pre-dates diagnosis in 20% [12]. The quality-of-life impact relates to the time spent toileting, dependence on carers, fears of – and actual – faecal incontinence and disruption to routine.

It is important to recognize that whilst constipation and incontinence are the focus of most consultations, the term neurogenic bowel dysfunction (NBD) includes other gut problems occurring with increased frequency in patients with neurological disease: haemorrhoids, anal fissure, rectal prolapse, megacolon, and colonic volvulus [13]. Management of these

complications falls outside the scope of this chapter. The overall burden is that there is a more than doubling of the rate of hospitalization in neurological disease patients with NBD compared to those without [14]. This is especially relevant as the length of survival after spinal injury or neurological diagnosis increases [15].

The symptoms of bowel dysfunction in an individual depend upon the location and severity of CNS damage, essentially relating to partial or complete impairment of sensory and/or voluntary motor function to the hindgut and pelvic floor [1]. The result is alterations in gut transit and anorectal sensory awareness of urge and ability to void the bowel. Lesions above the level of the termination of the spinal cord – supraconal lesions – result in what is termed a *reflex bowel*. Essentially, loss of supraspinal inhibitory control leads to a hypertonic, hyperreflexic distal colon and rectum [1, 16]; this tends to cause difficulty with voiding with possible reflex voiding in response to digital stimulation of the anus. By contrast, lesions of the conus medullaris or the cauda equina result in a *flaccid bowel*, with hypotonia and hyporeflexia of the colon and reduced anal sphincter pressure [1, 16]; this tends to cause faecal impaction and a tendency to faecal soiling.

The actual symptoms experienced also relate to a balance between other aspects of the underlying CNS disorder – altered mobility, spasticity, altered cognitive function, adverse effects of medication, and co-morbid illnesses (e.g., the increased prevalence of coeliac disease in patients with MS [13]).

19.2 Treatment: General

A logical approach to therapy is based on addressing the factors listed earlier in each individual and, as such, therapy is informed by evidence rather than being rigidly protocoled. Careful clinical assessment is therefore critical: history should document current bowel pattern and the particular steps required, premorbid bowel function history, medication usage, and impact on quality of life [13]. This can be complemented by use of a diet and bowel diary. The dataset required for such an assessment in patients with SCI has been developed [17]. To quantify symptom severity the neurogenic bowel dysfunction score has been developed [18], primarily for SCI but latterly also used in patients with MS.

Digital anorectal examination is mandatory, to assess anal tone, voluntary contraction, and sensation in addition to rectal fullness. This can be quantified in specialist centres or with treatment of refractory patients, by anorectal physiology testing [13, 19]. In such situations, assessment of whole gut transit time (most commonly with abdominal X-ray after ingestion of radio-opaque markers) can complement the assessment [13]. The place for anorectal physiology studies has not been established, but the assessment may help in defining the level and completeness of spinal injury [19]. In patients with multiple sclerosis, such testing may even help determine treatment [20].

In the absence of definitive controlled trials in the management of neurogenic bowel dysfunction, an empirical approach to therapy is usually adopted in a rehabilitation setting. This stepwise approach has been crystallized in the treatment pyramid (Figure 19.1), which argues for conservative therapy as a starting point, and for refractory patients to progress through more interventional approaches, including transanal irrigation and even consideration of surgery [21]. Another key factor in the general approach to bowel management in patients with neurological disease is that studies often compare different bowel regimes as a whole rather than individual

drug or non-pharmacological components of that regime [22]. As such, therapy tends to be empiric and tailored to the individual, with rigorous controlled trials not being feasible given the heterogeneous patient population.

19.3 Treatment: Non-Pharmacological

19.3.1 Structured assessment
Harari et al. reported a study of 146 patients following a stroke who were randomized to standard bowel care versus a nurse-led structured assessment dictating a patient education [23]. There was a short-term increase in bowel frequency and satisfaction with bowel function, but this did not persist at one year. What was clear at one year was that patients in the education group were more likely to be using diet, fluid intake, and laxatives to manage their bowel than those in the control group [23].

19.3.2 Timing of bowel regime
A bowel-opening regime aimed at voiding in the morning is effective more rapidly than a regime aimed at voiding in the evening [24]. This study of 39 post-stroke patients showed that optimal continence when timing for bowel management was matched to pre-stroke bowel habit.

In another small study of 35 chronic SCI patients [25] it was suggested that standard bowel care was preferable to stepwise care in terms of faecal incontinence and time spent on bowel care.

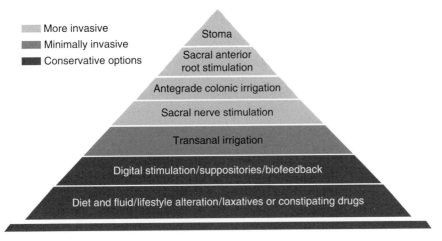

More invasive
Minimally invasive
Conservative options

Stoma
Sacral anterior root stimulation
Antegrade colonic irrigation
Sacral nerve stimulation
Transanal irrigation
Digital stimulation/suppositories/biofeedback
Diet and fluid/lifestyle alteration/laxatives or constipating drugs

Figure 19.1 Treatment pyramid for the management of neurogenic bowel dysfunction

19.3.3 Abdominal massage

A randomized study of the additional benefit of abdominal massage over the effect of lifestyle education was undertaken in 30 patients with MS [26]. After four weeks there was an improvement in constipation, but this was not maintained and not associated with improved quality of life.

19.3.4 Dietary intervention

Only one randomized controlled study of fluid intake appears in the literature. In 40 post-stroke patients, it was shown that carbonated drinks improved overall constipation scores compared to tap water, although there was no actual increase in stool output [27].

With regard to dietary fibre, a crossover trial of fibre-fortified drinks versus unfortified control in 15 institutionalized adults [28] suggested that enema use was reduced with fibre supplementation. There was, however, no alteration in stool output [28]. An uncontrolled study of patients with Parkinson's disease [29] suggested that insoluble fibre supplementation resulted in less constipation and improved L-dopa kinetics (and hence motor function). A similarly uncontrolled study of 11 SCI patients showed that fibre *prolonged* transit and did not improve stool output [30].

19.3.5 Biofeedback

Anorectal and pelvic floor biofeedback was studied in 21 SCI patients with constipation [31]. Patients with incomplete SCI responded as well as functional controls, and demonstrated improved sensorimotor function and balloon expulsion.

19.3.6 Summary

While there is little evidence to support most lifestyle modifications, they are commonly used as first-line therapy. This approach is most often supplemented by digital anal stimulation to trigger voiding [32].

19.4 Treatment: Pharmacological

19.4.1 Laxatives

Two different eight-week placebo-controlled trials in patients with Parkinson's disease have shown that bulking laxatives (fibre) improve stool output and frequency [33] and that osmotic laxatives increase bowel frequency, albeit at the cast of looser stools [34]. For these commonly used drugs no data remain in SCI or MS.

19.4.2 Prokinetics

The cholinomimetic neostigmine, given intravenously in a placebo-controlled crossover study of SCI patients, was found to increase rectal evacuation, as assessed by proctography [35]. A more practically usable therapy, oral prucalopride (a 5HT-4 receptor agonist) was shown in 23 SCI patients to be associated with accelerated transit and increased bowel frequency [36]. Note that five patients had to discontinue therapy due to adverse effects (mostly gastrointestinal, i.e. loose stool, nausea, and abdominal cramp).

19.4.3 Suppositories

There is only one study in the neurogenic bowel literature, in 15 SCI patients, showing that PEG-based bisacodyl suppositories were more effective than normal bisacodyl suppositories in terms of speed of onset of evacuation [37].

19.4.4 Summary

While laxatives and suppositories are the most commonly used pharmacological options, there is little published evidence of their efficacy [32].

19.5 Treatment: Instrumental and Surgical

19.5.1 Transanal irrigation

Following a definitive randomized controlled trial of a large cohort of SCI patients [38], transanal irrigation has become established as a key option in managing NBD [21]. Long-term cost-effectiveness has been demonstrated (primarily related to reduced hospitalizations, reduced urinary tract infections, and reduced stoma surgery) [39]. The key to optimizing outcomes is careful patient selection, taking indication and contraindications into account, directly supervised training of the patient by experienced healthcare personnel, and sustained follow-up to improve adherence. A tailored, stepped approach to care is advocated to maintain outcome.

19.5.2 Neuromodulation

Sacral nerve stimulation has been proposed in a single publication of 13 SCI patients with incomplete injuries as being of potential value, especially when faecal incontinence is the dominant symptom [40]. However, no long-term data support this costly and invasive procedure, and the technique is not used in NBD to any extent [13].

19.5.3 Antegrade irrigation surgery

The Malone appendicostomy for antegrade colonic enema (ACE) administration has been a key therapy for children with faecal incontinence secondary to spina bifida [41]. Improvement in bowel function (voiding and continence) is seen in up to 87% of patients, and a decision analysis concluded that ACE is the best long-term treatment modality for NBD [42]. As with transanal irrigation, careful patient selection and training are key to longer-term success.

19.5.4 Somato-autonomic reflex arc surgery

Pioneered in China as a therapy for neurogenic bladder dysfunction, the technique was suggested as a possible therapy for bowel symptoms, but has not been found effective in a study of 10 patients with complete SCI [43].

19.5.5 Stoma formation surgery

When conservative therapies and transanal irrigation fail to improve symptoms, stoma surgery is an option for NBD patients [13]. A range of studies have shown that colostomy reduces bowel symptoms and time spent on bowel care, as well as improving independence from carers, and hence improving quality of life [44, 45]. Safadi et al. showed in a study of 45 SCI patients that outcomes were functionally equivalent whatever surgery was done, whether right-sided colostomy, left-sided colostomy, or ileostomy [45].

References

1. Craggs MD, Balasubramaniam AV, Chung EAL, et al. Aberrant reflexes and function of the pelvic organs following spinal injury in man. *Autonomic Neuroscience* 2006; 126–7, 355–70.

2. Glickman S, Kamm MA. Bowel dysfunction in spinal cord injury patients. *Lancet* 1996; **347** (9016): 1651–3.

3. Byrne CM, Pager CK, Rex J, et al. Assessment of quality of life in the treatment of patients with neuropathic fecal incontinence. *Dis. Colon Rectum* 2002; **45**: 1431–6.

4. Stone JM, Nino-Murcia M, Wolfe VA, et al. Chronic gastrointestinal problems in spinal cord injury patients: A prospective analysis. *Am. J. Gastroenterol.* 1990; **84**: 1114–19.

5. Krogh K, Nielsen J, Djurhuus JC, et al. Colorectal function in patients with spinal cord lesions. *Dis. Colon Rectum* 1997; **40**: 1233–9.

6. De Loose D, Van Laere M, Muynck De, et al. Constipation and other chronic gastrointestinal problems in spinal cord injured patients. *Spinal Cord* 1998; **36**: 63–6.

7. Faaborg PM, Christensen P, Finnerup N, et al. The pattern of colorectal dysfunction changes with time since spinal cord injury. *Spinal Cord* 2008; **46**: 234–8.

8. Lie HR, Lagergren J, Rasmussen F, et al. Bowel and bladder control of children with myelomeningocele: A Nordic study. *Dev. Med. Child. Neurol.* 1991; **35**: 1053–61.

9. Krogh K, Lie HR, Bilenberg N, et al. Bowel function in Danish children with myelomeningocele. *APMIS Suppl.* 2003; **109**: 81–5.

10. Preziosi G, Raptis DA, Raeburn A, et al. Gut dysfunction in patients with multiple sclerosis and the role of spinal cord involvement in the disease. *Eur. J. Gastroenterol. Hepatol.* 2013; **25**: 1044–50.

11. Nortvedt MW, Riise T, Frugard J, et al. Prevalence of bladder, bowel and sexual problems among multiple sclerosis patients two to five years after diagnosis. *Mult. Scler.* 2007; **13**: 106–12.

12. Chen H, Zhao EJ, Zhang W, et al. Meta-analyses on prevalence of selected Parkinson's nonmotor symptoms before and after diagnosis. *Transl. Neurodegener.* 2015; **4**: 1–6.

13. Emmanuel A Managing neurogenic bowel dysfunction. *Clin. Rehabil.* 2010; **24**: 483–8.

14. Sonnenberg A, Tsou VT, Muller AD. The 'institutional colon': A frequent colonic dysmotility in psychiatric and neurologic disease. *Am. J. Gastro.* 1994; **89**: 62–6.

15. Biering-Sørensen F, Pedersen V, Clausen S. Epidemiology of spinal cord lesions in Denmark. *Paraplegia* 1990; **28**: 105–11.

16. Krogh K, Mosdal C, Gregersen H, et al. Rectal wall properties in patients with acute and chronic spinal cord lesions. *Dis. Colon Rectum* 2002; **45**: 641–9.

17. Krogh K, Perkash I, Stiens SA, Biering-Sørensen F. International bowel function extended spinal cord injury data set. *Spinal Cord* 2009; **47**: 230–4.

18. Krogh K, Christensen P, Sabroe S, et al. Neurogenic bowel dysfunction score. *Spinal Cord* 2006; **44**: 625–31.

19. Trivedi PM, Kumar L, Emmanuel AV. Altered colorectal compliance and anorectal physiology in upper and lower motor neurone spinal injury may explain bowel symptom pattern. *Am. J. Gastroenterol.* 2016; **111**: 552–60.

20. Preziosi G, Raptis DA, Raeburn A, Panicker J, Emmanuel A. Autonomic rectal dysfunction in patients with multiple sclerosis and bowel symptoms is secondary to spinal cord disease. *Dis. Colon Rectum.* 2014; **57**: 514–21.

21. Emmanuel AV, Krogh K, Bazzocchi G, et al. Consensus review of best practice of transanal irrigation in adults. *Spinal Cord* 2013; **51**(10): 732–8.

22. Coggrave M, Norton C, Cody JD. Management of faecal incontinence and constipation in adults with central neurological diseases. *Cochrane Database Syst. Rev.* 2014; **13**(1): CD002115.

23. Harari D, Norton C, Lockwood L, et al. Treatment of constipation and faecal incontinence in stroke patients: Randomized controlled trial. *Stroke* 2004; **35**(11): 2549–55.

24. Venn MR, Taft L, Carpentier B, et al. The influence of timing and suppository use on efficiency and effectiveness of bowel training after a stroke. *Rehabilitation Nursing* 1992; **17**: 116–20.

25. Coggrave MJ, Norton C. The need for manual evacuation and oral laxatives in the management of neurogenic bowel dysfunction after spinal cord injury: A randomised trial. *Spinal Cord* 2010; **48**: 504–10.

26. McClurg D, Hagen S, Hawkins S, et al. Abdominal massage for the alleviation of constipation symptoms in people with multiple sclerosis: A randomized controlled feasibility study. *Multiple Sclerosis* 2011; **17**: 223–33.

27. Mun JH, Jun SS. Effects of carbonated water intake on constipation in elderly patients following a cerebrovascular accident. [Korean]. *Journal of Korean Academy of Nursing* 2011; **41**: 269–75.

28. Dahl WJ, Whiting SJ, Isaac TM, et al. Effects of thickened beverages fortified with inulin on beverage acceptance, gastrointestinal function, and bone resorption in institutionalized adults. *Nutrition* 2005; **21**: 308–11.

29. Astarloa R, Mena MA, Sanchez V, et al. Clinical and pharmacokinetic effects of a diet rich in insoluble fiber on Parkinson's disease. *Clin. Neuropharmacol.* 1992; **15**: 375–80.

30. Cameron KJ, Nyulasi IB, Collier GR, et al. Assessment of the effect of increased dietary fibre intake on bowel function in patients with spinal cord injury. *Spinal Cord* 1996; **34**: 277–83.

31. Mazor Y, Jones M, Andrews A, et al. Anorectal biofeedback for neurogenic bowel dysfunction in incomplete spinal cord injury. *Spinal Cord.* 2016; **54**: 1132–8.

32. Coggrave M, Norton C, Wilson-Barnett J. Management of neurogenic bowel dysfunction in the community after spinal cord injury: A postal survey in the United Kingdom. *Spinal Cord* 2009; **47**: 323–3.

33. Ashraf W, Pfeiffer RF, Park F, et al. Constipation in Parkinson's disease: Objective assessment and response to psyllium. *Movement Disorders* 1997; **12**: 946–51.

34. Zangaglia R, Martignoni E, Glorioso M, et al. Macrogol for the treatment of constipation in Parkinson's disease: A randomized placebo-controlled study. *Movement Disorders* 2007; **22**: 1239–44.

35. Korsten MA, Rosman AS, Ng A, et al. Infusion of neostigmineglycopyrrolate for bowel evacuation in persons with spinal cord injury. *American Journal of Gastroenterology* 2005; **100**: 1560–5.

36. Krogh K, Jensen MB, Gandrup P, et al. Efficacy and tolerability of prucalopride in patients with constipation due to spinal cord injury. *Scandinavian Journal of Gastroenterology* 2002; **37**: 431–6.

37. House JG, Stiens SA. Pharmacologically initiated defecation for persons with spinal cord injury: Effectiveness of three agents. *Archives of Physical Medicine and Rehabilitation* 1997; **78**: 1062–5.

38. Christensen P, Bazzocchi G, Coggrave M, et al. A randomized, controlled trial of transanal irrigation versus conservative bowel management in spinal cord-injured patients. *Gastroenterology* 2006; **131**: 738–47.

39. Emmanuel A, Kumar G, Christensen P, et al. Long-term cost-effectiveness of transanal irrigation in patients with neurogenic bowel dysfunction. *PLoS One.* 2016; **11**(8): e0159394.

40. Jarrett ME, Matzel KE, Christiansen J, et al. Sacral nerve stimulation for faecal incontinence in patients with previous partial spinal injury including disc prolapse. *Br. J. Surg.* 2005; **92**: 734–9.

41. Koyle MA, Kaji DM, Duque M, et al. The Malone antegrade continence enema for neurogenic and

structural fecal incontinence and constipation. *J. Urol.* 1995; **154**: 759–61.

42. Furlan JC, Urbach DR, Fehlings MG. Optimal treatment for severe neurogenic bowel dysfunction after chronic spinal cord injury: A decision analysis. *Br. J. Surg.* 2007; **94**: 1139–50.

43. Rasmussen MM, Krogh K, Clemmensen D, et al. The artificial somato-autonomic reflex arch does not

improve bowel function in subjects with spinal cord injury. *Spinal Cord* 2015; **53**: 705–10.

44. Randell N, Lynch AC, Anthony A, et al. Does a colostomy alter quality of life in patients with spinal cord injury? A controlled study. *Spinal Cord* 2001; **39**: 279–82.

45. Safadi BY, Rosito O, Nino-Murcia M, et al. Which stoma works better for colonic dysmotility in the spinal cord injured patient? *Am. J. Surg.* 2003; **186**: 437–42.

Chapter 20

Management of Neurogenic Sexual Dysfunction

Gila Bronner and Tanya Gurevich

20.1 Introduction

Neurological disorders affect several aspects of sexuality, intimacy, and erotic experience for patients and their partners, and is often a source for discord and general dissatisfaction [1]. The myth that people with disabilities are less sexual than others has been proven wrong, and intimacy and sexual expressions have been recognized as important dimensions of quality of life (QoL) of people with neurological disorders [2]. For example, patients with spinal cord injury (SCI) rated sexual satisfaction as one of the five main long-term care needs required for rebuilding their lives [3], and patients with Parkinson's disease (PD) rated sexual dysfunction (SD) as the 12th out of 24 most bothering symptoms of their disease [4].

Rehabilitation aims at the restoration of human functions and QoL to the highest possible level in persons suffering from disease or injury, and to allow them to lead as normal a life as possible. Sexual rehabilitation is an integral part of rehabilitation. In patients with neurological disorders, it is designed (1) to help restore, wherever possible, their past sexual and intimate activities; (2) to provide alternatives for pleasurable sex (e.g., sexual aids, medical and technical solutions) whenever the neurological disorder imposes limitations and causes SD; (3) to provide appropriate information; (4) to give permission to exercise the restored or the new sexual alternatives.

A comprehensive approach is essential to achieve these goals according to the physical, emotional, and psychological characteristics of each patient. Sexual rehabilitation needs to be tailored to accommodate the individual patient's sexual problems, sexual history, and personal motivation [5]. The PLISSIT (see Section 20.1.4) model is a modular intervention tool that was designed to cope with the needs of persons with sexual problems [6].

However, sexuality is still bound by silence, and healthcare professionals find it difficult to routinely address sexual issues proactively. They describe barriers in discussing sexuality, such as lack of time, resources, and training; they voice concerns about their own knowledge and abilities, as well as worries about causing offense or personal discomfort, and they report a lack of awareness about patients' sexual needs [7]. Experts in sexology and sexual medicine are often not a part of the neurorehabilitation team.

This chapter provides health professionals with tools to perform primary sexual rehabilitation in the framework of neurorehabilitation clinics. These tools involve relevant information on sexual problems that can be used during discussions on sexual issues with patients and partners, on modular interventions that can be applied during the neurorehabilitation process, and on the indications to refer patients for further treatment by specialists.

20.2 Sexual Dysfunction in Neurological Disorders: Clinical Overview and Classification

Sexual problems may be a direct or indirect complication of neurological disorders involving the central, peripheral, or autonomic nervous systems. Moreover, medications used to treat neurological conditions may negatively affect various aspects of sexual function. The spectrum of SD includes direct damage to autonomic innervation (mono- and polyneuropathies, traumatic or inflammatory lesions of spinal cord, and others), peripheral neuropathy, spinal cord lesions, focal basal ganglia, or hemispheric lesions affecting central control of autonomic functions (e.g., impaired arousal), neuroendocrine disorders, and depression [1, 8]. Physical limitations can challenge the ability to touch and stimulate, as well as to find alternative positions for intercourse or any other intimate activity [9, 10].

Different neurological lesions may present with similar symptoms of SD. For example, erectile dysfunction (ED) may be a feature of a central nervous system lesion (SCI), autonomic neuropathy (amyloidosis), or vascular damage (diabetes). Arousal problems may be due to hemispheric lesions (ischemic strike, brain tumour), to a dopamine-dependent state (PD), as well as to psychological problems (anxiety, depression, low self-esteem, couple discord) [1, 11]. However, ED should be approached differently in these different situations, and therefore we suggest using a systems-based approach for the management of SD in patients with neurological disorders. In this chapter, SD is defined in terms of John Hughlings Jackson's hierarchy [12], according to low, middle, and high levels (Table 20.1). The treatments offered in this chapter are based on these three levels of SD. Additionally, the PLISSIT model (see Section 20.1.4) offers modular interventions, which enable practitioners to choose the extent of their involvement in sexual rehabilitation.

20.2.1 Level 1: The Low Level of SD

The low sensorimotor level of SD results from damage to the neural innervation responsible for controlling sexual functions. It is produced by disturbances of the peripheral nervous system (including motor function, sensation modalities, and autonomic nervous system), or disturbances of the spinal cord with a direct lesion of autonomic innervation. The consequent SD includes neurogenic ED in men, decreased lubrication in women, and decreased sensation, dysesthesia, and focal pain in both genders. The SD is easily diagnosed, and can be explained by clinicians in terms of lesion localization. Treatment of SD in the low level is directed towards restoration of the damaged function, or replacement with alternative compensating tools, aids, or mechanical devices.

20.2.2 Level 2: The Middle Level of SD

The middle sensorimotor level includes SD caused by indirect impairment of sexual function, such as neurologic or endocrine deficits, that modulate the sexual function. Included in this level are lesions at different areas of the central nervous system affecting cognition, hedonia, somato-sensory and emotional processing, or motor expression, as well as modulation of autonomic or endocrine elements, and factors causing spasticity [1]. Incontinence, both faecal and urinary, is frequently a result of neurological disorders, and is also included in the middle level. Side effects of various medications for conditions associated with this level may affect sexual function [13]. Treatment of middle-level SD should take into account the possibility of compensation or replacement of the neurological deficit or the cause of dysfunction, whereupon education and psychological treatments are integral parts of the therapeutic process. The PLISSIT model, especially the specific suggestions it provides, may be very useful when the aetiology is located in this level.

Sexual preoccupation behaviour [14] and hypersexuality are manifestations of the middle-level SD. They are caused by central nervous system lesions from traumatic brain injury, stroke, epilepsy, and dopaminergic treatment [13]. Unwanted hypersexuality may occur in men (rarely in women) with neurodegenerative disorders (PD, dementia), brain trauma, stroke, and epilepsy [11, 13, 15]. Sexual preoccupation-based behaviour patterns are confusing. Their clinical presentation is uniformly that of hypersexual behaviour, but they may have different aetiologies, which must be professionally assessed and treated accordingly [14]. For example, the behaviour of a man with ED might be perceived as hypersexual since he repeatedly attempts intercourse in order to demonstrate his masculinity, or he repeatedly discusses sex with others in order to share his frustration. He should be treated as a patient with ED according to the level of his neurological damage. Another example is a woman with restless genital syndrome (ReGS; also known as persistent genital arousal disorder [PGAD]). ReGS is a rare condition that is characterized by unwanted, uncomfortable, or painful genital arousal, spontaneous orgasms, or need for frequent sexual release to reduce discomfort in the genital area [16, 17]. Similarly, although the woman's sexual preoccupation will be erroneously diagnosed as hypersexual behaviour, her treatment should be determined by whether it is psychologic, pharmacologic, neurologic, or vascular in origin. It is also important to note that neurological patients with cognitive impairment may demonstrate otherwise appropriate sexual behaviours but that occur in the wrong time or the wrong place and are mistakenly regarded as hypersexual [18]. Such behaviour can also negatively affect their relations with caregivers and the rehabilitation team and increase the burden on partners and personnel [19]. Treatment of middle-level SD should enable compensation or replacement of the neurological deficit and, whenever possible, elimination of the causes for the dysfunction.

Table 20.1 Sensorimotor levels of sexual dysfunction and treatments for men and women with sexual dysfunction

Sensorimotor Levels of SD	Characteristics of the neurological disorder	Type of SD Men	Type of SD Women	Treatments Men	Treatments Women
Level 1: The Low Level of SD	Peripheral neuropathy: Autonomic disturbances – Sensory disturbances – Surgical disruption of the genital autonomic nerve supply – Surgical disruption of the genital autonomic nerve supply – Focal vascular problems or – Spinal cord injury or	– ED – Decreased sensation (Orgasmic disorder) – Dysesthesia) – Coital and non-coital pain	– Decreased lubrication – Decreased sensation (orgasmic disorder) – Dysesthesia) – Coital and non coital pain – ReGS	– ED treatments: Oral ICI Alprostadil intraurethral pellet Penile prosthetic surgery – Vacuum constriction devices – PLISSIT	– Pelvic floor physiotherapy – Vibrostimulation – Vacuum clitoral device – Sexual aids (vibrators) – PLISSIT
Level 2: The Middle Level of SD	– Basal ganglia disorders with dopamine deficient or dopamine excessive state Motor and other physical limitations preventing satisfying sexual performance – Neuroendocrinal disorders – Hemispheric disorders (limbic, occipital, etc.) – Medications side effects – Bladder, bowel dysfunction – Local genital pain or discomfort – Sexual preoccupation behaviour, including hypersexuality (unrelated to mania)-	– HSDD – ED – RE, DE – Sexual Preoccupation behaviour, including hypersexuality	– HSDD – Arousal disorder – Decreased lubrication – Orgasmic disorders – Sexual Preoccupation behaviour, including ReGS and hypersexuality	– Hormonal replacement therapy (testosterone) – Planning of sexual activity (timing, positions, etc.) – adjustment of medications, concerning medications side effects – PLISSIT	– Hormonal replacement therapy (Oestrogen, testosterone) – Planning of sexual activity (e.g., timing, positions, lubricants) – adjustment of medications, concerning medications side effects – PLISSIT

Level 3: The High Level of SD	– Depression – Anxiety – Fatigue – Psychological disorders – Generalized pain	– HSDD – ED – PE – Pain sexual disorder – RE, DE Sexual Preoccupation behaviour, including hypersexuality	– HSDD – Arousal disorder – Decreased Lubrication – Pain sexual disorder – Orgasmic disorders Sexual preoccupation behaviour, including hypersexuality	Psychological sexual therapies: – CBT – MBCT – Couple therapy – Sex therapy including: Sensate focus Systemic desensitization Stop-start and squeeze techniques Behaviour modification Intercourse-outercourse approach Catheter counselling – PLISSIT	Psychological sexual therapies: – CBT – MBCT – Couple therapy – Sex therapy including: Sensate focus Systemic desensitization Stop-Start and Squeeze techniques Behaviour Modification Intercourse-Outercourse approach Catheter counselling – PLISSIT

SD = Sexual Dysfunction; CSB = Compulsive Sexual Behaviour; ED = Erectile Dysfunction; PGAD = Persistent Genital Arousal Disorder; ReGS = Restless Genital Syndrome; HSDD = Hypoactive Sexual Desire Disorder; PE = Premature Ejaculation; RE = Retarded Ejaculation; ICI = Intracavernous Injection; DE = Delayed Ejaculation; CBT = Cognitive Behavioural therapy; MBCT = Mindfulness-Based Cognitive Therapy

PLISSIT Model [6] is a four step model for interventions with patient's sexual problems, offering Permission, Limited Information, Specific Suggestions, and Intensive Therapy.

20.2.3 Level 3: The High Level of SD

The high sensorimotor level includes SD that is not caused by a specific lesion of the central, peripheral, or autonomic nervous systems. It is the result of factors that accompany neurological disorders, such as fatigue, anxiety, depression, low self-esteem and other psychological problems, generalized and genital pain, and various physical limitations and disabilities. These symptoms can affect one or all the phases of the sexual response cycle (desire, arousal, orgasm, and ejaculation), and sometimes cause sexual pain. Treatment of the highest level of SD should include information and specific counselling, referral to experts in sexual medicine, prescription of psychiatric medication therapy, treatment by sex or couple therapists, and psychotherapy. All four steps of the PLISSIT model (see later in this chapter) can be integrated into the treatment of the highest level of SD.

20.2.4 The PLISSIT Model

The PLISSIT model can be easily implemented by healthcare professionals [6]. It is a four-step model comprised of four components – Permission, Limited Information, Specific Suggestions, and Intensive Therapy – all of which are relevant to the sexual well-being of patients with neurological disorders. The first step of this model, Permission, offers reassurance to patients that it is appropriate to discuss sexual difficulties in medical settings and to make necessary changes for a more satisfying sexual life. The next step, Limited Information, emphasizes the importance of providing information and explanations (e.g., description of the side effects of medications). The third step, Specific Suggestions, refers to practical advice and tips (e.g., lubricants for vaginal dryness, vaginal dilators to restore flexibility and reduce pain during intercourse, phosphodiesterase type 5 inhibitors [PDE5-inhibitors] for ED, and advising alternative positions to overcome limited mobility). Most patients will appreciate the first three levels of the model [20]. The fourth step of the model, Intensive Therapy, guides practitioners in referring patients for further counselling and treatment by experts in sexual medicine (e.g., urologists, psychiatrists, and gynaecologists), sex therapists, couple therapists, or psychotherapists. Our clinical experience of many years with neurological patients has demonstrated that many neurologists are able to provide the first three steps of the PLISSIT model and, to an extent, some

components of the fourth level. It is highly advisable that both partners attend the assessment and the intervention since sexual dysfunction in one partner is a risk factor for dysfunction in the other partner [21].

20.3 Treatment of Sexual Dysfunction in Neurological Disorders

Presuming that the choice of a compatible treatment for the SD in patients with neurological disorders might be easier when the appropriate level of SD is defined, we present the various types of sexual treatment according to the levels of neurological damage. Healthcare professionals can choose the most suitable treatment, as well as consider referrals to experts. In addition to the described treatments, the Permission and Limited Information steps of the PLISSIT model are relevant to every patient and partner and their application is highly recommended.

20.3.1 Treatments of Level 1 (Low Level of SD)

Treatment for low-level SD should be directed towards restoration of the damaged function or replacing it by alternative compensating tools, aids, and mechanical devices. They include treatments for men with neurogenic ED, physiotherapy of the pelvic floor, various devices and vibrostimulation. Sexual and psychological interventions as well as provision of information are integral parts of successful treatment. Step 3 in the PLISSIT model, Specific Suggestions, may also be highly relevant for better sexual rehabilitation at this level.

20.3.1.1 Treatment for Men with Neurogenic ED
Oral Treatment for Men with Neurogenic ED

PED-5 inhibitors comprise the first-line treatment for ED. They enhance erection mechanisms if the individual is sexually stimulated, and have been successfully used in men with diabetic neuropathy, multiple sclerosis (MS), PD, SCI, spina bifida, and familial amyloid polyneuropathy [12, 22]. PDE5 inhibitors can be taken daily or 'on demand', and they differ in time of onset, duration of action, and side effect profiles [23]. There are no data confirming that one is more efficacious than another; however, most of the studies in men with neurological disorders involved the use of sildenafil. Due to their vasodilatation effect and interaction with vasodilator drugs, they must be used with great care in the cardiac patient, and they are contraindicated in combination with vasodilator drugs that contain nitroglycerin. PDE5 inhibitors are mildly hypotensive and should be used cautiously in patients with autonomic neuropathy and orthostatic hypotension. Patients and partners can benefit from appropriate information and specific suggestions about the correct use of PDE5 inhibitors. For example, slowed gastrointestinal motility may diminish their absorption [24]; therefore, patients with diminished absorption (e.g., in PD) may need to wait longer than the recommended time following ingestion of the tablet for successful intercourse [10].

Local Therapy for Men with Neurogenic ED

Second-line treatment for men finding PDE5 inhibitors to be either ineffective or contraindicated include intracavernous injection (ICI) of vasoactive drugs. Alprostadil, papaverine, and the combination phentolamine plus vasoactive intestinal polypeptide are currently the licensed agents for ICI therapy. The medication is injected into the base of the penis approximately 5–10 minutes before sexual activity. ICI causes blood vessels within the penis to dilate, thus increasing blood flow to the penis and producing an erection. Erections resulting from ICI are commonly 30 minutes in duration [23]. Alprostadil is also available as an intraurethral pellet, but this route has lower success rates and some risk of hypotension as the drug becomes absorbed systemically. Both ICI and intraurethral therapy with alprostadil are effective and well-tolerated treatments for men with ED. Patients should be trained by a urologist or specialist nurse to perform self-injections. They should be informed that these treatments will create an erection independent of sexual arousal and that the erection may persist following orgasm and ejaculation (especially with ICIs). Comprehensive patient education and follow-up can minimize risks of priapism and penile fibrosis associated with ICI, or hypotension associated with intraurethral therapy. ICIs should not be used by men with conditions that predispose to priapism such as sickle cell disease, multiple myeloma, and leukaemia. The use of anticoagulants is not a contraindication to ICI, however [23]. Finally, partners may need to assist patients with physical limitations. Both partners often need help in getting used to this way of producing an erection, and follow-up visits are required to avoid early abandonment of the therapy.

Penile Prosthetic Surgery for ED

Insertion of a penile prosthesis is an effective treatment for ED when other less-invasive approaches fail or are contraindicated, or if patients are dissatisfied with the results of their ED therapy [25]. These devices provide the patient with the ability to engage in penetrative sexual activity without interfering with urination, ejaculation, sensation, or orgasm. The type of prosthesis is usually chosen based on the physician's surgical approach, assessment of the patient's manual dexterity, and overall cost. Patients with limited manual dexterity that makes it difficult to manipulate hydraulic devices may prefer the semi-rigid prosthesis unless a supportive and motivated partner is willing to handle the hydraulic device for the patient [23]. Preoperative consultation is vital for successful results. Patients must have realistic expectations and understand that penile implants only restore the ability to penetrate; however, other aspects of the sexual response (desire, arousal, sensations, or excitement) are unchanged. They need to know and accept that, unlike other approaches to ED, penile prosthetic surgery is irreversible. Additionally, penile rigidity in the post-implant erection is due to an increase in girth rather than enhanced length or size of the glans. Numerous studies on penile prosthetic surgery have reported high satisfaction rates for both patients and partners.

20.3.1.2 Physiotherapy of the Pelvic Floor

Physiotherapy of the pelvic floor aims to relieve pain during sexual activity, increase muscle relaxation and strength in men and women, and enable better arousal and lubrication in women. Physiotherapy of the pelvic floor often involves electromyographic muscle biofeedback and is an important component of treatment for sexual hesitancy due to incontinence, for women with sexual pain disorders (e.g., vaginismus and dyspareunia including vestibulodynia), and for men with painful ejaculation. The exercises may focus on either strengthening or relaxing the pelvic floor. Manual therapy, such as introital stretching techniques or pelvic floor massage, as well as the use of vaginal inserts (dilators), may be needed, with collaboration between the clinician, the physiotherapist, and the sex therapist for a simultaneous psychological and behavioural approach [26]. The physiotherapist may also advise in cases of physical barriers to sexual activity, including general pain and mobility restrictions, which affect comfort and positioning, and/or specific sexual functioning domains of desire, arousal, orgasm, and genital pain.

Devices and Vibrostimulation

Vibrostimulation is used for sperm retrieval when the neurological condition results in impairs ejaculation [27]. Following damage to spinal cord centres for orgasm or to neural bundles from the clitoris or penis, engorgement of the genital area by usual means of stimulation is no longer possible. A strong vibrator can add the necessary stimulation to reach the threshold of orgasm and also take over the function of weak muscles [28]. Eros clitoral therapy device (EROS-CTD; Clitoral Therapy Device, UroMetrics, Inc., St. Paul, MN) is a vacuum device designed to improve sexual responsiveness and orgasm in women with sexual disorders [29]. The woman places a flexible cap on the clitoris and the application of negative pressure through a battery-assisted pump causes the clitoral sinusoidal spaces to be engorged. The use of such a device was associated with significant improvement in genital sensation, vaginal lubrication, orgasm, and sexual satisfaction in women with arousal dysfunction unrelated to neurologic disease. Clinical observations suggest that women with SCI use the device to prepare the genitals for optimal congestion, but that they reach orgasm through other sources of stimulation, such as vibrators [8].

When using a vacuum constriction device (VCD) for treating ED, negative pressure results in engorgement of the penis, and constriction rings applied around the base artificially trap blood in the penis and keep it in place for up to 30 minutes [23]. VCDs can be operated by a hand pump or run on batteries. They are safe and effective, and may be considered first-line therapy for men with ED together with PDE5 inhibitors. The most common side effects of VCD are painful ejaculation, inability to ejaculate, generalized pain, petechiae, bruising, and numbness.

Potential VCD users should be carefully selected by the urologist, and special sessions should be dedicated to providing information and training to patients and partners. Devices with cuffs and elastic straps can hold objects, including dildos and vibrators, for patients with physical limitations.

20.3.2 Treatments of Level 2 (Middle Level of SD)

Treatments of SD in the middle level include hormones and medications, correct planning of sexual activities, and the use of lubricants. The assessment and the treatment of sexual preoccupation behaviour and hypersexuality are also relevant to this level. Various steps of the PLISSIT model (education, information, and psychological interventions) can be integrated to contribute to the success of the middle-level SD treatment.

20.3.2.1 Hormonal Replacement Therapy (HRT)

Hormone insufficiency (testosterone in men and oestrogen in women) was identified in patients with PD, MS, epilepsy, and Huntington's disease [28, 30–32]. Antiepileptic drugs, especially the older types (phenytoin, phenobarbital, primidone, carbamazepine and valproate), may lead to hormonal changes (particularly increased estradiol in women and decreased free testosterone levels in men), followed by decreased performance in both sexes [12]. Brain injury, especially with basal skull fracture, may interrupt gonadotrophin release, leading to a secondary low-testosterone state [1]. The typical symptoms of low testosterone are low desire, absent sleep-associated erections, delayed ejaculation, and low serum testosterone levels in the morning. In women, reduced desire and lubrication, difficulties to reach orgasm, amenorrhea, and infertility are the most common problems. If there are no contraindications (such as prostate cancer, cardiac failure, breast cancer, general frailty in older men, secondary hypogonadal state from pituitary tumour or hemochromatosis), hormone insufficiency should be investigated and treated in order to maintain better sexual and general wellbeing. HRTs have been used with success in the treatment of SD. For example, testosterone replacement therapy may improve sexual dysfunction (e.g., low libido) in men with MS [28].

20.3.2.2 Planning Sexual Activity

Neurological disease may impair mobility, making it difficult to caress, hug, hold, or stimulate a partner, to masturbate, to get into position for intercourse, and to rhythmically move the body. These mobility barriers worry patients with SCI, PD, MS, brain injury, and other conditions associated with immobility or abnormal movements [18]. Patients are advised to plan their sexual activities in time periods when 'they are at their best', and to choose comfortable positions ('side by side', 'spoons', or partner 'on top') that demand minimal effort and movement.

Devices (such as pillows and stabilizing straps) and muscle-relaxing strategies (massage and stretching exercises) can provide some solutions. Some patients need to warm up their muscles, whereas warmth may cause diminished neural function (the Uhthoff's sign) in others. Some devices, such as a rocking chair, can enable greater mobility and facilitate a pelvic thrust with minimal upper body effort. By allowing the user to have a dynamic sexual role, some devices can help overcome the mental barrier that the patient must assume a passive role during intimacy. Accessories like thigh slings can help patients maintain an elevated and open position for easy sexual contact [18, 28].

When patients suffering from tremor, rigidity, or difficulties in fine-finger movement wish to caress and arouse their partners effectively, they may use lubricants and massage oils. Vaginal penetration may become comfortable for both partners when they use water-soluble lubricants or almond oil on the penis. Some options to avoid or reduce incontinence during sexual activity include planning fluid intake, refraining from coffee and alcohol, emptying bowel and bladder before sex, catheterization before intercourse, or using a constriction ring around the base of the penis that closes the urethra.

20.3.2.3   Medications

Medications should be always be evaluated as a possible cause for sexual problems. For example, antidepressants are associated with decreased sexual desire, ED, and orgasmic dysfunction, and drug substitution or dose reduction may alleviate the associated sexual problems. Sildenafil treatment of SD in women taking antidepressants was associated with a significant reduction in adverse sexual effects, specifically, delayed orgasm responses and inadequate lubrication, while continuing stable-dose antidepressant treatment [33]. In countries where it is allowed, medical cannabis may reduce pain and limb spasticity, improve sexual sensations, and consequently increase sexual pleasure. These sexual benefits are dose-dependent and more consistent in females than in males [34]. The side effects of medical cannabis among patients with neurological disorders have not been investigated in depth.

20.3.2.4   Lubricants

Autonomic damage may impair lubrication, putting the woman at risk of painful arousal and intercourse.

The problem can be alleviated by external lubrication placed on the penis and in the vaginal or anal orifices. Lubricants should be carefully selected since sensitivities to parabens, alcohol, perfume, silicone, and glycerine are common. Water-based, silicone-based, and oil-based lubricants can be safely used with condoms and sex toys.

20.3.3   Treatments of Level 3 (High Level of SD)

Treatments of patients with a high level of SD include a variety of psychological and sexual therapies. The key for successful intervention in this level is the establishment of an open and relaxed communication on sexual and other intimate issues. The permission to frankly discuss sexuality enables patients to share their sexual concerns, personal needs, and intimate problems. Sex counselling, specific suggestions, and practical tips provide patients with new alternatives for 'pleasure-oriented' activities. This therapeutic approach equips patients with specific techniques to relearn new body sensations, reduce anxiety or depression, decrease pain, and cope with various forms of SD. Some of the interventions can be performed by the rehabilitation professional team, particularly that of offering permission and basic information (the first steps of the PLISSIT model). Anxiety can be treated using relaxation techniques (breathing, guided imagination, meditation), cognitive behavioural therapy (CBT), mindfulness-based cognitive therapy (MBCT), or prescribing appropriate medications. Other interventions should be practised with an expert in sex therapy, couple therapy, or psychotherapy.

20.4   Psychological and Sexual Therapies for SD

CBT, MBCT, and sex therapy are the essence of treatment of female SD and an important aspect in the treatment of male SD. These therapies are based on the concept of an interrelation between thoughts, physical or emotional sensations, and behaviour, and that a change in one can create a shift in the others [18].

CBT focuses on the role of thoughts in the multifaceted sexual behaviour, teaching patients to identify their thoughts and replace them with new, altered ones. Another goal of CBT is to increase patients' control over their sexual activity by increasing their awareness of all the contributing factors involved in the sexual response and pleasure, beyond the neurological illness. Patients are encouraged to choose whether they prefer to participate in intercourse or outercourse (sexual activity without penile–vaginal penetration), or in a non-erotic intimate pleasurable touch. The increased control provided by having a choice reduces anxious thoughts, increases sensual pleasure, and consequently enables a change in behaviour.

MBCT is a meditative and non-judgmental attention to the present moment, inspiring individuals to observe their thoughts, feelings, and physical sensations. MBCT encourages an acceptance of what is happening, rather than anticipating possible negative results. This is specifically relevant to men with performance anxiety and women who anticipate sexual pain. These negative expectations usually result in compromised ability to engage in sexual intercourse [18, 35].

Sex therapy comprises a synthesis of CBT and MBCT, with additional psychological interventions, use of practical techniques, and specific sex therapy tools, all tailored and adapted to each individual and couple. Sex therapy is often combined with sexual medical/surgical interventions (medications, surgery, etc.), thus providing care with a bio-psychosocial perspective. The sex therapist needs to consider the complex interplay of multiple factors in order to achieve the goal of the treatment – the restoration of lasting and satisfying sexual function. Sex therapy enables patients and their partners to discuss their concerns, assists them in adjusting to new sexual activities modes, and finds ways to increase their sexual arousal and satisfaction. Sex therapy employs practical interventions, such as behavioural experiments and structured assignments, which aim to help the patient or couple identify, analyse, and modify behaviour that has a negative influence on sexual encounters. These assignments are performed at home either alone or with a partner.

Sensate focus is one of the common structured assignments in sex therapy, originally developed by Masters and Johnson in 1970 [36]. Sensate focus assignments aim to restore pleasure and reduce anxiety in patients with neurological disorders by replacing intercourse with pleasurable touch. Assignments initially focus on sensual massage in non-erotic body zones. The couple then shifts to more erotic assignments. Sensate focus often accompanies other therapies used for the treatment of SD, such as those for ED, PE, and lack of desire disorders. It is a valuable tool for relearning altered body sensations. Men and women with SCI can explore their pleasure–pain continuum, and discover how to create a touch that will be pleasurable, as the skin near their injury can be hypersensitive or even painful to touch. The sensate focus assignments provide patients and their partners with positive and pleasurable experiences, which may contribute to the reduction of distress and increase the motivation for sexual rehabilitation.

Systemic desensitization is another common tool in sex therapy. It is designed to treat severe anxiety or phobic response to sexual stimulus, e.g., vaginismus in women or inhibited orgasm and inability to ejaculate during intercourse. Relaxation techniques, including training in breathing and muscle relaxation, are helpful in reducing distress. Gradual exposure to non-sexual and sexual activities is planned according to the patient's needs and ability.

The stop-start and squeeze techniques are traditional sexual assignments for men with premature ejaculation (PE) [37]. These assignments are done by the man alone, and are later implemented in intercourse. Men with PE gradually learn to control ejaculation by training techniques combined with psychotherapy, CBT, and MBCT. The application of local anaesthetics to the glans to delay ejaculation continues to be used both in medical practice and as an 'over-the-counter' remedy, and can be combined with the other therapies for PE. Medications such as non-selective serotonin reuptake inhibitors (such as clomipramine) and selective serotonin reuptake inhibitors (such as paroxetine, fluoxetine, and sertraline) have been recommended.

Behaviour modification follows the identification and assessment of specific sexual behaviours that negatively affect sexual function and satisfaction. Discussing these findings may help in choosing alternative sexual options. For example, when physical and mental fatigue interfere with the ability to get aroused, persons with MS may change the timing of their sexual activity. In addition, using strong vibrators to stimulate the clitoris in women with SCI may enable orgasm, and planning more comfortable positions may assist men with PD to maintain their erection.

Outercourse is lovemaking without penile penetration into a vagina or an anus [9]. Various methods of touching and pleasurable activity can be used during outercourse, including oral or manual stimulation of the genitals or other sensual parts of the body. Partners can stop at any level of excitement that satisfies them, or try to reach an orgasm. They can enhance the sexual atmosphere, use fantasy, or masturbate together or separately. The intercourse–outercourse options of sexual activities can be discussed with the couple, giving them permission to choose their specific type of pleasure, and to find better coping methods to overcome the SD. They can have intercourse with or without medical treatment for their SD, or enjoy outercourse. Outercourse can be a good option for pleasurable activity for women with an indwelling catheter and for men with partial erections.

Counselling with regard to catheter use is an important aspect of patients' sex education [9, 38]. In cases of women with an indwelling catheter, it is important to emphasize that the catheter is not in the vagina. Due to social taboos, women and men are often not familiar with genital anatomy. A mirror can be used to identify the location of the urethra and the vagina in order to emphasize that they are separate orifices. Decreasing fluid intake a few hours before intimacy, removing a catheter, or taping it to the thigh can minimize the effect of bladder dysfunction on intercourse. Men with a catheter are advised to use a condom over the penis. For a patient requiring long-term catheterization, using a suprapubic catheter has distinct advantages over a urethral catheter in facilitating sexual activity. There are comfortable positions that enable intercourse with an indwelling catheter in women or men (side, spoons, and 'man on top' positions). It is essential to discuss such sensitive issues candidly with the couple. When these alternatives are unacceptable, the physician can suggest outercourse as an alternative for pleasurable intimate activity.

Couple therapy is often integrated into sex therapy. It focuses on issues related to the couple's relationship. It is well known that sexual problems of one partner impact the other partner [21]. Therefore, SD is always perceived as a couple problem, and sex therapy is relevant to both. In sexual rehabilitation, the partner's assistance and cooperation is needed for successful and satisfying sexual function. Better couple relationships, including improvement in the ability to listen, share, understand, and be empathic, can reduce disharmony and increase the couple's motivation for sexual rehabilitation.

20.5 Basic Principles of Sexual Rehabilitation: Discussion and Recommendations

1. **Address** sexuality and SD in patients with neurological disorders. Sexual health issues should be routinely assessed since neurogenic sexual dysfunction often severely disrupts the QoL of patients and their partners.

2. **Assess** sexual problems according to the three sensorimotor levels (low, middle, and high).

3. **Use** the PLISSIT model, which enables practitioners to choose the extent of their involvement in sexual rehabilitation.

4. **Plan** an individually tailored treatment based on the patient's age, other demographic factors, and existing co-morbidities (such as depression, cardiovascular disease, hypertension, diabetes, medications, and alcohol or drug abuse).

5. **Try** to understand the patients' and partners' attitudes towards sex, their sexual orientation, and their cultural and spiritual issues. This information should be taken into consideration for adequate sexual therapies.

6. **Equity** in sexual healthcare: all patients, regardless of age, gender, origin, and type of neurological disorder, should be offered education, information, and choice to receive sexual rehabilitation.

7. **Start** with the education of patients and their partners about the impact of their neurologic disability on sexual functioning. The more informed they are, the greater is the chance that they will regain sexual function.

8. **Information** can be provided along the rehabilitation process, through individual counselling, written material, during specific lectures or seminars, and referral to websites and Internet videos.

9. **Readiness** to participate in sexual activity should not be the criterion to give or postpone the provision of sexual information.

10. **Involve both** patients and partners. It is preferable that both partners attend the intervention to better ensure application of the information and suggestions.

11. **Consideration of partners** is crucial, since they face the challenge of continuously supporting

the patient and adjusting their own lives accordingly.

12. **Professional training** aimed at increasing awareness to the sexuality of people with chronic illness and understanding sexual rehabilitation and treatment modalities can make a significant difference for patients and partners.

13. **Simply asking** sex-related questions and responding in a thoughtful, empathic and non-judgmental way to the patient's (or the partner's) concerns can be remarkably therapeutic.

14. **Referral to experts** for intensive therapy is appropriate when an individual or couple requires therapy beyond the physician's expertise.

15. **Cooperate with other experts.** Sexual rehabilitation is a series of multidisciplinary interventions, including medical, psychological, sexual, and behavioural therapies. Therefore, it is essential to cooperate with experts from all professions, including those outside the rehabilitation unit.

References

1. Rees PM, Fowler CJ, Maas CP. Sexual function in men and women with neurological disorders. *Lancet* 2007; 369(9560): 512–25.

2. Welsh M, Hung L, Waters CH. Sexuality in women with Parkinson's disease. *Mov. Disord.* 1997; **12**: 923–7.

3. Chang MY, Chen HY, Cheng ML, Liu HY. Rebuilding life: Investigating the long-term homecare needs of clients with spinal cord injuries. *J. Nurs. Res.* 2016, **2** Aug. [Epub ahead of print]

4. Politis M, Wu K, Molloy S, Bain PG, Chaudhuri KR, Piccini P. Parkinson's disease symptoms: The patient's perspective. *Mov. Disord.* 2010; **25**: 1646–51.

5. New PW, Seddon M, Redpath C, Currie KE, Warren N. Recommendations for spinal rehabilitation professionals regarding sexual education needs and preferences of people with spinal cord dysfunction: A mixed-methods study. *Spinal Cord* 2016, May 10. doi:10.1038/sc.2016.62. [Epub ahead of print]

6. Annon JS. The PLISSIT model: A proposed conceptual scheme for the behavioral treatment of sexual problems. *J. Sex. Educ. Ther.* 1976; **2**: 1–15.

7. Dyer K, das Nair R. Why don't healthcare professionals talk about sex? A systematic review of recent qualitative studies conducted in the United Kingdom. *J. Sex. Med.* 2014; **10**(11): 2658–70.

8. Winder K, Linker RA, Seifert F, Deutsch M, Engelhorn T, Dörfler A, Lee DH, Hoesl KM, Hilz MJ. Neuroanatomic correlates of female sexual dysfunction in multiple sclerosis. *Ann. Neurol.* 2016; **80** (4): 490–8.

9. Courtois F, Charvier K. Sexual dysfunction in patients with spinal cord lesions. *Handb. Clin. Neurol.* 2015; **130**: 225–45.

10. Bronner G, Elran E, Golomb J, Korczyn AD. Female sexuality in multiple sclerosis: The multidimensional nature of the problem and the intervention. *Acta Neurol. Scand.* 2010; **121**: 289–301.

11. Bronner G, Aharon-Peretz J, Hassin-Baer S. Sexuality in patients with Parkinson's disease, Alzheimer's disease, and other dementias. *Handb. Clin. Neurol.* 2015; **130**: 297–323.

12. Taylor J, Holmes G, Walshe FMR, eds. *Selected writings of John Hughlings Jackson*, vol. **2**. London, UK: Hodder and Stoughton,1932.

13. Lundberg PO, Ertekin C, Ghezzi A, Swash M, Vodusek D. Neurosexology: Guidelines for neurologists. *Eur. J. Neurol.* 2001; **8**(s3): 2–24.

14. Bronner G, Hassin-Baer S, Gurevich T. Sexual preoccupation behavior in Parkinson's disease. *J. Parkinson Dis.* (2017); **7**(1): 175–82.

15. Morrell MJ, Guldner GT. Self-reported sexual function and sexual arousability in women with epilepsy. *Epilepsia* 1996; **37**: 1204–10.

16. Facelle TM, Sadeghi-Nejad H, Goldmeier D. Persistent genital arousal disorder: Characterization, etiology, and management. *J. Sex. Med.* 2013; **10**: 439–50.

17. Waldinger MD, Venema PL, Van Gils APG, Schweitzer DH. New insights into restless genital syndrome: Static mechanical hyperesthesia and neuropathy of the nervus dorsalis clitoridis. *J. Sex. Med.* 2009; **6**: 2778–87.

18. Basson R, Bronner G. Management and rehabilitation of neurologic patients with sexual dysfunction. *Handb. Clin. Neurol.* 2015; **130**: 415–34.

19. Ahmed RM, Kaizik C, Irish M, Mioshi E, Dermody N, Kiernan MC, Piguet O, Hodges JR. Characterizing sexual behavior in frontotemporal dementia. *J. Alzheimers Dis.* 2015; **46**: 677–86.

20. Khakbazan Z, Daneshfar F, Behboodi-Moghadam Z, Nabavi SM, Ghasemzadeh S, Mehran A. The effectiveness of the Permission, Limited Information, Specific Suggestions, Intensive Therapy (PLISSIT) model based sexual counseling on the sexual function of women with multiple sclerosis who are sexually active. *Mult. Scler. Relat. Disord.* 2016; **8**: 113–19.

21. Fisher WA, Eardley I, McCabe M, Sand M. Erectile dysfunction is a shared sexual concern of couples I:

Couple conceptions of ED. *J. Sex. Med.* 2009; **6**: 2746–60.

22. Xiao Y, Wang J, Luo H. Sildenafil citrate for erectile dysfunction in patients with multiple sclerosis. *Cochrane Database Syst. Rev.* 2012; **4**: CD009427.

23. Montorsi F, Adaikan G, Becher E, Giuliano F, Khoury S, Lue TF, Sharlip I, Althof SE, Andersson KE, Brock G, Broderick G, Burnett A, Buvat J, Dean J, Donatucci C, Eardley I, Fugl-Meyer KS, Goldstein I, Hackett G, Hatzichristou D, Hellstrom W, Incrocci L, Jackson G, Kadioglu A, Levine L, Lewis RW, Maggi M, McCabe M, McMahon CG, Montague D, Montorsi P, Mulhall J, Pfaus J, Porst H, Ralph D, Rosen R, Rowland D, Sadeghi-Nejad H, Shabsigh R, Stief C, Vardi Y, Wallen K, Wasserman M. Summary of the recommendations on sexual dysfunctions in men. *J Sex Med* 2010; **7**: 3572–88.

24. Pfeiffer RF. Gastrointestinal dysfunction in Parkinson's disease. *Lancet Neurol.* 2003; **2**: 107–16.

25. Levine LA, Becher E, Bella A, Brant W, Kohler T, Martinez-Salamanca JI, Trost L, Morey A. Penile prosthesis surgery: Current recommendations from the international consultation on sexual medicine. *Sex Med.* 2016; **13**: 489–518.

26. Rosenbaum T, Vadas D, Kalichman L. Sexual function in post-stroke patients: Considerations for rehabilitation. *J. Sex Med.* 2014; **11**: 15–21.

27. Phillips E, Carpenter C, Oates RD. Ejaculatory dysfunction. *Urol. Clin. North Am.* 2014; **41**: 115–28.

28. Lew-Starowicz M, Gianotten WL. Sexual dysfunction in patients with multiple sclerosis. *Handb. Clin. Neurol.* 2015; **130**: 357–70.

29. Billups KL, Berman L, Berman J, Metz ME, Glennon ME, Goldstein I. A new non-pharmacological vacuum therapy for female sexual dysfunction. *J. Sex. Marital Ther.* 2001; **27**: 435–41.

30. Okun MS, McDonald WM, DeLong MR. Refractory nonmotor symptoms in male patients with Parkinson disease due to testosterone deficiency. *Arch. Neurol.* 2002; **59**: 807–11.

31. Luef G, Madersbacher H. Sexual dysfunction in patients with epilepsy. Handb. Clin. Neurol. 2015; **130**: 383–94.

32. Reininghaus E, Lackner N. Relationship satisfaction and sexuality in Huntington's disease. *Handb. Clin. Neurol.* 2015; **130**: 325–34.

33. Nurnberg HG, Hensley PL, Heiman JR, Croft HA, Debattista C, Paine S. Sildenafil treatment of women with antidepressant-associated sexual dysfunction: A randomized controlled trial. *JAMA* 2008; **300**: 395–404.

34. Gorzalka BB, Hill MN, Chang SC. Male-female differences in the effects of cannabinoids on sexual behavior and gonadal hormone function. *Horm. Behav.* 2010; **58**: 91–9.

35. Brotto LA, Basson R, Luria M. A mindfulness-based group psychoeducational intervention targeting sexual arousal disorder in women. *J. Sex. Med.* 2008; **5**: 1646–59.

36. Masters W, Johnson V. Eds. *Human sexual inadequacy*. Boston, MA: Little, Brown & Company, 1970.

37. Riley A, Segraves RT. Treatment of premature ejaculation. *Int. J. Clin. Pract.* 2006; **60**: 694–7.

38. Aisen ML Neurological rehabilitation: Sexuality and reproductive health. *Handb. Clin. Neurol.* 2013; **110**: 229–37.

Index

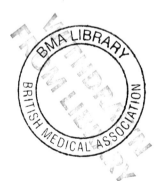